G·R·E·A·T EXPECTATIONS

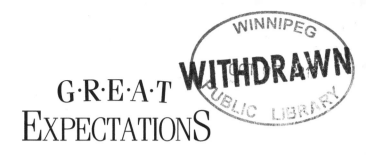

D1173709

Pregnancy & Childbirth

Marcie Jones & Sandy Jones

with Peter S. Bernstein, MD, MPH, FACOG and
Claire McCamman Westdahl, CNM, MPH, IBCLC, FACNM

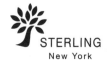
STERLING
New York

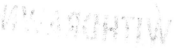

STERLING
New York

An Imprint of Sterling Publishing
387 Park Avenue South
New York, NY 10016

© 2004, 2012 by Marcie Jones and Sandy Jones
Illustrations by Stephen Tulk and Nicole Kaufman
Illustrations by Laura Hartman Maestro, p. 56, 183–184, 240

ISBN 978-1-4027-8185-8

Distributed in Canada by Sterling Publishing
c/o Canadian Manda Group, 165 Dufferin Street
Toronto, Ontario, Canada M6K 3H6
Distributed in the United Kingdom by GMC Distribution Services
Castle Place, 166 High Street, Lewes, East Sussex, England BN7 1XU
Distributed in Australia by Capricorn Link (Australia) Pty. Ltd.
P.O. Box 704, Windsor, NSW 2756, Australia

For information about custom editions, special sales, and premium and corporate purchases,
please contact Sterling Special Sales at 800-805-5489 or specialsales@sterlingpublishing.com.

Manufactured in the United States of America

2 4 6 8 10 9 7 5 3 1

www.sterlingpublishing.com

Acknowledgments

Many thanks to Peter Bernstein, MD, MPH, FACOG and Claire McCamman Westdahl, CNM, MPH, IBCLC, FACNM, Katherine Gallo, and Miriam Schecter, MD, who ensured the book was accurate and provided valuable insights. And to the hundreds of pregnant women and new moms who took the time to share their hopes, their dreams, and their day-to-day realities with us.

Contents

Introduction: A Word from the Authors

It's been almost a decade since the first *Great Expectations: Pregnancy & Childbirth* came out, and a lot—and yet little—has changed. Screening and diagnostic test technology have leapt forward, with crisper images and more precise results, but pregnant women still worry. Parenting roles have shifted slowly but surely—1 in 5 babies with a stay-at-home parent are now home with dad. Fewer parents are opting to be married, too, with nearly 40 percent of babies born to single moms.

On the health front, understanding of the roles of certain vitamins, minerals, macronutrients, and fatty acids has grown, and so has the average mom's weight at conception, along with increases in related health conditions. In happier news, we grow ever closer to unraveling some health mysteries, like the genetic origins of traits and abnormalities, the causes of SIDS, and the impact of prenatal exposures on a child's life. For better or worse, it becomes increasingly more apparent that what a mom-to-be eats, the chemicals she's exposed to, and even her moods during pregnancy can have a lifelong effect on a baby's health and temperament.

In between editions, we've also had the opportunity to add research on the physiology of baby sleep, the economics of child care, and, because readers requested it, expand on detailed weekly fetal-development information, so you can come as close as possible to knowing what your little peanut is doing every second. And we worked hard to arrange everything in a comprehensive way to make the information easy to access. We hope you enjoy this new edition.

CONGRATULATIONS—YOU'RE PREGNANT!

Three little words, or a line on a little wand, and you'll find yourself in a strange new world. There's no way to be prepared for carrying another person inside of your body, someone you are responsible for, body and soul, as long as you both shall live—even if this isn't your first pregnancy. While the changes in your body may be easy to see and feel, the changes that happen to you as a person, in your heart, mind, and hormones are just as momentous.

We wrote this book as a travel guide to this journey. A lot of pregnancy books seem to be written by people who have never been pregnant before, or who have forgotten what it's really like.

The books we studied seemed to go no deeper than the message "don't worry, you're normal." While you probably shouldn't worry, and chances are you are normal, we wanted to give you more than simple reassurances. We assumed that, like us, you want to know why and how things happen.

Equally as important, we wanted you to have a book that would give you information without being judgmental about it. We know all too well there's nothing more annoying than the chorus of people telling pregnant women what they should do. The truth about being pregnant (or being a parent) is that no matter what choice you make, there will always be someone who thinks your choice is wrong.

You can't please everyone, try as you might to be the "perfect" pregnant woman with the "right" kind of delivery. But if you've done your research, you can separate real risks from imagined ones and make choices based on evidence, not opinion.

Finally, we have tried to create a book that would present pregnancy as realistically as possible. There's a lot more to pregnancy than just glowing! Sure, it's a miracle and everything, and you're probably excited about having a baby, but sometimes, frankly, pregnancy can be uncomfortable, undignified, and yucky. It can feel like a boot camp of learning how to surrender to discomfort and unpredictability, and finding balance between self-caring and self-sacrifice. No matter what other books tell you, it's okay to not enjoy the experience all of the time.

Even when pregnancy isn't fun, or even when things don't go as planned, it is always meaningful. You will never be the same after this. It may feel like an endless sacrifice, but in the final analysis, what you will have lost in muscle tone, you'll gain tenfold in heart, courage, and humanity. You can do it, you will do it, and we're rooting for you, no matter how you do it!

INSIDE OUR BOOK

Our first chapter, "Your Pregnancy Week by Week," is an easy-to-navigate map that says "you are here" and carries you from the first day you discover you're pregnant through your final weeks until labor. It shows you how you and your baby change and grow and directs you to all the information you'll need when you're most likely to need it.

The second chapter, "What (and What *Not*) to Worry About," formerly "Managing Your Pregnancy," lists alphabetically women's most common concerns, from "Age over 35" to "Yoga," and offers practical, evidence-based solutions for practical problems during pregnancy.

Chapter 3, "Managing Your Nutrition," helps you untangle the many vitamins, minerals, macronutrients, and dietary recommendations for pregnant women, and offers information on weight gain and food safety.

The fourth chapter, "Birth," kicks off with frequently asked questions about going into labor. What are the odds of your water breaking spontaneously? How do you know when you're really in labor?

You'll learn all about the process of labor, what your pain relief options are, and the latest research on the most commonly used medical interventions. We offer you both the benefits and the risks of routine procedures such as epidurals, induction, labor augmentation, and cesarean sections, and tell you how they feel.

Chapter 5, "You and Your Baby," will help you in recovering physically and emotionally from pregnancy and childbirth. It also offers hundreds of practical suggestions for taking care of your newborn during the first 6 months.

The sixth chapter, "Baby Gear Primer," is an A-to-Z guide to buying safe, durable baby products. It will guide you in what to buy and what to avoid, and give you helpful information on all major baby product categories, including cribs, car seats, and strollers.

In the back of the book, the "Resources" is chock-full of reliable Internet pregnancy and baby resources. And the "Pregnancy Dictionary" is a basic reader on hundreds of pregnancy and medical definitions that have been translated by us into easy-to-understand concepts. It also offers page references throughout the book for more discussion on a given topic.

We have gathered the information presented in *Great Expectations* from hundreds of recent medical studies; from the wealth of wisdom and knowledge in the fields of obstetrics, family practice, midwifery, and nursing; and from the shared experiences of childbirth educators and doulas. In addition, we have incorporated wisdom from the numerous mothers who have shared their pregnancy, birth, and childrearing experiences with us. And of course, we have used our own experiences of pregnancy, labor, and infant care to guide us.

FINDING YOUR WAY AROUND

Great Expectations is designed to be a "30-second" reference book for busy mothers just like you. We want you to have the choice of dipping into topics based on your specific concerns or to read the book from cover to cover.

Throughout the text of each section, you'll find references to specific pages elsewhere that discuss the topic you are currently exploring.

Medical terms throughout the book are set in italics and bold the first time they appear in any section. That signals that you'll find them defined in the "Pregnancy Dictionary."

The index at the end of the book speeds your journeys into the book. Throughout, we've translated the latest, most comprehensive research findings into easy-to-follow "flash facts" that will help you be an informed consumer.

When it comes to talking about your baby, we've tried to remain gender neutral by giving equal weight to the possibility of your baby being a boy or a girl. So, you will find that we have alternated throughout the book "he" and "she" to allow for both possibilities for the sex of your baby.

YOUR HEALTHCARE PROVIDER

Also, because nearly one-third of pregnant moms don't have husbands, we refer to your companion as your "partner," who may be your husband, your baby's father, a dear friend, your mother, or someone else you've chosen to accompany you through your pregnancy experience. While this book is the most comprehensive out there, you're going to need more help and human support than any bound volume can offer during your pregnancy. That's why we consistently recommend that you seek the advice of your healthcare provider throughout the book. Although most women in the U.S. use obstetricians for prenatal care and delivery, we purposely refer to the professional you've chosen to help you with your birth as "your healthcare provider." We recognize that you have the option of delivering your baby with a family care medicine physician, midwife, or nurse-midwife too. An experienced healthcare provider can play an important role in supporting you and guiding you through your birth and delivery. At best, he or she will be present to assist you in weighing a wide range of options every step of the way, will keep your preferred strategies for pain relief and your birth preferences in the forefront, and will refrain from recommending any medical tests or interventions that aren't totally in the best interest of you and your baby. (Information on how to choose a healthcare provider can be found on pages 7–12.)

Also, we can't overstress the importance of having someone in the room during birth to support and assist you. Recent research shows that women who have active support during labor feel less pain, have less anxiety, and experience better outcomes, such as fewer cesarean sections. We suggest using a combination of both your chosen birth partner and a labor assistant (doula) to accompany you through labor.

A NOTE ON EVIDENCE-BASED MEDICINE

The factual findings on medical practices are based on evidence-based medicine, the use of research from a variety of clinical studies of large numbers of pregnant women and babies, in order to recommend only practices that have been solidly proven to be beneficial.

Thanks to this exciting revolution in medicine, tests or interventions that have been shown to be of limited benefit, or no benefit at all, are being discontinued. However, sometimes there can be a time lag between the publishing of scientific findings and changes in the practices of healthcare providers, particularly when findings contradict routine procedures.

Healthcare practitioners, who are only human, tend to rely on what they've been taught and to trust routines they've become used to. And like everyone else in the world, they're more likely to believe information that seems to confirm what they already believe and find flaw with things that conflict with these beliefs. If you or your baby's safety and well-being are at stake, we suggest being a well-informed medical consumer, which may include seeking a second opinion.

About Us

Great Expectations: Pregnancy & Childbirth has been created by two mothers for all mothers. Veteran writer Sandy Jones has a master's degree in psychology and has been authoring books and articles for parents for 35 years. She is the author of six other books on babies and child care, including *To Love a Baby; Crying Baby, Sleepless Nights;* and *The Guide to Baby Products* from Consumer Reports. She is the mother of Marcie Jones, a writer, writing teacher, and mother of two with a master's degree in publications design.

Our ultimate hope is that *Great Expectations* will make the process of moving through your pregnancy, having your baby, and taking care of yourself and your baby easier and less intimidating. Our plan from the beginning has been that the book's progressive design and clarity will make it easy for you to access exactly the right piece of information you need when you need it.

Marcie Jones & Sandy Jones

Foreword: A Note from Dr. Peter Bernstein

In 1989 a United States Public Health Service expert panel issued a report on prenatal care in the United States. While they acknowledged the progress made over the past century in the modern medical care of pregnant women and their newborn children, they also indicated that there were significant areas that needed greater attention, specifically the psychological, social, and educational aspects of pregnancy. *Great Expectations: Pregnancy & Childbirth* by Marcie Jones and Sandy Jones goes a long way to answer this need.

While modern medicine has made great advances in prenatal care, more and more research is demonstrating that those expectant couples who educate themselves and actively partner with their prenatal care provider have the best outcomes. The more fully informed a pregnant woman is, the more she can completely participate in her care. Unfortunately, too often care providers do not have the time to educate their patients on many important components of prenatal care, such as good nutrition, the importance of breastfeeding, contraceptive options, and caring for newborns.

Here's an example of the power that knowledge can provide to a pregnant woman. For a woman who is uninformed about the natural process of labor, every contraction can be a terrifying experience, making her feel like her body is out of control. All the fear she experiences can even make her labor more painful. For the woman who is prepared, the onset of contractions signals that labor has begun, which is exciting, less scary, less painful, and more fulfilling.

Great Expectations: Pregnancy & Childbirth provides the expectant couple with many of the tools they'll need to prepare for the pregnancy, delivery, and initial care of their newborn.

I like the systematic and complete way this book approaches all aspects of pregnancy. It carefully covers pregnancy from start to finish and beyond, as well as from head to toe. It helps women to understand what is happening to their bodies, prepares them emotionally for changes of pregnancy, and gives them the knowledge they need to be active participants in their prenatal care. And then the book goes one step further by helping the new mother to prepare for the early days of parenthood. This is all done in a clear and easy to understand way.

Pregnancy is an exciting time for a woman—but it is also an important opportunity for her to refocus on her own health and the health of her family. Armed with the knowledge contained in this book, she will be in a great position to make a genuine difference in creating a strong foundation for herself and her family.

Peter S. Bernstein, MD, MPH, FACOG; Medical Director of Obstetrics and Gynecology; the Comprehensive Family Care Center at Montefiore Medical Center; Associate Professor of Clinical Obstetrics & Gynecology and Women's Health; Albert Einstein College of Medicine

Foreword: Pregnancy for the Twenty-first-Century Woman . . . 6 Years Later

So much has changed; so much has stayed the same. The heartfelt comments I made for the first edition of *Great Expectations: Pregnancy & Childbirth* are as relevant and pertinent today as they were 6 years ago. Since the first edition, digital media has exploded. One result of that explosion is that there is often too much information and from too many sources. The challenge for expectant parents is to sift through the information, judge its quality, and then apply that information to make critical decisions about pregnancy health, genetic testing, birth options, feeding choices, and parenting styles, and so much more. Marcie Jones and Sandy Jones make this daunting task possible with an authoritative book that is both easy to navigate and trust.

The last few years have brought an explosion of information about fetal origins, a pioneering field that recognizes that the time spent in utero is the most consequential period of our lives. Normal development of all the fetal organs depends on adequate nutrition, hormones, and blood flow to the uterus. The impact of poor nutrition and stress during pregnancy can predispose an infant to diabetes, anxiety, depression, and other chronic diseases. *Great Expectations: Pregnancy & Childbirth* informs the decisions a woman needs to make during pregnancy to be well nourished, achieve appropriate weight gain, and create a healthy environment for her baby to grow and develop. The information in this book will help her—and you—achieve that, as well as prepare you for breastfeeding and parenting. This information is presented in a context that is *reassuring* during a critical time in a woman's life—and her baby's.

So, for all women who will be pregnant during the second decade of the twenty-first century, *Great Expectations: Pregnancy & Childbirth* is the best resource for up-to-date, current information for decision making, as well as support for those decisions, based on the belief that pregnancy can be a safe, healthy, and enjoyable transition in the life of women and their families.

Claire McCamman Westdahl, CNM, MPH, IBCLC, FACNM

Your Pregnancy Week by Week

In this section, organized by week, you'll find out how many days you've been pregnant, how many days you have to go, and details your baby's height, weight, and physical and mental development. You can read about what's happening to your body, what you should worry about, and what's normal. Every week you'll find information about risks you should be aware of, choices you may need to make and situations you may find yourself in as your pregnancy progresses. Specific medical and pregnancy terms are in bold and italic, which will let you know that a more thorough and specific definition can be found in the Pregnancy Dictionary at the back of this book.

You can begin reading the Week-by-Week Guide at the specific week you're in if your care provider has given you a *due date*. Or if it's too soon to even have a due date—you're waiting until it's time to test, or you have a feeling you might be pregnant but you aren't sure—start reading right here!

Are You Pregnant?

Just How Easy Is It to Get Pregnant?

It's actually pretty easy for most women to get pregnant, especially in the most-fertile late teen and early 20-something years.

If you have regular periods you can expect to be fertile for about 24 hours of any given cycle. But the catch is, if conditions are optimal, sperm can live for as long as 3 or 4 days, waiting for *ovulation*. So while it might seem like the odds of getting pregnant by having unprotected sex once on any random day of your cycle would be 1 in 28 (or however many days your cycle typically is), really the odds can be as low as 1 in 7 while you're in your peak *fertility* years.

It can be hard to know when you're fertile. Periods happen 13 to 14 days after ovulation—not the other way around—so you can still get pregnant if your periods are irregular. It's even possible to get pregnant during your period if you have a short or irregular cycle, and you can also get pregnant after giving birth and before your period returns. And even predictable cycles can change up from time to time, which is why calendar or rhythm methods of birth control have about the same failure rates as no birth control at all. (For more on birth control, see page 108.)

If there's a chance you're pregnant, the only way to really know for sure is to take a pregnancy test. To reduce the chance of a false negative (when the test says you're not pregnant but you really are), wait at least until the day your period is due to take a urine test. Even if the test is negative, if your period is due but doesn't arrive, test again in a few days, and in the meantime, look out for these pregnancy signs:

- You feel like you have PMS, but your period hasn't come. Cramps, bloating, achy or sensitive breasts, fatigue, headaches and crankiness are all early pregnancy symptoms, but can also be symptoms of some combination of PMS, a cold, or mild food poisoning. But if you have some or all of these symptoms for more than a day or two and still no period, take a test.
- Your sense of smell is sharper. For some women, the first sign of pregnancy is their ability to suddenly detect odors that

they couldn't before. The stink of exhaust fumes, cigarette smoke, incense, frying food, or other airborne odors may offend you to the point of queasiness. The intensity of your reaction will typically intensify as your *hormone* levels rise and start to ease after the first *trimester*, though for some women lasts for the entire pregnancy.

- Something's different about your breasts. Your breasts may simply feel tender or more sensitive, as if you had PMS. But sometimes pregnancy breasts are more extreme: even early on they may suddenly appear larger, fuller, and perkier. Some women may even experience nipple tingling.
- You feel bloated. Your underwear, rings, and bracelets may feel like they've shrunk, and you have to suck in to zip up the tighter pants and skirts in your wardrobe.
- You feel queasy, either when you smell, eat, or even think about certain foods, or for no reason in particular. (For more on pregnancy-related *nausea*, see page 18.)

WHAT IF I THINK I'M PREGNANT, BUT THE TEST IS NEGATIVE?

Pregnancy-test false negatives are really common, in spite of what their boxes might claim. One study in the *American Journal of Obstetrics and Gynecology* found that only one of eighteen brands tested were sensitive enough to detect pregnancy at 4 weeks from LMP (last menstrual period).

If you get a negative result on

a home pregnancy test, but your period is still late, test again 24 to 48 hours later. In early pregnancy, a woman's hCG levels will double every 2 to 3 days. Most tests are able to detect pregnancy between 12 to 15 days from implantation, but remember it can take as many as 4 days after sex for conception to happen, then 3 or 4 more days after that for the fertilized *egg* to implant. No test can detect pregnancy before implantation. So it might take from 5 to 12 days total after intercourse for a fertilized egg to implant and hCG production to begin, and plenty of pregnant women still may not have levels of hCG high enough to be detectable by some over-the-counter tests until as late as 6 weeks after their last periods.

The most sensitive tests can detect as low as 6.5 mIU/ml (thousands of an International Unit per milliliter), sensitive enough to detect a pregnancy a day after implantation. The least sensitive tests detect 100 mIU/ml, which means the test may not be able to accurately detect pregnancy even a week after implantation. Consumer Reports, the nonprofit consumer advocacy organization, reviews the effectiveness of pregnancy tests. Search "Consumer Reports pregnancy test" to find the most recent report on what brands of test proved most sensitive.

If there's a possibility you could be pregnant—you've had unprotected sex at least once since your last period—even if you've gotten a negative test, if you still haven't gotten your period, play it safe and act "as if" with the tips below.

THE TEST IS POSITIVE, NOW WHAT?

- Sit down for a moment to take in the news.
- Call your healthcare provider to make an appointment.
- Decide who to tell and when.
- Review "Things to Avoid" during pregnancy, below, and all of Chapter 2.

HEARING THE NEWS

Women's reactions to positive pregnancy tests can range from denial to unmitigated glee to hyperventilating horror. Don't blame yourself for your emotions—there's no wrong way to react to such major life-changing news. It's also totally normal to have lots of mixed feelings at once, like happy about the baby, but not thrilled about the prospect of pregnancy, *labor*, or the costs of raising a child.

If your pregnancy was unplanned, you'll probably have a very different reaction than someone who's been trying to get pregnant for a long time. Everyone's different, and you have 9 months (and 18 years!) to figure out how you feel about parenthood.

If you get a positive pregnancy-test result, you'll want to call your family doctor, gynecologist, healthcare provider, *midwife*, or a clinic right away to schedule a check-up and get independent confirmation of your results. As excited and panicked as you might be, your healthcare providers will probably have a more blasé reaction. Most will wait until between the sixth and eighth week after the first day of your last period to book your first prenatal appointment.

It's okay to make prenatal appointments with your current doctor now and to politely cancel them if you find a different care provider in the meantime. (See later in this chapter for details on different types of care providers.)

Until your appointment, take a daily multivitamin. It's ideal to take one before you conceive, but if you weren't already in the habit, start now. Your nutritional needs go up while you're pregnant, and while it's best to get nutrients from quality food, a vitamin and mineral supplement can act as an insurance policy against deficiencies. If you're too nauseated, though, you can skip the vitamin and opt for a nutritionally optimized diet instead. (For recommended daily allowances of vitamins and minerals in pregnancy, see page 157.)

A vitamin doesn't need to be labeled "prenatal," but you want to be sure you get all of your recommended allowances of vitamins and minerals every day, especially folate (400 to 600 mcg), iron (30 mg), vitamin D (200 IU), and calcium (1,000 to 1,300 mg).

Things to Avoid:
- **Using any medication, topical cream, or dietary supplement** without checking its safety with your healthcare provider or a pharmacist. Many over-the-counter and prescription drugs have been linked to pregnancy complications, and most medications simply haven't

been tested for safety during pregnancy at all. The first 14 weeks are when all of your baby's major organ systems form, so you want to be particularly cautious during this time.
- **Drinking alcohol.** Many, many links have been found between maternal drinking and lifelong physical and mental disabilities in children. Alcohol disrupts the formation of fetal brain cells, and some studies have shown as little as a drink and a half a week can lead to a baby with symptoms of *Fetal Alcohol Syndrome*, such as being born shorter and with a smaller head circumference, and having learning and behavioral problems later. Other studies have contradicted this finding, showing that one to two drinks a week are okay. There seems to be a strong genetic component, with some women able to drink and cause no harm to the *fetus*, and others causing harm with as few as two drinks a week. With so much at stake, and no way to know what sort of *genes* you have, your best bet is to abstain completely. (For more on alcohol, see page 104.)
- **First- and secondhand cigarette smoke and smokeless tobacco or nicotine replacement products.** It's also no secret that tobacco can be very dangerous to fetuses and has been linked to a variety of bad outcomes, including *birth defects* and even fetal death.
- **Ingesting more than about 150 to 200 mg of caffeine per day.** That's one to two cups of coffee, or three-quarters of an energy drink. Higher amounts of caffeine

have been linked to a slightly higher rate of *miscarriage* early in the first trimester. Some fetuses are also particularly sensitive to caffeine, and for them even small amounts of caffeine can cause heart *arrhythmia*s. If an *ultrasound* detects any kind of fetal heartbeat irregularity, you will need to cut out caffeine completely.

- **Germs, within reason.** Beware of other people's bodily fluids—avoid sneezers on the subway and don't have unprotected sex if you are not in a monogamous relationship. Wash or sanitize hands often and/or wear gloves if you work where you might come into contact with other people's fluids, like at a hospital, day care center, bank, or tollbooth. Always wash your hands thoroughly before putting on contacts or eye makeup. Call your healthcare provider if you experience any symptoms of *infection*, such as a *fever*, inflammation, or pain.
- **Exposure to high levels of radiation.** Airport scanners are safe, as are routine dental X-rays, but if you work as an X-ray technician or in some other job that requires ongoing exposure, take precautions to limit how much your fetus is exposed to.
- **Poorly handled prepared foods.** Avoid unheated cured or smoked meats, raw fish and shellfish, hot dogs, deli or lunch meats, unpasteurized dairy products and juices, and unwashed vegetables or sprouts, because of the risk of food poisoning. (See "Listeriosis" in the Pregnancy Dictionary for more information.)

- **Extremely hot baths, saunas, or electric or heating pads on your lower abdomen.** Exposure to heat in excess of 102°F in the first trimester has been linked with an increased rate of miscarriage, and communal hot tubs can also carry some rather nasty *bacteria* (see page 131).
- **Eating a strictly vegan diet without nutritional supplements.** (See the nutrition chapter.)
- **Handling dirty cat litter, soil, or dead rodents without gloves.** (See "Cat Litter Boxes" on page 114.)
- **Certain types of fish.** Fish is one of the healthiest foods around, low in fat, high in *protein*, and full of omega-3 fatty acids. But some species of fish contain high levels or *mercury* and/or other pollutants. The Environmental Protection Agency's Web site, *www.epa.gov*, lists updates on contaminated fish. If you limit your fish intake, consider purified fish oil capsules as a source of DHA. (See more about mercury and pollutants on page 125 and more about DHA on page 161.)

  Have more:
- **Exercise.** Conventional wisdom used to hold that pregnant women should avoid exerting themselves, but research has shown the opposite to be true: women who are in shape and stay active during pregnancy have shorter labors, fewer complications, and quicker *postpartum* recoveries.

  Fit women are less likely to suffer depression during pregnancy and after birth. When you find out you're pregnant, there's no need to stop exercising unless you want to or your healthcare provider tells you to stop (though do avoid really vigorous exercise in the last trimester, and also activities that risk *trauma* to your lower abdomen). Keeping active will help your body be more able to cope with the stress of carrying around the extra weight you'll be gaining.

If you're out of shape or have never exercised before, start gently when you feel physically up to it. Try a simple 30- to 60-minute walk, swim, or prenatal exercise class three to seven times a week, adding more frequency and/or distance as you're able.

- **Colorful vegetables and leafy greens, fruit, whole grains, and other plant foods.** In particular, cruciferous vegetables, such as cabbage, broccoli, cauliflower, and Brussels sprouts, have lots of nutrients and fiber, and research has found that eating these vegetables during pregnancy may protect your offspring from cancer later in life.
- **Omega-3 and vitamin D supplements, or small fish.** Small, low-on-the-food-chain fishes like anchovies, sardines, and herring are all very low in contaminants and a great source of healthy fats, protein, and vitamin D. If you can't (or don't want to) eat at least 12 ounces of little fatty fish a week, take supplements to make sure you get enough fatty acids and vitamin D.
- **Water.** Your body's fluid needs go way up in early pregnancy, and not getting enough water can cause more headaches, fatigue,

nausea, and mood swings. Later in pregnancy, *dehydration* can affect your *amniotic fluid* volume. Drinking water will also make you less likely to retain water.
- **Rest.** Though you may feel like your normal self, your body is doing a lot of work. Take whatever chances you can get to catch a few Zs.

TELLING THE NEWS

Your Partner

After a pregnancy test confirms that you're pregnant, you get to tell your partner, unless he or she was standing next to you as you stared at the stick. Will you say two words, or put on an elaborate production number? As you try to decide, keep in mind that a reaction of disbelief, shock, and terror is as common as whoops of joy. Your partner is normal if he doesn't believe it at first ("Are you sure?") or expresses his misgivings ("How are we going to afford it?"). This reaction is just as legitimate as one of joy, and it doesn't mean your partner won't blossom into a wonderful parent.

Your Parents and Close Friends

Of course you'll tell your parents, best friends, and close relations right away. Not everyone has a partner to share the news with, and if this is the case you'll need to reach out for extra support to the other important people in your life.

Your Healthcare Provider

Call your women's healthcare provider's office on the next business day to make your first prenatal appointment.

If you work, it's good sense to wait to make your announcement until at least after the first trimester has passed and you've done some quiet research about your company's leave policies and treatment of previous pregnant employees. Pregnancy-related job discrimination does still happen in this day and age, and if you know your employer has a history of forcing out or "mommy tracking" pregnant employees, you'll probably want to delay your announcement as long as possible.

THE WHO, WHY, AND WHEN OF PRENATAL CARE

Your usual women's healthcare provider does not need to be the person who delivers your baby. It's a good idea to do a little homework to find out the best local doctors, midwives, and birth facilities in your area.

Seeing a healthcare provider (*obstetrician*, family practitioner, or certified *nurse-midwife*) regularly is important during pregnancy, because catching health issues early can prevent major problems.

The usual schedule for *prenatal care* is an appointment once a month for the first 28 weeks, then every 2 weeks between weeks 28 and 36, and then once a week after that, for about fourteen appointments total. That's a lot of time to spend with someone, so it's important to have a care provider you like and respect and trust to give you good information.

What Makes a Care Provider Good?

Are you sure that your current care provider is the right person to deliver your baby? Do you like only one provider in an eight-person practice? Does the hospital where your provider delivers have a soaring cesarean section rate? If you have any kind of healthcare choices, now is the time to be choosy. If you have health insurance, talk to your insurance company about your options, and schedule consultations with care providers to find out what their birth philosophies are. With a good care provider:

• You feel comfortable discussing intimate subjects.
• You feel comfortable asking questions, and your questions are answered thoroughly and with respect.
• Exams and procedures are clearly explained.
• You like and respect all of the other doctors, midwives, and nurses in the practice.
• Your care provider offers any specific options that you want during labor, such as alternative pain relief, a water birth, or a home birth.
• The office staff is pleasant and helpful.
• Someone is available at all times (at least by phone or e-mail) to address any health concerns you have.
• You don't feel rushed during visits.

Doctor or Midwife?

Which kind of care provider should you choose? You have many choices.

Obstetrician. Unlike midwives, obstetricians are able to perform surgical interventions, such as c-sections, should one be necessary.

OB/GYNs may have their offices in a hospital, arranged in a group practice with other doctors, or with doctors and midwives. As babies can be born any time of the day or night, it's uncommon to find an OB/GYN who works solo (unless you live in a very, very small town). If your OB/GYN works in a practice, consider making appointments for prenatal checkups with other members of the practice as your pregnancy progresses. This way, you'll be familiar with the partner who's on call when you go into labor.

Pros:

OB/GYNs all have advanced medical training and skills for dealing with emergency situations, including surgical skills.

Cons:

Statistically, OB/GYNs are more likely than midwives to intervene medically in your delivery, and patients of obstetricians are more likely to experience a c-section, episiotomies, labor stimulated with medication, continual fetal monitoring, and the use of instruments such as vacuum extractors and *forceps* during delivery. (Though OBs also are more likely to have higher-risk patients, too.)

OB/GYNs tend to spend less time with you when you are in labor than a midwife.

Family physician. A family physician is a doctor who's spent at least 4 years in family medicine residency. They've been trained in not just *obstetrics* but also in pediatrics and adult medicine.

All family physicians (FPs) must be licensed as physicians and may be board certified in family medicine. Family physicians can preside over regular vaginal deliveries, and some with further training can do an *operative vaginal delivery*, such as those using forceps or *vacuum extraction*. You'll probably give birth in a hospital where your family physician will be able to consult with an obstetrician if the pregnancy or the labor becomes complicated. In addition to postpartum care, family doctors can also provide care to both you and your baby after birth.

Pros:

A family physician can provide a continuum of care, treating you and baby together.

Cons:

Family physicians who practice obstetrics are becoming increasingly rare, so you may not be able to find one.

Unlike obstetricians, a family physician may not be trained in surgical interventions.

Certified Nurse-Midwife (CNM). A *certified nurse-midwife* is a registered nurse with a minimum of 2 years of advanced training on normal obstetrics and women's healthcare. A certified midwife (CM) is a professionally educated midwife who was not first educated as a nurse.

CNMs and CMs usually practice in collaborative relationships with physicians. They provide care for normal pregnancies, provide support during pregnancy and labor, and manage labor and deliver babies with the backup of an obstetrician in case surgical intervention becomes necessary or other complications arise.

Midwives do not perform cesareans and many don't accept patients that they believe to be at high risk for needing surgical intervention, such as patients with serious health conditions. CNMs and CMs also attend to patients after birth, conduct postpartum exams, and advise patients about proper aftercare at home. Midwives also attend to women's ongoing health needs, such as annual exams and birth control. Some midwives provide a wide range of pain-relief options during birth, such as water birthing, massage, or TENS machines. If they attend births in hospitals, most will have access to medically based labor pain management, such as *epidurals*. (Epidurals are discussed on page 189.)

Be sure to ask your midwife about the types of pain medication and comfort measures available to you. You can find CNMs/CMs in your area on the ACNM Web site at *www.acnm.org*.

Pros:
Most CNMs/CMs will stay with you from your arrival at the hospital until the baby's born.

Midwives are more likely than physicians or OB/GYNs to have knowledge and experience with alternative pain-relief and labor-encouraging measures.

Some CNMs/CMs will also offer postpartum care, which might include house calls and *lactation* consulting.

Most CNMs/CMs have designated obstetrical backup in case of complications.

Cons:
CNMs are not trained or authorized to perform surgical interventions except episiotomies.

CNMs may not accept certain high-risk patients, such as women with serious chronic health problems. If you develop complications during pregnancy or delivery, your care may have to be handed over to an obstetrician.

Certified Professional Midwife (CPM). A CPM, also known as a *direct-entry midwife* (DEM), is someone certified by the North American Registry of Midwives (NARM). For *certification*, NARM requires that midwives have graduated from an accredited school or served as an apprentice midwife.

CPMs must pass a national certifying exam, be periodically reviewed, and have experience attending births in out-of-hospital settings.

CPMs are less likely to work in hospitals and more likely to be found in *birth centers* or attending to home births. This means that they may not have direct access to a backup physician in case of complications, which could mean that you have to take an ambulance to a local emergency room should something go wrong during delivery.

CPMs tend to work either in communities underserved by physicians or with women who want to avoid technological interventions such as continuous fetal monitoring, epidural pain relief, and surgical interventions.

Pros:
Midwives can offer a more intimate atmosphere for delivery, such as a birth center or your home.

If you don't have health insurance, a CPM may be the least expensive option.

Cons:

Without a nursing degree, CPMs are not allowed to deliver in hospitals, though some may have a hospital affiliation that enables them to admit patients and attend births on an as-needed basis. CPMs may not have adequate medical backup if a medical complication arises.

CPMs may not be licensed to work in all states.

QUESTIONS FOR A PROSPECTIVE OBSTETRICIAN OR CERTIFIED NURSE-MIDWIFE

Keep your list of questions, a pen, and a notebook in hand when you interview obstetricians or nurse-midwives over the phone and in person.

Over the phone:

- Are you taking new patients, and do you accept my insurance (or offer deals to uninsured patients)?
- Is this a solo or group practice?
- What are the healthcare practitioners' credentials? Are they board-certified obstetricians, certified midwives, or a combination? Does anyone in the practice have specialty training?
- At what hospital or birth center do you deliver?
- Can I schedule a consultation? Can I bring my husband/boyfriend/partner/other support person to the consultation with me?

- (If you've previously had a c-section) Should I attempt a *vaginal birth* after my cesarean (a *VBAC*), or would you recommend a repeat c-section?

At a consultation:

- How long have you been in practice?
- How many babies do you and your practice deliver per week/month/year? (Fewer than twenty deliveries per provider per month is best.)
- Who are the other professionals in the practice? Will I see them also? Who will deliver my baby if you're not available? Do I have a choice about who in the practice delivers my baby?
- How often will I see you? Who will handle my non-urgent questions?
- Can I e-mail questions? How long should I expect it to take before I get a response to a call or e-mail?
- Who should I call if I experience bleeding or premature labor after office hours?
- What percentage of your delivering patients have: c-sections (see page 193), induced labor (see page 98), episiotomies (see page 179), epidurals (see page 189)?
- Do you think expectant parents should write *birth plan*s? Do you read them?
- What happens during a typical visit?
- What prenatal tests do you recommend, and when should they be scheduled? Are there any prenatal screening tests you *don't* recommend?
- Do you also offer patients alternative pain relief techniques

Preconception Care

About one-third to half of all pregnancies in the United States are unplanned. But if you know that you want to get pregnant (or you're not trying to avoid it), there are things you can do before you get pregnant that can help improve your chances of a healthy outcome:

- Take a prenatal or multivitamin with at least 400 micrograms (mcg) of folate (also known as *folic acid* or vitamin B9). There is evidence that folate also prevents chromosomal defects in sperm, so ask your partner to do the same for about 3 months before you begin trying to **conceive.**[1]
- To make it easier to conceive and to lower your risk of potential complications during pregnancy, do your best to get to a healthy weight before you conceive.
- If you smoke, quit. Also stop any medications, drugs, or dietary supplements not cleared for safety or recommended by your healthcare provider.
- If you drink alcohol consider stopping before you conceive. While there isn't clear evidence that an occasional drink is harmful, alcohol use early in pregnancy is the leading cause of preventable mental retardation, and many professional medical organizations recommend complete abstinence before trying to conceive.
- Make an appointment for a pre-**conception** checkup. This is vitally important if you have had a previous miscarriage, **stillbirth**, or **preterm delivery**, or if you have a pre-existing condition like **diabetes**, high **blood pressure**, seizures, or an autoimmune disorder. Make sure your healthcare provider knows about any medications or supplements that you take on a regular basis.
- Consider making an appointment for yourself and your partner with a **genetics** counselor to identify if either or both of you are carriers for certain genetic diseases or belong to a group with a high frequency of carrying genetic diseases (e.g., African-American, Ashkenazi Jewish).
- If you're using hormonal **contraception** or an **IUD**, ask your healthcare provider if you need to wait a certain amount of time before stopping birth control and trying to conceive.

to epidurals, such as water birth or continual pain-management support with a labor assistant? (For more on pain management during labor, see page 188.)
- Do you recommend that your patients use a professional labor assistant (*doula*) during delivery?
- Do you use continuous or intermittent fetal monitoring?
- Do you recommend patients take childbirth classes (or does the practice offer classes)?
- How do you deal with post-date pregnancies, and at what point would you strongly urge labor *induction*?
- At what point during labor will you meet me at the hospital? Do you stay at the hospital throughout a patient's labor?

   Ask yourself:
- Am I comfortable with this person and practice?
- Was the support staff helpful?
- Does this practice meet my practical needs? (For example, the practice and delivery facilities are reasonably close to your home, and the facility accepts your insurance plan.)

Before you settle on a provider, it's also a good idea to take a tour of the hospital or birth center where any prospective healthcare provider delivers. Your individual doctor or midwife will only be one part of the whole birth, delivery, and recovery experience. Most hospitals have regularly scheduled tours of their maternity wards for parents-to-be. If you love the provider but the only hospital where she has privileges smells funny or has women delivering in the halls from overcrowding, that's not good. (For more on hospital tours—what to look for and questions to ask—see page 64.)

The First Trimester

Weeks 1 through 13

During these next 13 weeks, your future child will grow from two cells into a recognizable human shape about the height of your thumb!

Your baby will be building basic body structures according to a standard genetic blueprint. While all of the genes for individual characteristics are in your baby's every cell, in the formative first few weeks, your baby will look like the *embryo* and fetus of every mammal.

Yet by the end of the first trimester, he or she will have a face, arms, legs, and the beginnings of all major organ systems. And you will have grown an entirely new organ, the *placenta*.

For you, the first trimester can feel like a real roller-coaster ride. Pregnancy changes every cell in your body.

You may lose the shape of your waist, and your breasts may grow an entire cup size. Your ribs and hips will widen. By the end of the first trimester, you'll feel and look more padded all over, though probably not so much that people on the street will know your condition.

Your body and head hair, complexion, and the pigment on your nipples and body will be different 3 months from now. Your breasts will be preparing to make milk, with systems that have been in place since you yourself were a fetus. During this trimester, you may even find that your breasts begin to leak drops of **colostrum**, or pre-milk, though usually not enough to soak through your bras or shirts.

By your second trimester your hormone levels will have stabilized, your condition will be known, and your friends and family will be well on the way to adjusting to their new roles. By the time you go into labor, you'll probably feel more than ready for the baby's arrival! That may seem like a pretty far-fetched notion right now, though.

Some women love the physical experience of pregnancy. They love the excitement, anticipation, attention, and healthy glow, and the feeling of growing a little life inside.

Other women hate everything about pregnancy, dreading labor and feeling ungainly and oppressed by their tiny slave driver downstairs. Love or hate pregnancy, lots of women find the first trimester the most difficult, for a number of reasons.

- You feel awful. Eighty percent of women experience nausea and/or vomiting. Even if you can keep your food down and aren't in a constant state of disgust, you still will certainly experience fatigue, bloating, crabbiness, and achy breasts.
- It's the biggest news of your life, and you have to keep it secret. Well, you don't *have* to, but most women do wait at least until they hear a heartbeat, because of the 10 to 25 percent risk of miscarriage before a heartbeat is detected. (After the heartbeat is detected the risk drops to 4 percent for moms 35 and younger, and about 10 percent for moms between 35 and 40.) Keeping the cat in the bag can be especially tough if you're nauseated.
- Your relationships are changing and may be tested. Your partner is going to be "dad" (or "other mommy") and your mother will be "grandma." You're now closer to some friends, and others you may have a harder time relating to.
- Your future has changed. Any plans you had for moving to a foreign country or touring small clubs with your band may have to be put on hold for the time being.
- Crazy-making hormones. Combine the mental stress of pregnancy with your surging hormones, and you might feel like you're losing your mind sometimes. One minute, elation, the next, deep despair, and it can be hard to tell sometimes if what you're feeling is real and reasonable or just a by-product of what's going on with you physically.

Drops and jumps in your blood sugar and blood pressure can make you nauseated. Aches and pains can make you cranky. All of the extra *estrogen* in your system can make you feel weepy and sensitive.

- You may also frequently feel "out of it." As your veins expand and your blood pressure goes down, there actually is less blood than usual making it to your brain. You may find yourself having moments of feeling dizzy or "fuzzy minded."
- If you focus too much on negative news stories it can make you feel vulnerable to a world full of dangers—pollutants, contaminants, germs, electromagnetic fields, etc., etc. Of course you want to stay informed, but don't let yourself feel disempowered by whatever latest health panic is on the news.

Just take common-sense steps to reduce your exposure to common things that have potential to cause harm: quit smoking, wear your seat belt, clean out your medicine cabinet, and give yourself license to throw away anything in the refrigerator that's old or smells funny. Leaf through Chapter 2 if you have a particular worry, and ask your healthcare provider whatever questions you have, even if you think they sound minor or silly (we promise you they will have heard sillier). Accept that there is a certain amount of risk involved in getting out of bed every day, and trust that you will be able to deal with any crisis that comes your way.

NAP

The first trimester is for resting. Sleep as much as you need to. It'll keep your mood up.

EAT RIGHT

Now is the time to focus on healthy eating habits. Eating small, low-sugar, high-protein snacks during the day can help quell fatigue and nausea. (See Chapter 2.)

RESEARCH

You'll be seeing your care provider about once a month until your last month of pregnancy, when you'll see him or her once a week. Use your appointments to ask plenty of questions—the more you know and the more confidence you feel in your provider's abilities, the less frightening the whole pregnancy, birth, and labor process will be. Also don't be afraid to call the office for any question you may have, even if you just want advice about nutrition or safe foods.

ADJUST YOUR LIFESTYLE

Does this describe you? You're of ideal weight. You eat at least five different fruits and/or vegetables every single day, drink nothing but milk or water, don't touch caffeine, exercise for at least an hour 5 days a week, and never smoke or so much as look at a white wine spritzer. You're so healthy you don't even need to keep aspirin in your medicine cabinet. But if you're like most of us, you're in for some major lifestyle changes if you want to give your baby the best start in life. It's really hard to change your every habit overnight, but small changes can make a big difference.

KEEP A JOURNAL OF YOUR HABITS

As you probably already know, smoking and drinking are bad, exercise and a nutritious diet are good, and you want to gain enough, but not too much, weight. But how do you translate this information into real-life action? One way is to start keeping a journal. To establish better habits, it helps to know what your current habits are. For a week, write down everything that you put in your mouth and every physical activity you engage in. You'll see in black and white if you need to eat less candy, get more calcium, drink more water, exercise more often, and so on. Set small and manageable goals, and phrase them positively. Don't try to stop eating candy forever, for instance. Instead, set a goal to eat smaller portions less often, and think of ways to substitute better alternatives to your habits. Try to isolate exactly what it is about a bad-habit food that you love so much, and see if you can satisfy your craving in a healthier way. For instance, if you notice that you can't go a day without potato chips, think of ways to feed the craving for a salty crunch without so many calories, like vegetable chips, or carrot sticks or celery with hummus. After you've looked over habits and thought about alternatives, start afresh.

Don't worry about individual days, but whether by the end of the week you're eating and living a little bit healthier on average than you did before. Your pregnancy can be an opportunity to establish lifelong healthy habits.

START OR CONTINUE EXERCISING

Pregnancy, labor, birth, and your baby's infancy and toddlerhood are physically challenging, and the more fit you are, the easier they'll be for you. Women who are in shape and keep fit during pregnancy have shorter labors, fewer complications, and quicker postpartum recoveries. Fit women are less likely to suffer depression during pregnancy and after birth.

If you're already exercising regularly and feel up to it, pregnancy itself is no reason to change your routine or cut back. Just use commonsense to avoid dehydration, overheating, and injury. If you're out of shape or have never exercised before, start gently when you feel physically up to it. Try a simple 30-minute walk, swim, or stretch or *yoga* session three times a week, adding more frequency and intensity as you progress.

WEEKS 2 AND 3

Fetal Age: 1 to 14 days

38 to 36 weeks, 266 to 252 days until your EDD

Baby

Size: Fits on the head of a pin.

Development: Though some women swear that they were aware of the moment of conception, most are oblivious. Hormonal changes don't kick in until after the fertilized egg implants. But incredible things have happened in your *fallopian tubes* and *uterus*.

At the moment of conception, two single cells, his sperm and your egg (otherwise known as gametes), merge. The conditions that allow this to occur are extremely specific.

Twelve to 24 hours prior to conception, your estrogen levels will have reached their monthly peak, triggering a release of an egg from one of your *ovaries*. Your *cervix* softens and lifts and begins to secrete a slick fluid that contains microscopic fernlike ladders. Before ovulation, the cervical mucus is dense and impenetrable to the sperm. But during ovulation, the mucus becomes more watery, and the sperm travel up the ladders it forms, swimming upward at a rate of 7 inches in half an hour.

Sperm work in teams and are somehow aware of one another. They organize into scouting parties to find the egg. If another man's sperm is around, some sperm will form a kamikaze army and beat them back, fighting to the death for domination. Like bicyclists in the Tour de France, sperm form protective, defensive groups that help each other maintain speed and edge out competitors.

If there's no egg, the sperm will rest their heads on the walls of the fallopian tubes, waiting like groupies. An exceptionally strong sperm in optimal conditions can wait for up to 4 days for an egg to appear.

If a group of sperm finds an egg, the sperm get "hyperactivated," and the ramming begins. Sperm whack at the egg's outside with their thick, enzyme-coated heads.

The enzymes actually can weaken and dissolve the egg's outer shell (called the zona). The winning sperm, the 1 in 200 million, is the one whose head first penetrates the egg's outside. At that nanosecond, the egg absorbs the winning sperm's head, the egg shuts down completely, and no more sperm will be admitted.

Inside the egg, the two sets of cell nuclei lie side by side. Each cell has half of a set of *chromosome*s, and the moment of conception is the moment they fuse together and unite them. At this moment your future baby is assigned a gender, eye color, hair color, and thousands of other characteristics.

The cell that results is called a *zygote*, which rapidly divides into two, four, eight, and then sixteen cells and eventually into a tiny fluid-filled ball of cells that travels down the fallopian tube and into the uterus and lands along the uterine wall. About 3 to 5 days after conception, and 8 to 10 days after ovulation, the *blastocyst* will burrow into the lining of the wall of the uterus (the *endometrium*)

and will be known as an embryo from that point until about 8 weeks after conception, when it earns the title of fetus (Latin for "little one"). It's estimated that about 30 to 50 percent of fertilized eggs do not successfully implant, though, and are instead passed within 12 days of conception.

It takes about 12 to 15 days from implantation for a urine pregnancy test to detect hCG.

WEEK 4

Fetal Age: 2 weeks (15 to 21 days)

36 to 35 weeks, 251 to 245 days until your due date

Baby

Size: Barely visible to the naked eye.

Development: During the short window of time that implantation in the uterus is possible, the zygote, or mass of cells, is passed down the fallopian tube by tiny hair-like projections called cilia. The zygote has a coating of protein called selectins, which latch onto carbohydrates. After ovulation, the lining of the uterus develops carbohydrate molecules that reach out to these selectins, and that causes the egg to stick to the side of the uterus.

The synchronization of these two events means that when the zygote descends into the uterus, it can firmly take hold of the uterine wall, burrow beneath the surface, and start forming a placenta using tiny, fingerlike projections called *villi* to dig in and set up the baby "nest." A majority of pregnancy losses occur during this very sensitive implantation process.

Within your embryo, cells are lining up to create a central streak that will turn into the neural tube.

You

The fertilized egg burrowing into your uterus can make you shed a few spots of pink or light-brown blood about 5 to 12 days after conception. Bleeding or spotting that's heavier than a dot or two or happens any other time during pregnancy should always be reported to your healthcare provider right away, though, because it could be a sign of infection, *ectopic pregnancy*, or impending miscarriage. (For more on miscarriage, see page 23.)

Any pregnancy symptoms you have will be barely, if at all, noticeable. If you're very sensitive, you may notice feelings of fatigue, queasiness, bloating, and breast tenderness, and changes in your skin and hair. If you take a super-sensitive test, such as a blood test at your doctor's office, it's possible to get a positive result a week after conception. If you test at home this early, know that it's more probable that you'll get a false negative at this stage.

How you feel: It can seem difficult to believe the news, especially if you look and feel exactly the same as you did before.

You may be worried about the living it up you did before you knew you were pregnant. Don't. For better or worse, at this early pregnancy stage it's all or nothing: if anything you ingested was toxic enough to harm your pregnancy, the zygote would not have

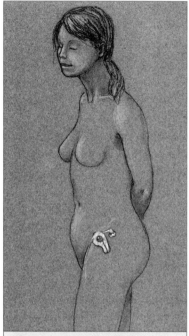

Uterus, 2 weeks post-conception

implanted, or the embryo would have been lost early on.

If you took a pregnancy test, and it was negative (very likely at this stage), but your period hasn't come, and you feel like you have PMS that just won't go away, then take another test, waiting at least 24 to 48 hours between tests to give pregnancy hormones a chance to build to detectable levels.

When you get the news that you're pregnant, accept your emotions, and don't worry about how you "should" feel. No one knows what you're going through but you.

WEEK 5

Fetal Age: 3 weeks (22 to 28 days)

35 to 34 weeks, 244 to 238 days until your due date

Baby

Size: The embryo is about 2 millimeters long, about the size of a grain of sand.

Development: Your embryo transforms into a bundle of cells organized in a C-shape with a top, bottom, front, and back. A groove has developed on the embryo's back, which will seal and develop into the neural tube (which later will become the spinal cord). At this point, the tube already has a wider, flatter top that will grow into your baby's brain. A bulge has developed in the center of the embryo, which will soon become a tiny U-shaped tube that will form the heart. This tube will start beating between days 21 and 24, and is circulating the embryo's own blood, which is nourished and cleansed by nutrients from the placenta. On about day 26, arm buds form, looking like knobs on the side of the body. Your embryo is encased in protective *membranes* and attached to a yolk sac, which manufactures the embryo's own unique blood cells.

You

Now and for the next 6 weeks, your body is producing large amounts of pregnancy hormones. Hormones are chemical signals that circulate in your body fluids and cause physical effects in your cells. These hormones are the unsung heroes of pregnancy. They actually affect the cells in your body—changing you at the most elemental level. Their powerful effects include:

• Keeping your uterus from shedding the embryo as it naturally would during your monthly cycle.
• Stimulating your breasts' milk production.
• Widening your blood vessels to bring more blood to the baby and less to your brain, possibly making you feel dizzy when you stand up quickly.
• Making your digestion more efficient by slowing down your metabolism.
• Affecting your brain chemistry, causing mood swings. Estrogen, in particular, can make you feel weepy, sensitive, and vulnerable.
• Sharpening your sense of smell.
• Making the ligaments in your hips soften to widen and make room for pregnancy and birth.

How you may be feeling now and for the rest of your first trimester:
• **Nauseated.** As pregnancy hormones start to kick in, so does pregnancy-related nausea. At any time of the day or night, you may have a vaguely queasy stomach or full-on vomiting bouts. Keep your stomach lined with small, healthy meals. If your prenatal vitamins are making you sick, try taking them at night, and/or talk to your healthcare provider about trying a different vitamin formulation, or if you have a healthy diet, skipping the vitamins altogether. Note that from now until the second trimester is a very sensitive time of fetal development, when vitamin deficiencies or exposure to toxins can cause the most

long-term harm, so contact your healthcare provider right away if you can't keep food down for more than a day.

- **Feisty.** The first trimester can feel a lot like an extended case of PMS, and you may frequently feel cranky and irritable (or not—everyone's different).
- **Moody and emotional.** You may feel a whole range of emotions—joy, excitement, weepiness, irritability— sometimes in quick succession. One minute you find yourself enraged by dirty socks on the floor, the next sobbing at a diaper commercial. Sometimes mood swings are triggered by pregnancy-hormone or blood-sugar shifts; sometimes they're circumstantial (people really *should* pick up their own socks, after all). Just take it an hour, day, or diaper commercial at a time. If you find yourself flying into a rage, try drinking a little water and eating something before going ballistic.
- **Tired.** Growing a baby takes a lot of energy, so don't feel guilty about taking as many naps as you feel like. Take a pillow to work and use your first 15 minutes of your lunch hour for quiet time. At home, the dishes can wait. Or better yet, somebody else can do them.
- **Crampy.** Generalized pain in your *pelvis*, akin to menstrual cramps, is normal. Any one-sided sharp pain is a potential warning sign of ectopic (tubal) pregnancy and should be reported to your doctor right away.
- **Bloated.** Your clothes may feel unusually tight. To people who see you in clothes, though, your body won't look any differently until sometime in the late second trimester.

- **Obsessed with food.** You may be having strange cravings for, and aversions to, foods that you may have never given much thought to before.
- **Disgusted** by smoke, alcohol, and odors. Your disgust can be expressed in any number of ways, like feeling short of breath, nauseous, dizzy, having dry heaves, or straight-up barfing. On the bright side, this means your body's embryo-protecting mechanisms have kicked in. Avoid being exposed to whatever disgusts you—even if it doesn't make sense to you at the time, your body's clearly trying to tell you something.
- **Like you gotta go.** Pregnancy hormones can make your *bladder* seem to shrink in half, as increased blood flow to your kidneys increases the amount of urine you make. In about 2 months, the pressure will ease. It can help if you lean forward when you pee to empty your bladder more completely.
- **Sexy.** Increased blood flow to the pelvis can make sex more fun.
- **Chesty.** Your breasts can get seriously uncomfortable, tingly, and achy as they swell. Your nipples are also sensitive and tender. If going down the stairs, running, or jumping hurts, try a snug sports bra, or even two, one on top of the other. Many women even sleep in a bra, French style, to avoid having their nipples rubbed by a nightgown or bed sheets.
- **Drooly.** Pregnancy makes you produce more saliva. It's not uncommon to wake up from a nap and find a puddle on the pillow. You may also start to spit when you talk.
- **Gassy.** Nothing complements spitting when you talk like having

copious amounts of gas, which is the by-product of your slowed-down intestinal tract. Some foods may cause more gas than others, like dairy, beans, and vegetables in the cabbage family.

WEEK 6

Fetal Age: 4 weeks (29 to 35 days)

34 to 33 weeks, 237 to 231 days until your due date

Baby

Size: A month after conception, your embryo looks something like a newt or a tadpole, and it has gills like a fish! Right now, the embryo of your future baby looks much like the embryo of any other animal—a bird, rabbit, or monkey. It has two tiny cups of pigment on the side of its head that will develop into eyes.

Development: Tiny buds that will form the lungs have appeared. The neural tube has closed. One end is flattening and expanding to become the brain, and the other end will become the spine. It's already ten thousand times larger than the fertilized egg. The embryo doesn't have gender characteristics yet, but has little dots where the nipples will be, whether it's a boy or a girl.

The heart, a tiny U-shaped tube, will start beating between days 21 and 24, and is circulating the embryo's own blood.

It has a small mouth and lips and fingernails are forming.

You

Your production of pregnancy hormones (hCG) continues to increase, making you susceptible

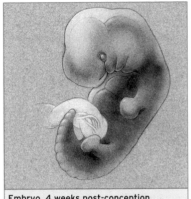

Embryo, 4 weeks post-conception

to nausea and fatigue. Your blood pressure is lower than it was before you were pregnant, which can make you light-headed and dizzy.

Early miscarriages are common. If you experience more than a few dime-sized drops of blood, call your healthcare provider, who will likely schedule you for an ultrasound to check for a fetal heartbeat. If you have a miscarriage this early on, you'll experience menstrual-period-level bleeding. (For more on miscarriage, see page 23.)

Things to Do

Clean out the fridge. If you're not feeling too queasy, now is a good time to clean out your refrigerator. Pregnancy gives you a free pass to throw away any food that's old, unappealing, or suspect. Foodborne bacteria are never something you want to take lightly, and avoiding food poisoning is particularly important while you're pregnant because there are harmful bacterial strains, such as Listeria, that can make both you and the baby sick. (For more on food safety, see Chapter 3.)

Bad bacteria can come into your life on raw food products, especially meat and dairy, though produce can also be contaminated. They can also thrive in cooked food that's been improperly heated and stored.

So kick off your new, food-safety-conscious lifestyle with a fridge party with a big new garbage bag. Patrol the shelves for:

- Any foods older than the "use by" or expiration date, or a week or more past the "sell by" date
- Leaky containers
- Fish or shellfish more than 1 day old
- Raw poultry or ground uncooked meat more than 2 days old
- Cooked leftovers, cold cuts, salads made with mayonnaise that are more than 3 to 5 days old
- Uncooked fresh beef, pork or lamb chops, steaks or roasts more than 3 to 5 days old
- Fresh vegetables more than 1 week old
- Mayonnaise and dressings more than 2 months old

Probably needless to say, don't test a suspect food by tasting it, and heed the adage, "if in doubt, throw it out."

When you're finished purging the fridge of old food, clean the shelves with warm soapy water and sanitize them with a solution of 1 teaspoon of bleach to a quart of water. While you're in there, leave a thermometer so you can make sure that the refrigerator is maintaining a temperature between 34°F and 40°F. Colder temperatures don't kill bacteria, but do make them reproduce more slowly. Bacteria multiply most quickly in food at a temperature of 40°F to 140°F and are killed at 165°F.

When you go grocery shopping:
- Avoid slimy or wilted produce.
- Check sell-by and use-by dates on packages to pick the freshest food, and pick and meat and dairy from the back of the case.
- Avoid any undated meat or dairy products.
- Check bread, produce, and dairy for signs of mold.

When you cook:
- Thoroughly rinse all of your produce, even the prewashed kind.
- Avoid transferring bacteria by keeping your hands, utensils, and food prep surfaces clean.
- Rinse surfaces with bleach-and-water solution after they come into contact with raw meat or dirt from vegetables.
- Use a meat thermometer when you're cooking hamburgers or roasts.

When you go out:
- Avoid buffets that have been sitting out for more than 3 hours.
- Avoid eating at restaurants with dirty bathrooms. To paraphrase a famous chef, if a restaurant can't keep clean the areas that customers see, the parts customers don't see are surely even filthier. And use a paper towel to open the bathroom door, so as not to re-dirty your hands with germs from the bathroom patrons who didn't wash.

Mental Health Tips

Emotionally, hormonally, and lifestyle-wise, there is no bigger change of life than pregnancy (especially a first one). So many changes all at once can make you feel like you're going crazy, and it can be hard to tell if it's hormones, or pregnancy symptoms, or if you're freaking out for a completely justified reason. Some coping tips:

- Sleep whenever you can. Getting enough sleep can make the difference between being able to cope and being miserable. Try going to bed an hour earlier, and don't be afraid to turn off your phone and nap when you can. As pregnancy progresses, a lot of women start to develop sleep cycle changes. Expect that before the pregnancy is over you'll have more than one night where you go to bed straight from work or school, get up to eat in the middle of the night, go back to bed until 4 a.m., and then doze on and off for the rest of the morning until baby kicks, responsibilities, or body aches rouse you again.

  Do let your healthcare provider know if you're sleeping excessively on a regular basis (like more than 10 hours per day, 5 days a week), as that could be a sign of *anemia* and/or depression.

- Seek professional help if your negative feelings overwhelm you, or you feel depressed and down for more than a day or so.

- Be candid about your needs with friends and family, and be honest about what they can do to help you feel better, be it "please wash the dishes in the sink because they're making me gag" or "please just be quiet and listen."

- Find other moms-to-be, and keep learning. Ask your care provider any and every question you have, and consider taking a childbirth class with real people (as opposed to using DVDs or an app).

- Avoid (or at least take with a grain of salt) Internet message boards, which tend to be full of horror stories and half-baked or biased information.

- Scale down stresses. Evaluate all of your commitments to see if there are any you can scale back on to give yourself more downtime.

- Practice deep breathing and relaxation. Take time out to just sit (or lie down) and focus on your breathing, and take breathe-and-stretch breaks to send your baby and your body a rush of oxygen.

- Keep a journal—a private one on paper. Writing down your experiences will help you put them in perspective over time. One journaling trick can be useful: divide your journal page into two columns. In the left column, write down every negative thought you have, and don't stop until you've gotten every feeling out. In the right column, force yourself to write down the exact opposite of those feelings. For example, if you have recurrent fears the baby will be born deformed or die, write that on the left side and on the right put that the baby is healthy, beautiful, and perfect. Positive thoughts can be powerful too.

How You're Feeling: The extra *progesterone* and other hormones may be making you feel tired, achy, nauseated, and cranky, or you not may be feeling much different than normal. You might have an ultrasound as early as this week to determine fetal age or if you've had multiple miscarriages in the past.

You'll start noticing babies more and may start to wonder if yours will be as funny-looking as the ones you see on the street. Don't worry, your baby will be the cutest ever born (or at least, you'll think so).

About Miscarriage

Should you worry about having a miscarriage? Miscarriages aren't the most pleasant thing to talk about, but they are common in the first trimester.

Your chances of having one increase as you age: studies have found that about 9 percent of recognized pregnancies for women ages 20 to 24 ended in miscarriage. The risk rises to about 20 percent at age 35 to 39, and more than 50 percent by age 42.

For women with no vaginal bleeding, most estimates suggest that the odds or having a miscarriage after seeing a heartbeat are about 4 percent. For women with vaginal bleeding but also a detected heartbeat on ultrasound, risk of miscarriage is about 13 percent according to one study.

WHAT IS A MISCARRIAGE?

A miscarriage is a pregnancy that ends before the twentieth medical week. After week 20, the loss of the fetus is classified as a stillbirth or a preterm delivery. Eighty percent of miscarriages happen in the first trimester. They commonly occur around the time the woman's menstrual periods would have—around the fourth, eighth, twelfth, and sixteenth medical weeks of pregnancy. Miscarriages that happen in the first few weeks of pregnancy are referred to as *blighted ovums*, or *anembryonic gestations*, which means that the fertilized egg simply fails to develop for unknown reasons. Many women miscarry more than once in their lives. About one in thirty-six women will have two miscarriages due to nothing more than chance. Most often they are unpreventable, and no cause is found.

WHY DOES MISCARRIAGE HAPPEN?

Most of the time, for no reason other than bad luck, some chromosomal or genetic information is lost during conception. When the needed genetic information isn't there at the developmental point when the fetus needs it to continue growing, you will miscarry. By eliminating about 95 percent of fertilized eggs or embryos with genetic problems, nature ensures that any offspring you have will have the best possible chance for long-term survival. Certain infections also appear play a part in some miscarriages.

WHAT HAPPENS?

Miscarriages early in pregnancy often happen in the form of a heavy, late period, and if you don't know that you're pregnant, you won't even be aware you're having one. Spotting and light bleeding is common in early pregnancy, but the longer the bleeding lasts and the more cramps you feel, the more likely it is that you're experiencing a miscarriage. The bleeding associated with miscarriages lasts for about 7 to 10 days.

WHAT TO DO

If you experience blood spotting during your pregnancy, call your care provider immediately. Your practitioner will probably perform an ultrasound exam.

If you have indeed miscarried, your healthcare provider will determine if the miscarriage is complete (all fetal tissue has been passed) or incomplete.

If you haven't miscarried, your healthcare provider may test the hormone levels in your blood and will continue to monitor you with ultrasound. Some healthcare providers may order bed rest. (See "Bed Rest" on page 107.) If your progesterone levels are low, you may be given suppositories of progesterone to help maintain your pregnancy, although this is of no proven benefit. Incomplete miscarriages, when some but not all of the pregnancy tissue is passed, are more common the longer you've been pregnant. In the case of an incomplete miscarriage, your healthcare provider may order a D&C (*dilation and curettage*). This procedure reduces the likelihood of infection. If you have an incomplete miscarriage and are under the supervision of a midwife, you'll be put under the care of her attending obstetrician for this procedure. During a D&C, you will be given general or local anesthesia, your cervix will be dilated, and any retained fetal or placental tissue will be removed. The D&C doesn't weaken your cervix or make you more likely to miscarry in subsequent pregnancies. Very rarely, a D&C can cause an infection in your uterus, which is treated by a course of antibiotics.

An alternative, which many providers are starting to use, involves the use of the medications *misoprostol* and mifepristone to trigger the uterus to start cramping and cause the remaining tissue from the pregnancy to be expelled.

HOW DOES A MISCARRIAGE FEEL?

Any of the following symptoms may signal that you are possibly having a miscarriage: your abdomen rhythmically tightening and releasing (*contraction*s) every 10 minutes or more often; a feeling of pelvic pressure as though your baby is pushing down; a low, dull backache; abdominal or menstrual-like cramps with or without diarrhea; and the discharge of fluid, blood, or clots.

Emotionally, things may be difficult, particularly if you've been trying hard to get pregnant for a long time, or a lot of people know your baby news. The loss of a baby is not something you get over, and family and friends may not know how to support you in a helpful way.

Since miscarriage is so common, you may find you're not alone if you share your experience with friends or family members—it's a secret that a lot of women out there share. If you don't want to talk about your experience with anyone you know, there are also Internet and hospital support groups, should you ever want to share about your experience or help support someone else.

If you worry that drinking, smoking, or staying out late caused your miscarriage—don't. Unless you're a chronic alcoholic or crack addict or smoke five packs a day, your behavior is not the cause.

HOW TO HELP SOMEONE WHO'S HAD A MISCARRIAGE

If you're a partner, relative, or friend it can be tough to know what to say to someone who's had a miscarriage. On the other hand, you certainly don't want to carry on like nothing's happened, or avoid a person because you feel awkward. Some ideas:

- "I'm so sorry for your loss."
- "I don't know what to say, but I'm here for you. Please let me know if there's anything I can do to help."
- "Can I babysit/help clean house/run errands while you rest?"
- "Do you want to talk about it? If you ever do, please know I'll always be here to listen, even if it's 3 a.m."
- Check back in. The pain doesn't go away in a few days or weeks. The baby's due date can be an especially tough time, as can the anniversary of the loss.
- Avoid at all costs saying any of the following: "but you can have more," "one miscarriage isn't so bad, so-and-so has had three," "at least you weren't that far along," "it wasn't meant to be," "it was God's plan," "the baby probably had some kind of defect and wouldn't have survived anyway," "you need to ___" (fill in the blank: "cry," "cry less," "move on," "try again," "focus on the kids you do have," "take a class," or any other unsolicited advice on how to grieve).
- Know that while some people might want to talk, others will need space, and it's okay and normal if your friend or partner doesn't want to talk about it, or even cuts you off if you

bring it up. Everyone mourns in a different way. Often the most and best you can do is to let someone know you care about them and you're there for them and willing to listen and help, if needed.

A NOTE ON ECTOPIC PREGNANCY

In about one out of a hundred pregnancies, the ovum doesn't implant in the wall of the uterus where it should, but migrates and implants in the wrong place, such as the side of a fallopian tube or, extremely rarely, in the abdomen. With rare exceptions, ectopic pregnancies are not *viable*. Furthermore, they are dangerous for the mother, internal bleeding being a common complication. If the embryo is in the fallopian tube, this can cause the tube to rupture. Removal of the embryo often requires surgery (although it is sometimes possible to treat this condition with a medication called methotrexate). In such cases, saving the pregnancy is not possible. The signs of an ectopic pregnancy are severe abdominal pain, bleeding, and severe cramps, and you may possibly experience faintness, nausea, dizziness, and vomiting. The chances of having an ectopic pregnancy are ten times higher for women who have had Pelvic Inflammatory Disease (PID) due to the scarring it causes.

WEEK 7

Fetal Age: 5 weeks (36 to 42 days)

33 to 32 weeks, 230 to 224 days until your due date

Baby

Size: Your baby enters its second month of development weighing no more than a chocolate chip or a berry. It's about 5 to 13 millimeters long (less than half an inch), and weighs less than a gram (0.8 g), or less than one-twentieth of an ounce.

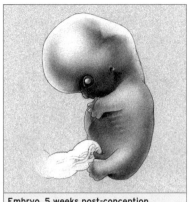

Embryo, 5 weeks post-conception

Development: It has only been a little more than a month, and the human blueprints are already visible. Your embryo is beginning to form a digestive tract, lungs, nostrils, hands and feet, and a bump of a mouth. The liver, tongue, and lenses of your baby's eyes are forming. There are beds for your baby's fingernails, and the buds of teeth are forming in the gums.

If you could take a picture, your baby would look a little more like a baby and less like a reptile, though it still has a tail. The baby's nerve channels and muscles are connecting, and the body can wiggle when the cells communicate. In just 2 days, from days 31 to 33, the brain becomes one-quarter larger.

If you were to have an ultrasound, it would be able to detect the beating U-shaped tube that will become the heart, which shows up looking like a tiny flashing light.

You

The mucus on your cervix is thickening, forming a plug that will keep your uterus sealed until you give birth.

How you're feeling: You might be feeling tired, achy, and cranky—or not. You might be feeling queasy, or you may never feel queasy. A lack of symptoms doesn't mean that there's anything wrong with you or the baby, though pregnancy-related nausea has been linked to a lower rate of miscarriage.

You've probably experienced one of pregnancy's first psychological changes: You relate everything you eat, drink, or experience to how it may affect your condition. Your baby is smaller than a fingernail, so she doesn't need lots of calories right now, but she does need to have certain nutrients available for cell division and communication.

Prenatal vitamins will help prevent deficiencies, but your body uses nutrients most efficiently if you get them through the foods you eat. A diet with plenty of fiber, vegetables, and fluids will also help keep you from gaining too much weight. Fortified cereals, big salads with colorful vegetables, and vegetable soups are good choices that will help you get enough folic acid and B vitamins as well as calcium and fluids.

Your First Visit to Your Doctor or Midwife

After a review and discussion of your medical history, your care provider and his or her staff will:

- Create a medical record that will be checked at every visit to make sure that you're gaining weight at a healthy pace.
- Measure the height of your uterus to confirm how far along you are and to create a growth chart for your uterus.
- Take a blood sample from your arm. Blood samples are used to check all sorts of things, including:
  - Finding out if you're potentially a carrier for certain genetic disorders, such as **cystic fibrosis** or **hemoglobin** disorders. (See "Cystic Fibrosis Screening" and "Birth and Genetic Defects" in Chapter 2).
  - Determining your blood type (A, B, AB, or O), and whether or not you are Rh positive or negative (see "Rh Screening" in Chapter 2).
  - Checking glucose and hemoglobin levels.
  - Checking for the presence of infections such as **syphilis**, **hepatitis B**, and **HIV**.
  - Seeing if you have antibodies to **rubella** (German measles). If you were vaccinated or had the disease as a child, there's no need to worry. If you don't have antibodies, however, you'll need to be careful to avoid exposure to anyone with the infection, because it can cause birth defects. (See "Immunizations" on page 256.)
- Some care providers also may check to see if you have immunities to **toxoplasmosis**, a parasitic disease. (See page 114 for more about toxoplasmosis.)

If your care provider doesn't have a lab on site to draw and test blood, ask him to recommend a diagnostic lab where the phlebotomists are experienced enough to draw blood with the first stick. You may have quite a few vials drawn from you during the first trimester.

Your care provider will also take a urine sample to check your levels of protein, sugar, and bacteria. Protein and/or the presence of red and white blood cells could be a sign of high blood pressure or a urinary tract or kidney infection.

Later in pregnancy, protein may be a sign of **preeclampsia**, also known as toxemia. Your care provider might check your urine at every visit. (For more information, see "Preeclampsia" in the Pregnancy Dictionary.)

You'll also receive a physical exam, where your care provider will:

- Measure your height, weight, and blood pressure.
- Possibly check out your eyes, gums, and skin.
- Listen to your heart and lungs to check for abnormalities or congestion.
- Palpate your abdomen for tenderness or unusual lumps.
- Conduct a pelvic exam. Your caregiver will inspect the color of your cervix and the size of your uterus. If you're pregnant, your cervix will have a bluish tint, and your uterus will be heavy and firm. Your care provider may also take swabs from your cervix for a Pap test to screen for cervical cancer and to check for infections.

And, last but not least, your care provider will give you a due date and, based on that, help you schedule any additional tests, such as a

YOUR FIRST VISIT TO YOUR DOCTOR OR MIDWIFE, *CONTINUED*

first-trimester blood screen or an ultrasound. Most healthcare providers routinely schedule blood serum testing and an ultrasound between weeks 9 and 13, and a second ultrasound between weeks 18 and 20. (For more information, see "Ultrasound" in the Pregnancy Dictionary.)
Remember to ask:
- What is my due date?
- Do I have any health issues I need to be concerned about?
- Do I need to avoid any specific medications, dietary supplements, or activities?
- Should I pay attention to weight gain? How often should I exercise, and what kind of activities do you suggest?
- What kind of options do I have for prenatal vitamins? Should I take any additional supplements, like extra vitamin D, calcium, iron, or DHA?

Kegel Who?

It's never too soon to start doing *Kegel exercises*! This miraculous exercise, "invented" by California gynecologist Arnold Kegel, strengthens urogenital and *pubococcygeus muscles*, which support the pelvic floor. If you keep these muscles in shape you can prevent *urinary incontinence*, promote good blood flow to your pelvic floor, and more quickly recover your tone after childbirth.

To do a Kegel, you tighten the same muscles you would use to stop the flow of urine. Practice on the toilet, and after you get the hang of them, you can practice your Kegels while you're driving, at work, or even standing in the grocery line— no one will know what you're up to. Work on contracting the muscle as many times in a row as you can, contracting as tightly as you can, and holding the move for as long as possible. If you Kegel during every red light, boring phone call, and TV commercial, later in your pregnancy and after birth you'll be less likely to leak urine as you laugh or cough.

WEEK 8

Fetal Age: 6 weeks (43 to 49 days)

32 to 31 weeks, 223 to 217 days until your due date

Baby

Size: Your baby is now about the size of your thumbprint: one half to three-quarters of an inch.

Development: Six weeks is barely enough time to start a magazine subscription, but it's enough time for your fetus to develop limbs, tiny fingers and

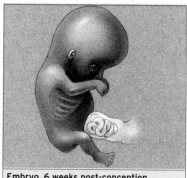

Embryo, 6 weeks post-conception

toes, the beginnings of external ear structures, eyelids, an upper lip, the tip of a nose, and intestines.

You

If you're going to get pregnancy-related nausea (aka *morning sickness*, aka all-darn-day sickness), it probably will have kicked in by now. Researchers don't know its exact cause, but it seems to play a role in protecting the baby from toxins during what is the most delicate and crucial time for development, when the brain and major organ structures are beginning to form.

Research has even found that pregnancy changes your sense of taste, with women in the first trimester finding bitter, citric, and salty flavors more intense and less appealing than women who were not pregnant. As pregnancy progressed, the more the women in

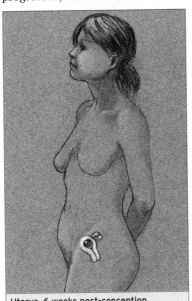

Uterus, 6 weeks post-conception

the study liked the salty and citric flavors, and they ranked the bitter flavors as less intense.

The intensity of nausea also seems to be related to hormone levels, since hormone levels and your level of nausea seem to rise and fall together, and women pregnant with multiples tend to feel more nauseated.

Whatever the exact mechanisms of nausea, there is an upside: the sicker you feel, apparently, the less likely you are to miscarry (which is not to say if you don't feel sick, you'll miscarry; you could just be lucky).

Because of nausea and vomiting, you may worry that you're not getting enough calories to your baby. Most of the time this is nothing to worry about, your embryo is tiny and doesn't need a lot of calories at this point. But if you throw up more than three times in a day or can't stand to eat or keep anything down for 12 hours (or longer), let your healthcare provider know: extreme queasiness can cause dehydration and other serious issues, and drug treatment is available.

Eat what you can stand, even if it's only one or two foods. Try to take a vitamin supplement if you can stand to.

You may also experience other gastrointestinal problems, such as *constipation* and/or diarrhea. The constipation is related to the slowing down of your digestive tract and the diarrhea appears to be your body's way of quickly moving out any food that isn't good for your system.

How you're feeling emotionally: Worried. Are you worrying about all of the living it up you did before you knew you were pregnant? You probably have nothing to worry about. To be blunt, if you'd done any damage at this early stage, the embryo probably would not have survived to this point.

If you've been trying to conceive for a long time and have had miscarriages in the past, this can be a particularly harrowing time. Even if your provider offers a weekly ultrasound and frequent blood tests to check your hormone levels, consider that this plan won't prevent or stop an impending miscarriage and may actually increase your stress level.

What you can do: As soon as your underwear is tight, treat yourself to stretchy cotton bikini-style maternity underwear. You don't want a *urinary tract infection* (UTI). Toss your thongs—they help *E. coli* bacteria migrate to your urinary tract and *vagina*, which can cause potentially dangerous (and painful) UTIs and vaginal bacterial and *yeast infection*s. Thongs made of synthetic materials can also cause tiny cuts, which provide a place for bacteria to grow. You're more susceptible to infections while you're pregnant, and any infection is potentially dangerous to the baby.

While you're at it, also toss any scented toilet papers, perfumed bubble baths, or feminine deodorant sprays you have. Soaps, sprays, and scented products can upset the balance of "good" bacteria in your vagina, making you more prone to yeast infections, *vaginitis*, and UTIs. It is normal to have more discharge than usual during pregnancy, but nothing in your vaginal area should hurt, burn, or have a foul odor. Discharge that smells funny, has an

unusual texture, or is any color but white is not healthy. (See more on discharge in Chapter 2.)

If you do get a yeast infection or experience any kind of vaginal itching, burning, unusual discharge, or painful urination, tell your care provider right away, and don't try to self-diagnose or medicate, because other conditions like vaginitis can have similar symptoms. Also, some yeast infection treatments shouldn't be used during the first trimester, and urinary tract infections can only be treated with prescription *antibiotics*.

TIP

To prevent injury, muscle pulls, and fatigue, strengthen the muscles in your back with a program designed by a personal trainer, or swim laps to build strength, endurance, and flexibility.

Strategies for Coping with Nausea

Research has found that there's no one cure-all for pregnancy nausea: what works for one person, or with one pregnancy, won't help everyone. But most women are able to find one or two things that help a little. Some suggestions:
- **Listen to your body.** Never try to make yourself eat something that disgusts you.
- **Don't let yourself get too hungry.** Try to eat a small amount of something every 2 hours while you're awake.
- **B6.** With the approval of your

clinician, try to take 10 to 25 mg of B6 three times per day.

- **Ginger.** Drink ginger-infused tea, or eat ginger snaps. Ginger has been found to suppress vomiting. If you go for ginger ale, make sure real ginger is on the ingredients list—not all ginger-flavored sodas have it. One Chinese cure for morning sickness is lots of shredded fresh ginger boiled in water to make tea, sweetened with sugar or honey.
- **Tamarind.** The tangy legume is rumored to be one of the secret flavors of Coca-Cola, and is a popular pregnancy-nausea treatment in India. You may be able to find tamarind sodas, paste, or sweets in Asian or Latin American specialty grocery stores.
- **Seltzer.** Sip on seltzer water or club soda.
- **Lemon.** Make lemon zest from the peel of a whole lemon, keep it in a baggie, and sniff it when nauseous feelings start to rise. Lemon-flavored hard candies may also help.
- **Yogurt.** Eat yogurt to encourage the friendly bacteria in your digestive system.
- **Black licorice.** If you like licorice, try strings, twists, or drops.
- **Bouillon.** Sip on a cup of warm beef or chicken bouillon or miso soup. The warmth can be soothing, and the salt will help replenish you after bouts of vomiting.
- **Sports drinks.** If you throw up a lot, sports drinks can help replace electrolytes. Avoid drinks that contain caffeine.
- **Water.** Stay hydrated by sipping water throughout the day. Drink between meals and not with meals to prevent your stomach

from becoming overfull.
- **Crackers.** Try saltines or other crackers. If an empty stomach makes you queasy, keep a couple of crackers by your bedside.
- **Acupressure.** Wear acupressure bands, usually displayed in pharmacies next to the seasickness medications. The bands fit around your wrists and have a small knob on the underside that presses into the area beneath your thumb about 1 inch below the inside of your wrist bone. This specific pressure point is thought to curtail nausea (and seasickness).
- **Avoid caffeine.** Cut out coffee, tea, chocolate, and soda, which can exacerbate nausea and vomiting.
- **Indulge.** Give in to food cravings (in moderation).
- **Change or skip the vitamins.** If your prenatal vitamins make you sick, take them at night or switch brands. Children's chewables with iron can work too, as long as they contain enough B vitamins. Or, if you are able to get in all of your nutrients from food, skip the vitamins entirely. (See Chapter 3 for more on nutrients and supplements.)
- **Protein.** Avoid processed sugars, and eat frequent small, high-protein snacks instead, which will help keep your blood sugar levels steady.
- **Sleep.** Nap frequently. Fatigue makes stomach upset worse.
- **Close your nose.** Stay away from offending odors. Cover your nose with your hand or a tissue.
- **Be prepared.** If you're prone to spontaneous bouts of vomiting, keep a plastic bag and a few paper towels in your purse and/or car.

WEEK 9

Fetal Age: 7 weeks (50 to 56 days)

31 to 30 weeks, 216 to 210 days until your due date

Baby

Size: Your baby is now about three-quarters of an inch long, about as tall as a thumbnail.

Development: At the end of this week your little passenger graduates from "embryo" to "fetus."

A membrane lid covers your baby's eyes. Muscles are beginning to develop, and she can make tiny movements. Limbs are growing, but her arms and hands are forming more quickly than her legs and feet. The hands are actually still known as "hand paddles" and look just like they sound. Ridges have formed on the paddles, which will soon become well-defined fingers. Your baby is developing little dimples where her knees and ankles will go, and her elbows are becoming visible. This week is when sex characteristics begin to assert themselves, and ovaries or testes will soon appear (though most ultrasound machines won't be able to detect specific sex organs for another month or so). Your baby's brain waves can now be detected.

You

Your nauseating hCG levels are at their peak this week. The good news is that starting next week, as your hormone levels stabilize, you'll start feeling a lot better. The bad news is that this week may be rough. If you're throwing up a

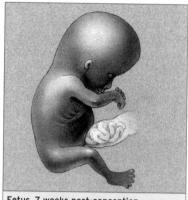

Fetus, 7 weeks post-conception

lot, drink plenty of water to keep yourself from dehydrating.

Your uterus has doubled from pre-pregnancy size and is now about the size of a tennis ball. The area under your navel is definitely firmer than usual. Many women report being too tired and queasy to be interested in sex at this stage, though some women also report being more interested than usual.

It's common at this stage to have sharp pain on either side of your pelvis, especially when you twist or stand up after sitting for a while. Your uterus is becoming heavy, and this can strain your round ligaments, which are the muscles that hold your uterus in place. Let your healthcare provider know if the pain is constant and/or doesn't change when you move around.

You may begin to notice changes in your hair and skin. Your hair might feel thick and lustrous—or greasy, thin, and limp. Resist the urge to try to dye, perm, or highlight your hair—it may not take to the chemicals evenly. Do switch your shampoo and conditioner to suit your new hair texture.

How you're feeling: It's tough to be upbeat while you're feeling sick. It's also hard to keep your pregnancy a secret at work if you're constantly nauseated. Take care of yourself and have faith you'll feel better soon. If you're lucky, you have a co-worker you can trust to keep your secret, who can cover for you on your many trips to the bathroom. It can also be tough to keep your pregnancy a secret if you were once a social drinker and now, suddenly, you aren't.

Pregnancy can make you feel like you're all alone in the world, no matter how many billions of women have been in your condition. It also doesn't help that your condition is invisible to your partner—he just sees that you're moody, tired, and queasy and may be wondering when you're going to be back to your old self again.

Things to organize: If you haven't already visited your care provider, make an appointment now. The earlier you can be tested for certain conditions and infections, the more likely you are to deliver a healthy baby. Your first ultrasound may be performed as early as this week. While you may be anxious to get an ultrasound, remember that they are expensive medical tests. You probably won't be offered one unless you can't remember when your last menstrual period was, if multiple births run in your family, or if you've had unusual bleeding. It's important to note that much is still unknown about the effects of ultrasound. (For more on this, see "Ultrasound" on page 149.)

WEEK 10

Fetal Age: 8 weeks (57 to 63 days)

30 to 29 weeks, 209 to 203 days until your due date

Baby

Size: Your baby is now about an inch long and weighs 5 g, or one-sixth of an ounce, roughly the size of a garden beetle.

Development: This end of the 2-month mark is a landmark date for your fetus. It's looking more human all the time. If you could look inside, you'd see a thumb tip–size, translucent creature that's unmistakably human. Kidneys, lungs, *genitals*, and the gastrointestinal tract are all present, though far from fully formed. Your baby's bones begin to form in his limbs, a process called ossification. The floor plan for your baby's structure has been laid down, and the next 30 weeks will be about expanding and developing on this blueprint.

If your baby is a boy, his testes are already producing testosterone. A *Doppler* handheld device can usually detect a fetal heartbeat by this point. Once the heartbeat is detectable, your chances of miscarrying in the first trimester are immediately lower: between 5 and 10 percent.

This and the following 4 weeks are an especially sensitive time for fetal organ development, when infections, nutritional deficiencies, radiation, alcohol, and medications can do the most serious damage.

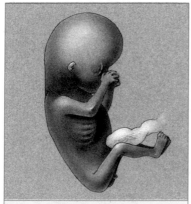

Fetus, 8 weeks post-conception

You

Congratulations, your uterus has swollen to the size of a softball! When you look in the mirror, your shape will have definitely changed, with a thicker waist and more chest.

You'll likely be offered the opportunity to take prenatal screening tests between weeks 11 and 14, usually a blood test that measures the levels of specific hormones and proteins, plus the **nuchal translucency** scan, which is an ultrasound to measure the folds in the fetus's neck.

When it comes to prenatal screening tests—blood screens, ultrasounds, and the more invasive ones—you can opt for some, all, or none. As you consider which tests to take, factor in what you would do with the results. Would you feel a whole lot better to know that your baby has lower risks of certain defects than other moms' of your age? If you find out 3 weeks from now that your baby does have a significant defect, would you terminate the pregnancy?

Some women decide simply to not undergo any testing at all—if you know you wouldn't terminate a pregnancy no matter what, there's a good argument to be made for saving yourself from the extra stress. You could also skip the early screenings but then get a detailed **sonogram** between weeks 18 and 20. Or opt to skip all tests of every kind and then hedge your bets by choosing to deliver in a hospital that offers the highest levels of care should the baby have a health issue.

Yet another strategy for prenatal testing is to opt to take the screening tests but decide beforehand how much uncertainly you're able to deal with. Would you want to undergo CVS testing if screening test reveals that you have a one-in-forty-seven risk of having a baby with **Down syndrome**? What about one in two hundred, four hundred, or seven hundred? While there's no such thing as being completely, totally reassured that nothing is wrong, it might be possible to decide at what point you're reassured *enough*. (For more on screening test results, see week 13.)

Or, finally, you can opt to go all-in and decide to have as much testing as you and your insurance company's money will buy. Forewarned is forearmed, and knowing as much detail as possible before birth about your baby will give you, your family, and your healthcare providers a better ability to prepare for the future.

Prenatal testing cuts to the very heart of personal, deep, and philosophical questions. The opinions of healthcare providers, your partner, and your family are all important, but at the end of the day, choosing to take prenatal tests and then how you deal with the results is your decision to make and to live with; you can only do the best you can to make choices that feel right given what you know and believe right now.

If you opt for the blood and ultrasound screening tests, your healthcare provider's office staff will help you arrange for the tests. Your healthcare provider may be equipped to draw and test blood in her office, or you may be sent to separate labs for the blood draw and ultrasound scan.

Then, after about a week after the blood and ultrasound tests your healthcare provider, a genetic counselor or a hospital OB will have a sit-down with you to discuss results. (For more detail on what to expect at this appointment see week 13.)

If you're over 35 or have a family history of genetic disorders, over the next 2 weeks, your care provider may offer a test called *chorionic villus sampling* (CVS), which uses a sample of tissue to screen for hundreds of genetic disorders. This test is highly accurate, but carries a significant risk of miscarriage.

How you may be feeling:
You may notice your weight gain picking up—though don't worry if you haven't gained any by now. If you've begun eating a healthier diet and exercising, you may have even lost weight. Bottom line, if your care provider isn't concerned about how much or little you've gained, you shouldn't be either.

Regardless of what the scale says, it can be helpful to write down what you eat for a week to see what nutrients you're getting, what supplements you may need to take, and how much of your typical weekly diet is empty

calories. If you gain extra weight during your pregnancy, don't try to diet it away—just make sure that you aren't going overboard on the sweets and processed foods. (See more in Chapter 3.)

What you can do:
- **Nap, eat, relax, and refuse to feel guilty.** Snack on foods rich in calcium, potassium, and magnesium. Try a smoothie made with skim milk, vanilla yogurt, and bananas.
- **Brush and floss for two.** Make sure you have a nice, soft-bristled brush, some appealing dental floss, and an antibacterial mouth rinse. Your gums may be softening and be more likely to bleed while you brush and floss. You also may be producing more saliva. Use a soft-bristled toothbrush, brush frequently (after every meal, if you can), floss daily, and avoid sticky sweets that can stay in the crevices of your gums. Now is a good time to make a dental appointment for a checkup and cleaning. Women with gum disease may run a greater risk of delivering a premature baby of low birth weight. Besides, you won't want to worry about going to the dentist for a cleaning in the next 6 months; you'll have other things to think about!
- **Wear your seat belt.** This is the single most important thing you can do for you and your baby's safety. Before the car even starts, buckle the lap portion of your belt around your hip bone. Wear it even if you're just going on a short trip. If your shoulder belt rubs your neck, buy a seat belt adjusting clip or panel (available in any auto-parts store, and at

most major discount stores), and use it to adjust the belt so it fits comfortably across your shoulder.

WEEK 11

Fetal Age: 9 weeks (64 to 70 days)

29 to 28 weeks, 202 to 196 days until your due date

Baby

Size: Your baby is about 1¾ to 2½ inches long and weighs about a third of an ounce, about as tall as a peanut.

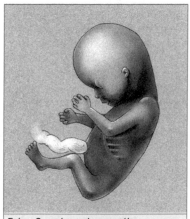

Fetus, 9 weeks post-conception

Development: This is a big week for your baby's growth—she'll double in height. At the end of the week, her head and body will be roughly equal in length. This week also starts an active phase for her—she can turn somersaults, roll over, flex her fingers, hiccup, and stretch. You won't be able to feel her movement for another month and a half. She's floating in lots of amniotic fluid.

Her limbs are developing from webbed paddles into arms and legs that have well-defined fingers and toes. Fingernails, toenails, and hair follicles are also beginning to form, and by next week her nails will be growing.

Your baby's testes or ovaries have developed, though the sex probably won't be visible on a sonogram for at least another month. Intestines have developed at the place where the **umbilical cord** meets your baby's body. The intestines are able to make constricting movements, though there won't be anything to digest until later.

You

Your body's expanding, inside and out. The next 10 weeks will be a period of rapid growth for you and the baby. You'll need more water as you produce more blood, sweat, oil, and amniotic fluid. You may feel desperately thirsty at times. It's a good idea to carry a beverage with you wherever you go, to keep your fluid levels up. Drink plenty of water, caffeine-free iced tea, and milk, but steer away from sodas and fruit juices, which may contribute to extra weight gain and swelling. The volume of blood in your body is increasing. An average woman with 9 pints of blood will have an extra 1.8 pints by the time she gives birth—a blood volume increase of almost 20 percent. As you make more blood, your blood pressure will return to normal, which will mean less dizziness, fatigue, and mental confusion.

It's also common to have headaches caused by dehydration

or sinus congestion. Your body needs a lot of water to make blood and amniotic fluid for the baby, and your sinuses have swollen to provide extra defense against germs. Other common causes of headaches are hunger and stress. If water, food, and relaxation don't work, take acetaminophen (Tylenol), not aspirin or ibuprofen. (See more on headaches in Chapter 2.)

You're burning calories in a hurry—up to 25 percent faster than you did before you were pregnant.

What you can do: Do you have the urge to eat dirt, cornstarch, cigarette ashes, or other weird non-foods? The urge is not as unusual as you might think. If you have weird cravings, tell your healthcare provider—it may signify a vitamin or mineral deficiency. Similarly, if you crave raw meat, you may be anemic. (See more on iron requirements in Chapter 3.) As your appetite increases, keep healthy snacks in your purse so you won't get ravenous and gorge on vending-machine food.

It's okay to be active: If you're in training for a marathon, ride horses, participate in contact sports, or even skydive, there's no reason to curtail your activities now. You don't need to worry about engaging in contact sports until your uterus tops your pelvic bones. Your baby is well protected by your abdominal muscles, your pelvis, and her amniotic fluid right now. With any physical activity, listen to your body. If you're just too tired, or feel faint, weak, or sick, don't push it. Next trimester, as your uterus emerges from your pelvis, sports that risk trauma to your abdomen won't be safe.

Are you feeling tired and weak? Try eating a high-iron food, such as linguine with clam sauce, a glass of prune juice, milk with a few tablespoons of blackstrap molasses, liver and onions, or a well-done hamburger.

Should you join a gym, pool, exercise group, or yoga studio? You certainly don't need an expensive membership to get exercise. Taking a walk is free. But it's not always easy to walk every day: it can get dull after a while, and the weather doesn't always cooperate.

In a perfect world there would be (free) gyms for expectant and new moms with a pool, pregnancy yoga, pregnancy massages, and clean showers with hot towels. However, if you can afford it and live in a larger-sized city, you may be able to find a pregnancy-friendly gym. Look for:

• **A pool.** In late pregnancy, it will feel wonderful to have a break from gravity, and swimming is an excellent low-impact exercise. Most YMCAs and YWCAs have pools. Some higher-end gyms may also have freshwater pools, which clean the water with oxidation and ionization, which means they don't have that chlorine smell or dry out your skin and hair as much.

• **Prenatal and postpartum personal trainers.** Look for a gym with personal trainers on staff who are certified and have experience working with pregnant women.

• **Nutritionists.** Some higher-end gyms have on-staff nutritionists, and your insurance company

may even foot the bill for you to consult with them.
- **A flexible contract.** Make sure that you can cancel or modify your membership if medical issues or complications arise that make it unsafe or inadvisable for you to work out (or if you just get bored of going).

WEEK 12

Fetal Age: 10 weeks (71 to 77 days)

28 to 27 weeks, 195 to 189 days until your due date

Baby

Size: Your baby's *crown-to-rump length* is about 2½ inches, or about the size of your thumb. She may weigh as much as half an ounce.

Development: With every passing day the fetus looks a little less like a wrinkly pink bean and more like a little Kewpie doll as its proportions change. The growth of the head slows down to let the rest of the body catch up, and the fetus goes from being half head to one-third head and two-thirds body over the next 2 weeks. What were little paddles a month ago have turned into arms and fingers, and your baby's posture is continually becoming less curled and more upright, a progression that will continue through babyhood.

You

You may get prenatal screening tests back this week.

It's a good idea to bring your partner or a friend for this appointment, for support and to

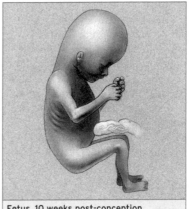

Fetus, 10 weeks post-conception

have a second set of ears. It can be helpful, too, to bring along a pen and something to write on, like your pregnancy journal, in case you have questions later.

The results of these tests is usually given as a ratio. Your healthcare provider should give you a single composite risk ratio that has your age and the results of your blood-chemistry screenings and various ultrasound measurements factored in. The risk can be as high as one in two or as low as one in ten thousand. Given these results, you can opt for CVS testing (which will have to be performed before week 14), or *amniocentesis* after 15 weeks.

When you get your results, you may also be given risk ratios for the individual factors that were screened for, sometimes broken down into "background risk" and "adjusted risk." The background risk is the risk any pregnant person of your age has for a particular defect, and the adjusted risk shows how new information changes these results. For instance, you might have a 1:122 background risk for Trisomy 21 (aka Down syndrome), then a 1:612 adjusted risk based on the ultrasound, a 1:47 risk based on your blood results, and finally an adjusted risk of 1:292. If your healthcare provider happens to give you all of these numbers, keep in mind that the number that matters is the composite, fully adjusted result, the 1:292 that takes all of the factors into account (and shows that you have less than half of the risk of the average person of your age).

Given these results, you can decide to have further testing, or not.

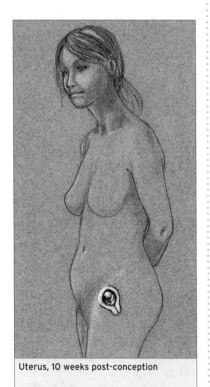

Uterus, 10 weeks post-conception

How you may be feeling emotionally: If you're waiting for prenatal test results you may find yourself frequently feeling like a nervous wreck. It's estimated that overall about 2 percent of babies will develop a defect that could affect their ability to function normally. For women over 35 the risk of defects rises about 1 to 2 percent. This is still very, very small. Picture a basket of a hundred Easter eggs, two or three of them with a million-dollar check stuffed inside. If you were completely logical, you wouldn't spend any more time worrying about birth defects than you would mentally spending the money before you stuck your hand in the basket. But it's human nature to worry, and a certain amount of worrying is probably inevitable. Finding other pregnant women online who are and have been through the same thing can be really helpful and reassuring.

What you can do: Take brisk walks (aim for 15 to 60 minutes each day), eat high-fiber foods, and drink plenty of water to help keep your intestinal tract moving. If your breasts hurt, try a new sports bra, or even two sports bras for super support, or consider swimming, riding a stationary bike, stair-stepping, or using a cross-country ski machine or, if you're in good shape already, a rowing machine.

If you have a desk job, try to arrange to work standing up and/or take frequent stretch breaks.

If you find yourself exceptionally gassy, check your food journal and see what you ate earlier in the day. You may be able to pick out certain "trigger foods" to avoid.

If you feel your sex drive coming back, take advantage now, because your partner's sex drive may decrease as the weeks go by: studies have found that living with a pregnant woman can actually cause a man's hormones to fluctuate, sometimes causing a decrease in testosterone.

WEEK 13

Fetal Age: 11 weeks (78 to 84 days)

27 to 26 weeks, 188 to 182 days until your due date

Baby

Size: Your baby is 2½ to 3 inches long, the size of a medium goldfish. She weighs about 1 ounce.

Development: Your baby is shorter than a finger, but her face is already showing individual features and characteristics. Her ears are now developed enough that she may be able to hear when you sing, hum, or talk.

And her vocal cords will form this week. Babies do mimic crying movements in the *womb*, though no sound will come out without air to transmit it. Your baby spends her time in your womb flexing her new and developing muscles and joints. Bouts of prenatal hiccups are strengthening your baby's *diaphragm*, which is preparing her respiratory system for breathing.

Less glamorous but highly necessary organ systems for making hormones, absorbing nutrients, and filtering waste are also in place this week. The pancreas, gallbladder, and thyroid have developed, the kidneys can make urine, and her bone marrow is making white blood cells to help fight infection after she's born.

You

Physically you may start to feel less queasy and more energized with each passing day as your placenta takes over hormone production. In 2 weeks or less, you might just be nausea-free, though some women experience queasiness their whole pregnancies.

However, you may still have several weeks of nausea before you get relief. Your smell and taste aversions may stick with you for the rest of your pregnancy, but unless you're very unlucky, the spontaneous throwing up will ease. Tell your care provider if it doesn't. If you haven't felt queasy by now, you've probably successfully avoided morning sickness.

It may be time for a shoe check—shoes that fit pre-pregnancy will start feeling tight as your feet swell and hormones and pressure make your foot bones spread out. Now is a good time to invest in a pair that can accommodate your widening feet. Soon it won't be easy to tie your shoes, and you'll appreciate a pair that slips on and off easily. Shoes made for doctors and nurses are good for pregnant feet. They're designed to be lightweight and to support you while standing. Cork-soled sandals, pool shoes, and canvas sneakers are also comfortable. Avoid high heels and platform shoes, because your sense of balance will start to be thrown off by your changing weight.

Pregnancy makes your digestive muscles slow down, while at the same time making you prone to harder and drier stools and making you gassier.

Your uterus has gotten too big to fit in its usual spot—your pelvis. It's now pushing into your abdomen, though not yet in any uncomfortable way. Your heart rate may speed up because of the extra volume of blood in your body. As you breathe in, you're taking 40 to 50 percent more air into your body than normal. Your rib cage has expanded, which may mean your bras need to be a size larger than usual.

As your ligaments soften, you may experience pain in your tailbone (coccyx), especially if you spend much of your day sitting down. Your hips are actually widening to make more room for your uterus to grow. Apply heat or ice (whichever feels better) to your tailbone area for 15 minutes at a time, or try a warm bath.

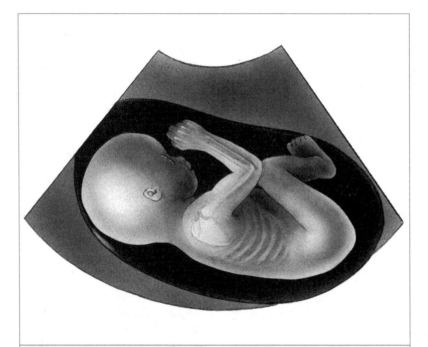

A sonogram is an image produced by ultrasound. Most ultrasound machines render sonograms with baby's bones as white and tissues as gray. Newer machines capable of real-time volume rendering ("4-D" machines), however, can produce images in a variety of tints. For more information on ultrasound, see page 49.

The Second Trimester

Weeks 14 through 27

Most moms agree that the second trimester is the highlight of the pregnancy experience. Your chances of carrying your pregnancy to term have gone from 80 percent to higher than 97 percent. Your nausea eases, you have almost as much energy as a non-pregnant person, and some women report that their sex lives during these 3 months are better than ever.

During this trimester you'll start to look pregnant instead of just padded, but you're not so pregnant that it's become difficult to put on your socks or get out of a car. You may even get the "glow of pregnancy," a kind of radiance that comes from extra blood flow to the capillaries of your skin, and if you were plagued with acne, it may ease up. The second trimester is a great time to travel, to decorate, and to take care of projects that need your attention. As you enter the third trimester, weight and fatigue may slow you down again. The second trimester is also a great time for your baby. Organ systems are fully in place, and by the end of the trimester, they'll be developed to the point that the baby could possibly survive outside of the womb with medical intervention. In the meantime, your body will nourish, protect, and keep her clean as she goes from being the size of a fist to the size of a football. She already looks human and will grow from being scrawny with a huge head to looking more like a *newborn*.

Another highlight of the second trimester is feeling movement—if you've had a baby before, you may feel wiggling any day now. If this is your first child, you may have to wait for another month or so before you feel anything. What starts as a feeling of fluttering will turn into poking, and even sharp kicking, by the end of this trimester. The odds of your baby being born healthy are tremendously in your favor, even if your pregnancy has been labeled high risk. Moms who are obese or whose babies have implanted on the front of their uteruses may take longer to feel kicks.

At this point in your pregnancy it may seem like you have a long time left to wait before it's over, but considering what goes on, pregnancy is so brief as to defy belief. There's never an idle moment in your uterus. Waste is moving in and out, neurons are forming, bones and tissues are building, and the baby is in almost constant motion. You can comfortably operate on the assumption that 6 months from now, someone's going to send you home from the hospital with a healthy baby.

The start of the second trimester is also a good time to find a childbirth class. Plenty of people don't take classes and go on to have a fine birth experience, but taking a class has advantages. It:

• **Increases control.** Studies have found that women who felt involved in the process, instead of feeling like birth was something being done to them, were far less likely to experience postpartum emotional disorders, such as depression and *post-traumatic birth disorder.*

- **Involves your partner.** Classes can help your partner know what to expect and how to be supportive.
- **Helps you make connections.** You'll get to meet other couples going through the same thing, a camaraderie that has forged many a lifelong friendship and/or toddler playgroup. Your unpregnant friends may be tired of tales of throwing up and *stretch marks*, but not this group. And childbirth educators themselves are a great resource. After meeting hundreds of couples, they know the real lowdown on all kinds of topics: where to get a good prenatal massage, who the best *pediatrician*s are in town, good lotions for an itchy belly, and sometimes even what other patients have had to say about your care provider.
- **Calms your fears.** Nothing is scarier than the unknown, and the more you know about birth and labor, the less anxiety you'll feel.
- **Helps to make you an educated consumer.** You'll learn what to expect from, and how to communicate with, your care provider and/or hospital.

You can ask your care provider for childbirth class recommendations, or you may have friends who've taken classes they liked. Depending on what's available in your area, you may be able to take a one-day seminar at a local hospital, or a much more detailed 13-week-long Bradley class.

The advantage of a longer class is that you'll have more of a chance to get to know other parents and to build confidence in the process. The downside to classes is that they may not be covered by your insurance. (See the Resources for common birth classes and their philosophies.)

WEEK 14

Fetal Age: 12 weeks (85 to 91 days)

26 to 25 weeks, 181 to 175 days until your due date

Baby

Size: Your baby is about 3½ inches long and weighs about 1½ ounces now—about the size of your fist.

Development: The past week has been one of rapid growth. The big development this week is the appearance of hair: *lanugo*, a covering of fine hairs that protects her skin, appears this week. Hair also begins growing on her head and eyebrows, and the hair may even have pigment in it if she has the genes for dark hair. Your baby's face continues to look more human, with individual characteristics becoming more pronounced all the time. Teeth have formed in your baby's gums. If you took a photo, you would be able to see her developing blood vessels, because her skin is very thin with no fat layer beneath it.

Her bone marrow has begun to produce blood cells, a chore previously performed by the yolk sac. Your fetus is rarely still. She's often wiggling fingers and toes, stretching, yawning, and hiccupping. If this is your first baby you may not be able to detect any movement for another month or so.

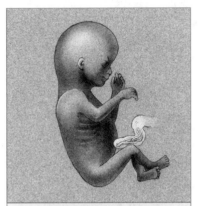

Fetus, 12 weeks post-conception

You

The amount of amniotic fluid that your baby is floating in increases dramatically this week, to about a quart. If you're going to undergo a diagnostic amniocentesis, it will likely be performed during the coming weeks.

Most moms find that their nausea, mood swings, exhaustion, and other hormonally related annoyances are easing up, though for some women symptoms may not completely disappear until after the baby is born.

Has the news of your pregnancy reached the far ends of your office and family yet? Almost certainly.

As far as gossip goes, pregnancy is everyone's favorite news. Now that everyone knows, you have an instant excuse to not do anything you don't want to do. For once, no one will be offended if you turn

down socializing by saying, "I just don't feel up to it."

If you're still feeling tired this week, make sure you're getting enough iron. The National Institutes of Health recommend that expectant moms take a daily iron supplement containing 30 mg. Try to get your extra iron from other sources besides iron supplements, because the mineral is much better absorbed through food. Eat clams, red meat, liver, leafy green vegetables, and acidic foods such as tomato sauce that are prepared in an iron frying pan. (The acids actually erode the pan a little bit, so that you get extra iron in your diet.) Take iron supplements with a glass of orange juice, because acid breaks down the iron so it is absorbed more readily. If you've started suffering from pregnancy-related **heartburn**, however, acidic juices and sauces may not be what you want. This annoying symptom can kick in as your digestive system slows down.

You may have plenty of cravings and food aversions by now. Give in to cravings, but with moderation. If you crave meats, dairy, or vegetables, consider that your diet may be deficient in certain vitamins or minerals, so by all means send your partner out in the driving snow for that pork chop or milkshake.

What you can do: It's not too soon to think about your birth philosophy and give some thought to who will be on your **birth team**. You've probably already picked out a physician or midwife to deliver your baby, but who else do you want in the room? What do you want your baby's birth to be like? What will your partner's role be?

You're probably now wearing

the more forgiving items in your wardrobe. You may as well shop for maternity clothes as soon as you feel like it—or at least maternity underwear and big cotton bras. If you can borrow from your relatives or friends, so much the better. You'll only be wearing this stuff for the next 6 to 9 months, and you're going to get a whole lot bigger, so a custom-tailored suit is not a good purchase right now.

Loose dresses, big shirts, and stretchy pants are good values. If you're planning to breastfeed, opt for button-down shirts that you can wear after the baby arrives.

WEEK 15

Fetal Age: 13 weeks (92 to 98 days)

25 to 24 weeks, 174 to 168 days until your due date

Baby

Size: About 4 to 4½ inches and about 1¾ of an ounce.

Development: This week your fetus will start to show his own distinct personality: facial muscles are developing and flexing, and fetuses begin to show distinct facial expressions such as smiles and grimaces. Some 13-week-old fetuses even suck their thumbs. All of his tiny organs, nerves, and muscles are starting to function, and all of the brain structures are in place. His neck is straighter and longer than it was last week, and he can turn his head from side to side.

The intestines have moved farther into the baby's body; his liver begins to secrete bile, which will later aid in the digestion of fats; and his pancreas begins to produce *insulin*, a hormone that turns sugar into energy.

You

Your womb is now starting to grow up and out of your pelvis, so you may have a neat and noticeable little bump below your belly button.

Your milk glands may already be kicking into production. You may sometimes notice what looks like water sitting on the tips of your nipples, or nipple-level wet spots on your sheets when you wake up in the morning. If you need to, put breast pads (or trimmed panty liners) inside your bra.

You may begin to feel *Braxton-Hicks contractions*, which get your uterus in shape to give birth. These "practice" contractions feel like a tightening in your uterus or abdominal area. Your uterus is the strongest muscle in your body, and these usually painless contractions are the way it stretches and expands its fibers to accommodate your growing baby. You may get them more frequently after exercise, and they usually go away if you drink water or change position. If you have regular contractions (more than four or five an hour) that get stronger over time, uncomfortable pelvic pressure, pain that starts in the back and moves toward the front like a tightening rubber band, or discharge lots of fluid or mucus, contact your care provider. When you have an orgasm, you may notice that your uterus hardens for several minutes. This has always happened, but now that your uterus is bigger, you can feel it. These contractions are harmless to you and your baby.

Feeling crafty?

Some ideas for channeling your creativity:
• Start a scrapbook, and save mementos of your pregnancy.
• Make a journal out of a big blank book.
• Start a monthly video diary or take weekly photos of your expanding stomach.
• Videotape your friends and relatives delivering messages to your baby.
• Knit booties, socks, blankets, or caps.
• Sew stuffed animals, clothes, or light baby blankets.
• Sew curtains.
• Design a stenciled wall or border for the baby's room.

How to Find a Pediatric Healthcare Provider

The best time to choose a healthcare provider for your baby is by the beginning of your third trimester, or seventh month, of pregnancy, unless your pregnancy is considered at-risk. In that case, you may want to have your baby's healthcare provider on board much earlier. Plan to meet with several pediatric healthcare providers until you find one that feels right to you and your partner. There are several people and sources you can consult with as you make your choices:

• Friends and family members. Ask people you trust who have babies and young children whom they would recommend and why.
• Your insurance company. Contact your insurance plan to find a list of preferred providers; many plans have Internet Web sites

where you can do the search.
• The hospital. Check with the hospital where you plan to deliver; many offer physician referral services. It's helpful (though by no means required) for your pediatrician to have privileges at the hospital where you plan to deliver.
• Your favorite current healthcare provider. Your obstetrician, midwife, family care physician, or general practitioner may have suggestions for trustworthy pediatricians.

Pediatricians are the most common healthcare providers for babies and children, but you may also opt for a family practitioner (who sees patients of all ages), a pediatric *nurse practitioner*, or use a practice where routine care is overseen by a physician's assistant.

A pediatrician is a medical doctor who has completed 4 years of college, followed by 4 years of medical school and 3 years of supervised residency (on-the-job training) for providing medical care for babies and children. Some pediatricians also have advanced training in *neonatal* care, child cardiology, or other specialties.

If the initials FAAP follow the pediatrician's name, that means that he or she has passed a written exam, is considered to be board certified, and has become a *fellow* of the American Academy of Pediatrics.

You can check on any doctor's board certification for a small fee by going to *www.certifieddoctor.org*.

It's important to find someone with whom you feel comfortable. The nurse practitioner or physician you choose should be not only versed in treating childhood illnesses, but also knowledgeable in child development and child health. Determine if you want a male or female doctor, since some children feel more trusting of same-sex providers. Also decide whether you will be more comfortable in a small office practice or a larger group practice.

The ideal healthcare provider is warm, caring, and a good listener, and one with whom you feel confident sharing thoughts and concerns. If you feel cut off, rushed, or diminished from your interactions, then you should probably move on. You can speed up the doctor screening process by telephone.

Some simple but important questions to ask by phone are:
• whether the office accepts your health insurance
• the doctor's hospital affiliations
• the office hours
• if the doctor has regular, daily call-in times
• if there is more than one office, and how the doctor splits his time between them
• how many other providers there are in the practice
• how weekend and night calls are handled
• whether there is a separate waiting room for sick children
• if the office has laboratory facilities and can provide hearing and vision screening onsite.

If you're satisfied with the answers, ask if there is a charge for an initial, get-acquainted interview, and how soon you can get an appointment. If there will be a fee charged for your visit, ask if it can be applied to a future office visit, since it's not likely your health insurance will pay for it. The first interview is a good time for you and your partner to assess the pediatrician and his or her practice to see if they are aligned with your values and needs.

As a new parent, you'll need someone you feel completely comfortable with and who will be there to support you should your baby become ill. Take a few minutes to converse with the support staff, too, since they are the persons you will most often encounter first when you call with concerns or to make appointments.

More Questions to Ask

• Will you be the person we see each time we bring our baby in, or is there a pediatric nurse practitioner or other physician who will also be providing medical care?
• Do you have privileges at the hospital where I plan to deliver?
• Do you have a cell phone number that we can call if the baby has health issues after delivery?
• When should we schedule our first appointment after our baby is born?
• What is your recommended *immunization* schedule for infants?
• Can you give us some literature about *vaccinations*?
• How often should our baby visit you during his first year?
• How far in advance do you recommend we make appointments?
• On average, how long will we have to sit in the waiting room before we get see you? Can you

recommend certain days or hours when your schedule is less crowded?

- How much time do you typically spend with a baby and family on a routine visit?
- How quickly can we expect you to return telephone calls?
- How important is it for me to breastfeed for the first 6 months? Are there circumstances when you would recommend supplementing with formula? If I don't want to breastfeed at all could you be supportive of that decision too?
- (If you plan to breastfeed) Does the office provide the services of a *lactation consultant*?
- Do you offer Centering Pregnancy in your practice? (This is a model of care that involves private prenatal care plus group childbirth education.)
- (If you're having a son) What are your recommendations regarding *circumcision* and who would perform it? (For more on this issue, see page 216.)
- Let a prospective healthcare provider know if you have special circumstances or concerns. For example, if you are worried about the overuse of antibiotics, or you are in favor of complementary or alternative health approaches, then you may want to test out his or her acceptance of them. If you have important cultural, religious, or moral tenets that could affect your decisions about your baby's care, or if you are gay, or a single parent, or the baby is known to have pre-disposing conditions, then you will want to get a sense of his or her sensitivity to these issues.

You should walk away from the appointment feeling that you have a trusted ally on whom you can rely when you have any need or concern about your baby, no matter how insignificant it may seem.

WEEK 16

Fetal Age: 14 weeks (99 to 105 days)

24 to 23 weeks, 167 to 161 days until your due date

Baby

Size: At 79 grams, she is about 4½ inches from crown to rump—roughly the size of an avocado or gerbil, and weighs about 2½ ounces.

Your baby has plenty of room: At this point, she could fit in the palm of your hand. This is a great time to be a fetus.

Development: She's now able to grasp things with her fist, and at any given time, she might be playing with the umbilical cord, putting her thumb in her mouth, or kicking at the amniotic sac.

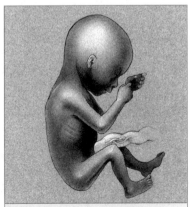

Fetus, 14 weeks post-conception

You

At any time, you will begin to feel fetal movement as your baby's bones begin to harden, and she starts a big growth spurt. Moms who have been pregnant before will tend to feel movement sooner, because they know what the sensation feels like, and also previous pregnancies will have made the uterine muscles more relaxed. It may take you longer to feel movement if you are overweight or if your placenta is positioned in the front of your uterus.

At 16 weeks post-conception, your uterus is outgrowing your pelvis. Since you have almost a cup of amniotic fluid in your uterus, your pelvic area will feel heavy and firm. You're also carrying all the extra poundage your body's putting on that can be attributed to extra blood and fluid volume, your placenta and baby's support systems, and enlarging breasts.

Extra blood and mucus will make you more prone to nasal congestion and nosebleeds. Try a humidifier or warm shower to open up your sinuses. Treat nosebleeds by pinching your nose with a tissue and tilting your head back. If you have an appointment this week, your care provider may recommend or offer these screening tests to detect the possibility of genetic defects:

Ultrasound. This painless test uses inaudible sound waves to create video images of your baby's anatomy. A radiologist or obstetrician uses these images to make sure your baby's organ systems are in place and to screen for signs of certain genetic defects. The test is usually best performed at 18 to 22 weeks, though some care providers give you the option of taking it earlier. If you're relatively young and have no family history of genetic defects, getting an ultrasound feels like more fun than a medical test should be.

For a lot of parents, the ultrasound is the first time that it really hits home that there's a little person in there. But the test can be stressful. For one thing, it's really hard to figure out what you're looking at, especially on older machines that render the image as gray and grainy. And with any ultrasound, the technician (called a sonographer) will be zooming in, out, and around. The blurriness has made many a mom shriek, "Oh my God! He has no hands!"

It's also important to note that most of the time your sonographer won't be able to make any diagnosis, unless he or she is also a *perinatologist* or radiologist. So though you may be frantically asking "Is the baby okay?" the person performing the test won't be able to tell you one way or the other. Instead, you have to wait for a radiologist, perinatologist, and/or your care provider to review images from the scan, which usually takes a few days. However, do ask the technician to point out body parts to you. And don't forget to ask for pictures!

Making a gender call isn't an official part of the ultrasound test, but most technicians will humor you and try to catch a peek at the baby's parts if you ask. Figuring out the baby's gender via ultrasound is basically a matter of seeing if there's a penis or not, but that's not always easy. The part in question is about the size of a grain of rice, and the baby has to be positioned just so. Even if your sonographer announces a gender with great confidence, don't print up the pink or blue baby announcements just yet. If you want to know your baby's gender, wait as long as possible before getting an ultrasound. While newer ultrasound machines may be clear enough that a technician can make a gender guess as early as 12 weeks, with an ultrasound machine that shows a gray, grainy, or blurry image, don't trust any guess made before 15 weeks.

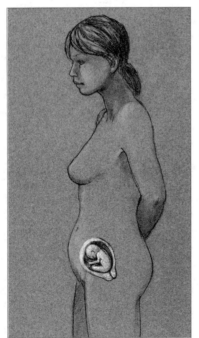

At 16 weeks post-conception, your uterus is outgrowing your pelvis.

Amniocentesis. This diagnostic test was once offered only to women over 35, women with a family history of genetic disorders, or women whose ultrasound or quad screen results revealed a possibility of a defect. These days the test is increasingly offered to all women.

This test analyzes a sample of your baby's genetic material, extracted from your amniotic fluid, for defects. Unlike screening tests that show indications that there might be an issue, amnio can conclusively diagnose a genetic defect.

Amnio is usually performed between this week and week 18.

While the quad screen and nuchal translucency scans have no known risks and minimal discomfort, amniocentesis comes with the very-small-but-real risk of inducing the *spontaneous abortion* of an otherwise healthy fetus—you will need to decide if knowing the results outweighs the potential risk. You can also decide to not undergo any screening tests at all, or only take first-trimester screening tests.

Some tests, such as an AFP blood screening test, have no known risks and minimal discomfort. Others, such as amniocentesis, have a level of risk and should only be undertaken if you feel it's important to know the results. Only you can decide if the risk involved to obtain the information is worth it.

Eight Indicators That You Should Change Care Providers

1. You spend a long time in the waiting room at every visit—a sign that your provider has more patients than he or she can comfortably handle.
2. Exams are rough or uncomfortable.
3. Your care provider dismisses, challenges, or demeans your questions or concerns.
4. Your care provider or the hospital where he or she has a cesarean rate of more than 30 percent, or your care provider or the hospital where he/she delivers won't let you attempt a VBAC (vaginal birth after caesarian) if you want one.
5. You feel like you can't be honest with your provider about your activities. (You feel uncomfortable talking to her about smoking, drinking, multiple partners, or drug use, for instance.)
6. When you telephone with a question, your call isn't taken or isn't returned promptly.
7. You don't like the other care providers in the group practice.
8. The hospital where your care provider delivers is far away from your home, crowded, or doesn't have features that are important to you (a high-level NICU or water birthing facilities, for instance).

WEEK 17

Fetal Age: 15 weeks (106 to 112 days)

23 to 22 weeks, 160 to 154 days until your due date

Baby

Size: She is about as wide as your palm, about 6 inches tall, and weighs about 4 ounces—about as much as a bar of soap. She now weighs more than your placenta.

Development: Your baby is now covered with a downy layer of lanugo, which swirls in fingerprint-like formations over her whole body. Her skin is still thin, but this week *brown fat*, a special type of fat that plays a role in body heat generation, begins to be deposited. Though she's had taste buds for a while, this week is when the ability to taste develops. She frequently swallows amniotic fluid, which is thought to carry traces of the stronger flavors of foods you've recently eaten, such as garlic or broccoli.

In the next few weeks, your baby's eyes will move beneath the lids in a side-to-side sweeping motion.

You

How you feel: Your sex drive, which probably took a backseat to your fatigue and nausea during the first trimester, may start coming back as you start to feel better. Many women report that sex during the second trimester is the best of their life! All of the extra blood flow to your pelvis may make arousal more frequent and intense than ever. But, like a great cosmic joke, for hormonal and psychological reasons, many men have feelings of apprehension about having sex with a pregnant woman.

Couvade syndrome is the medical term for when your partner starts showing pregnancy symptoms along with you. And it isn't just a psychological phenomenon—men who spend a lot of time with their pregnant partners can actually undergo hormonal shifts. The changes are in no way as dramatic as the ones you undergo, but your partner may indeed experience some nausea, indigestion, heartburn, loss of appetite for food, weight gain, and, notably, a loss of interest in sex.

Beyond hormonal changes, some men worry that they might hurt the fetus or that the fetus might be watching them (all untrue, but nevertheless not very arousing notions). Men can be unsettled by the realization that sex is for making babies, and breasts are for feeding them. Plus, because of hormonal changes, your vagina is darker-colored, has more discharge, smells different, and has more hair, which may disorient your partner.

How you may feel physically: As your breasts grow, they'll be sensitive and tender and sometimes just plain painful.

Your placenta is now a fully functional, well-established network of blood and tissue, distributing nutrients and removing waste. Now that this major construction project is complete, you'll have a lot more energy.

Your heart is now pumping 20 percent more blood. Your uterus is now about 2 inches below your navel and easy for you to feel.

When you move around, you may experience brief sharp pains around the front and side of your uterus, about where the leg holes of a high-cut bathing suit would be. These are called round ligament pains and are a result of your growing uterus straining the muscles that hold it in place. If the pain persists after a short rest or goes on when you're not moving, call your care provider.

What you can do: If your care provider tells you to avoid sex because you're at risk for preterm labor, be sure to ask exactly what he or she means by sex and which acts may be off limits.

WEEK 18

Fetal Age: 16 weeks (113 to 119 days)

22 to 21 weeks, 153 to 147 days until your due date

Baby

Size: She's about 5 to 5½ inches long from top to tail and weighs about 7 ounces, about the size of a lobster tail.

Development: While in earlier weeks, your baby may have been able to sense sound with her primitive ear structures, this week, the bones of the ear become fully formed and the nerves of the ear connect to the brain. She can hear your voice, your heart beating, stomach gurgling, and even the music you're listening to.

While there's no evidence that playing music, language tapes, or any other sounds to your baby will make her a genius, it can't hurt. Studies have suggested that babies will remember sounds that they have heard in utero and that they have a preference for known sounds. So a song you play for her now may help soothe her to sleep after she's born.

Hearing your voice will also influence her vocal development later: Research has found that newborns cry in the pitch structures of their native language, with German newborns starting out in a high pitch and becoming lower, and French babies' cries following the opposite pattern.

There's still plenty of room in your uterus, so your fetus can be quite active with her new muscles. She may change positions frequently, cross her legs, recline, suck her thumb, and turn somersaults. Her retinas have become light sensitive, and your baby will be able to detect a glow if you shine bright lights at your belly. Even though her eyelids are sealed, ultrasound pictures have shown fetuses moving their little hands to shield their eyes when bright lights are shined at the mom's belly.

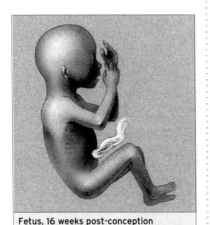

Fetus, 16 weeks post-conception

You

Space in the uterus gets tighter, and with every passing day the fluttery sensation of fetal movement will get stronger and more pronounced. The first sensations of movement are called **quickening**, and many cultures believe that this is when life begins. If you haven't felt any movement by 20 weeks, let your healthcare provider know.

You may have aches and pains in your legs, tailbone, and other muscles.

WEEK 19

Fetal Age: 17 weeks (120 to 126 days)

21 to 20 weeks, 146 to 140 days until your due date

Baby

Size: Your baby is between 5 and 6 inches long and weighs about 7 to 9 ounces, about the volume of a cup.

Development: If the baby is a girl, fallopian tubes are developing, and so are ovaries with *follicles* that are forming eggs. Soon, half of the genetic material for your potential future grandchildren will be formed.

Pictures of babies at this age show them touching the membrane of the amniotic sac, touching their own faces, reaching for the umbilical cord, pedaling their legs, and sucking their thumbs. If you're carrying twins, they may already be swatting at each other. Your baby may already have a preference for the left or right hand. In the brain, areas of nerve cells that serve the senses of touch, taste, smell, sight, and hearing are becoming specialized and are forming more complex connections. Loud sounds as well as any feelings you may have of stress or alarm may be communicated to the baby. The baby responds to these stresses by becoming more active.

You

You may experience shooting pains down your legs if your baby puts her weight on your *sciatic nerve*.

You may be popping out all over, with bigger breasts and a bulge above your pelvis, and you may experience back pain as the weight of your uterus makes your back work harder to keep you upright.

What you can do: Think about postpartum support. In the first few months after the baby's born, it's going to be virtually impossible for you to care for the baby and take care of household chores by yourself.

Until you establish a routine with your new baby, you'll be too occupied to cook meals, take care of pets, open the mail, pick up the phone, or do anything but breastfeed, soothe the baby, and sleep. We hope your partner is up to the challenge. If not, prepare to move your mother or another relative in for a time. Also consider hiring a postpartum doula or a baby nurse to help out.

WEEK 20

Fetal Age: 18 weeks (127 to 133 days)

20 to 19 weeks, 139 to 133 days until your due date

Baby

Size: Your baby is between 5½ and 6½ inches crown to rump, and between 9 and 10 inches from head to toe. She weighs about 9 ounces. Over the next month, she'll gain about a pound! Right now, she is about the size of a mango.

Development: Your baby's permanent teeth are already starting to form behind her baby teeth. These permanent teeth won't be mature for several years. By this point, your baby can move her eyes, though not always in tandem. What were sweeping left-right eye motions last week are turning into eye rolls. Eyebrows have formed, and hair is beginning to form on the scalp. Her skin is protected with a thin layer of *vernix*, a white, creamy substance with antibacterial properties that protects her in utero and will eventually help smooth her way through the *birth canal*.

From this point on, the baby seems to be able to differentiate between mornings, afternoons, and nighttime and starts to become active in cycles.

Your baby also has all of the neurons in her brain that she'll need, and the process of myelination begins in the brain. Walt Whitman was right—the body is electric, and myelin is a material that's mostly fat and acts as an electrical insulator for the nerve connections that conduct messages between parts of the brain. Like the covering of an electrical wire, the coating of myelin keeps the wiring of the brain from crossing signals or shorting out.

Building and insulating brain connections is an ongoing process, starting now and continuing on through the first years of your child's life. The myelin is about 80 percent fat, which is why you and later your baby and toddler

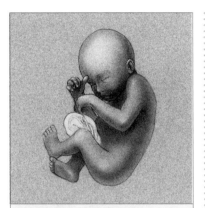

Fetus, 18 weeks post-conception

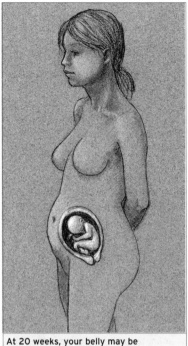

At 20 weeks, your belly may be outpacing your cleavage.

will need a higher-than-usual percentage of fat in your diets. (See Chapter 3 for more on this.)

You

Can you believe it? You'll be halfway to your due date at the end of this week!

Your belly may be horizontally outpacing your cleavage. Your care practitioner should begin monitoring your uterus's growth monthly with a tape measure or string and ruler. The top of your uterus should be now about in line with your belly button, and it will grow toward your rib cage at a rate of 1 centimeter a week from now until d-day.

What you can do: Now is a critical time for your baby's brain and a good time to make sure you get enough quality, non-hydrogenated fat in your diet, such as the fats found in olive oil, nuts, avocados, and fish.

Omega-3 fatty acids, found in oily fish such as salmon, tuna, and sardines, are great for your baby's brain. Some fish may be high in mercury, however, so consider limiting your intake

of oily fish to about 12 ounces a week and taking an omega-3 supplement instead.

Also good are the fats in nuts, avocados, and olive oil and the fats in dairy products. Still, try to limit your fat intake to one-third of your total daily calories.

Make sure that your diet contains plenty of B vitamins and good fats to support your baby's developing brain cells. When you exercise, work on your *cardiovascular* endurance, which will come in handy during labor and make it easier for you to carry your new baby wherever you go. Take long walks outside, walk on a treadmill with an incline, ride a stationary bike, use an elliptical trainer, and try these simple yoga poses:

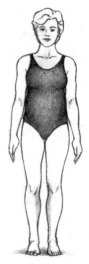

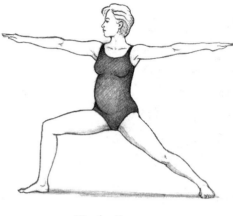

Warrior II
This pose helps stretch your groin
muscles. Step your legs apart, turn
one leg out and bend it at the knee
with your head vertically aligned to
your tailbone aligned and your arms
extended.

Mountain pose
Stand with your feet hip-width apart
and your feet parallel. Rest your weight
equally on the heels and balls of your
feet. Tuck your tailbone under. Bend
your knees slightly to release tension
in your back. Hold for 30 seconds.

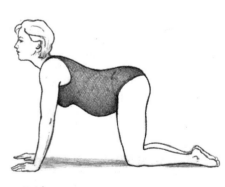

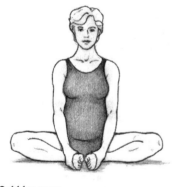

Cobbler pose
Sitting with a straight, long spine
and relaxed thigh muscles, press the
soles of your feet together firmly.
Concentrate on opening your hip and
groin muscles, lengthening your spine
while tucking your tailbone. While
keeping your spine extended, fold into
a gentle forward bend if you wish. Hold
for 30 seconds.

Cat/cow pose
Place your knees hip-width apart and
your hands shoulder-width apart.
Slowly flex and extend your spine
while breathing slowly and evenly.
Hold for 30 seconds.

WEEK 21

Fetal Age: 19 weeks (134-140 days)

19 to 18 weeks, 132 to 126 days until your due date

Baby

Size: She weighs about 10½ ounces, and her length from head to rump is 7 inches, about the length of a spoon.

Development: The biggest development this coming week will be swallowing: your baby will begin to drink amniotic fluid for hydration and nutrition, and her intestines also begin moving this week. The amniotic fluid actually develops flavor depending on what you eat, and babies have been observed swallowing more fluid following sweet foods and less after bitter or garlicky flavors. It takes about 15 minutes to an hour for the foods that you eat to reach the placenta.

Babies also urinate in the fluid, and breathe it in and out. Fortunately, the fluid pool is constantly changing and completely refreshes itself every 3 hours.

Your baby has begun her main project for the rest of your pregnancy: adding fat and putting on weight. Her liver and spleen are making blood cells, and so is her bone marrow.

Her eyelids, eyebrows, and eyelashes are fully developed. Her eyelids are still sealed, but her eyes are active.

You

Some women report feeling better and more energized at this stage of pregnancy than they have at any point in their life. We hope you're one of them!

Your uterus is now about a half an inch above your navel.

As your baby lays down her layers of fat, you're probably not going to be able to hide your expanding form for much longer. You need about 300 extra calories per day to support your active metabolism. Most women have gained 10 to 15 pounds by this point.

If you look in the mirror, especially if you're light-skinned, you'll be able to see blue veins all over your chest, supporting the maturing of your milk-making glands and tissues.

How you're feeling: Some women report a restlessness or even cramping in their legs at this point in their pregnancies. You might experience this too, in addition to the increased tiredness and irritability that may crop up.

On an emotional level, you might start thinking about strollers, swings, play sets, diaper disposal systems, and the myriad other gadgets that are on the market for infants. It's easy to see how parents can spend thousands of dollars on baby gear before the baby is even born!

And even though in the second trimester your odds of carrying a healthy baby to term are quite high, you may find that you can't force yourself to stop worrying that something will go wrong with your pregnancy.

What you can do:
• **Take stock.** As normal as worrying is, if you feel as if it's taking over your emotional life, it can help to pinpoint your worries, examine how likely they are to be true, and consider what you might

YOUR PREGNANCY WEEK BY WEEK • 57

do if they were. (For more on worry, see page 101.)

Pick a time during the day when the baby is normally active, perhaps drink a sip of juice, then sit or lie down in a quiet room or stand in the shower and count how long it takes for the baby to move 10 times. If all is well it should take about 20 minutes to feel 10 kicks and squirms; if it takes more than 2 hours you should let your healthcare provider know.

- **Stay calm.** If you're a first-time mom, remember that it's not necessary to go broke outfitting your nursery. It makes sense to wait to buy most things until after your baby shower, which is traditionally held around week 36 of pregnancy.

- **Look into childbirth classes.** There are many good reasons to educate yourself about the process of labor and birth. Studies have shown that women who felt that childbirth was something being done to them, as opposed to feeling involved in the process, were far more vulnerable to postpartum emotional disorders, such as depression and post-traumatic birth disorder.

- **Check your diet.** If your legs are restless at night, or you get sharp calf cramps, make sure that your diet and/or your prenatal vitamin regimen includes at least 400 mg of magnesium and 1,000–1,300 mg of calcium and that you are getting enough fluids.

If you find yourself getting irritable for what seems like no good reason, try a snack or a glass of juice or milk. Low blood sugar can make you tired and crabby.

WEEK 22

Fetal Age: 20 weeks (141 to 147 days)

18 to 17 weeks, 125 to 119 days until your due date

Baby

Size: Your baby is about 7½ inches from crown to rump and weighs between 13 and 16 ounces—about the size of a small grapefruit.

Development: Going into her fifth month of existence, your baby has fingernails and fully developed eyes, and her organ systems are becoming more functional and specialized. She has a distinct pair of lips, and her first teeth, canines and molars, are developing from hard tissue below her gum line. Her proportions have evened out and she now looks like a miniature newborn. Blood travels through the umbilical cord at 4 miles an hour, fueling her growth with oxygen and nutrients.

For boys, testes have developed and begun to descend from the abdomen.

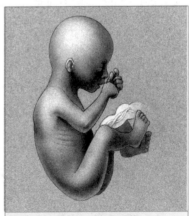

Fetus, 20 weeks post-conception

In girls, the development of the uterus and ovaries is complete, and she has 4 million immature egg cells.

You

If you haven't already noticed, you probably have a distinct little bump under your belly button, though you can still bend over or comfortably sleep on your stomach or back if you want to.

You may have increased vaginal discharge as your pregnancy progresses. Yeast infections during pregnancy are quite common, because pregnancy raises your body temperature. If you have vaginal itching, talk to your healthcare provider. Yeast infections are discussed on page 153.

What you can do: Your care provider should continue to monitor you for high blood pressure. Women who have no history of high blood pressure can develop what's called ***pregnancy-induced hypertension*** (PIH), which is dangerous if left untreated and may require medication. Tell your care provider if you experience dizziness, blurred vision, or swelling in your hands and feet. These all may be signs of PIH.

As pressure increases on your rear end, you enter the danger zone for constipation and hemorrhoids. Drinking water and getting enough fiber in your diet can help you with these. (See our discussion of constipation in the Pregnancy Dictionary at the back of this book.)

TIP

Have you considered a water birth? Many women have had safe, low-intervention births in tubs, either at home or at specially equipped hospitals. Search for online videos and local directories for care providers who offer water births.

Talking with Your Healthcare Provider About Pain

If you have an overriding fear of hospitals, procedures, or needles, discuss these in advance with your healthcare provider. Should you not feel heard or supported, consider changing providers or moving to an alternative healthcare system, such as a non-hospital-based birth center, which may feel less threatening.

- **Learn about drug benefits and risks.** Ask your healthcare provider for written materials about the drugs she commonly uses for pain relief during labor.
- **Tailor your use of drugs to your own philosophy.** If you have scrupulously avoided alcohol, caffeine, and cigarettes during pregnancy to protect your baby, or seldom choose to use medication for your own aches and pains, consider preparing for a non-medicated delivery. (See our list of alternatives on page 181.) If this path feels best to you, explore your healthcare provider's

approach to non-medicated labor and birth.

- **Ask about labor induction and augmentation.** Having your labor started or made stronger with synthetic hormones can increase the intensity and sometimes the pain of your labor. Ask your provider under what circumstances he uses *Pitocin* or other induction medications, and what percentage of his patients is given inductions and *augmentation of labor*. Find out if any of the pain relief medications recommended by your healthcare provider could potentially increase your risk of requiring augmentation of labor. Ask how he or she feels about *elective induction*s. (See our discussion of induction on page 98.) If you do have an induction, the contractions will be more bearable with pain relief.
- **Ask about epidurals.** Check to see whether your hospital provides 24-hour anesthesiology services for labor and delivery.

Questions to Ask Your Provider about Pain Relief Alternatives

If you hope to have a minimally medicated birth, it's useful to explore your healthcare practitioner's concepts and practices. Here are some questions to ask:

- What are your standing orders for your patients regarding pain relief measures?
- What are your thoughts about my not having a routine IV so I am free to move around?
- How many of your patients give birth without pain medication?

- What is your opinion of nondrug pain relief options such as self-hypnosis for birth, relaxation and breathing techniques, water birth, or other remedies?

WEEK 23

Fetal Age: 21 weeks (148 to 154 days)

17 to 16 weeks, 118 to 112 days until your due date

Baby

Size: Weighing in at about a pound, and at 8 inches long, your baby is starting to really look like a baby! You can compare her size to a box of sugar or a bag of coffee beans.

Development: Her skin is filling out as the first layers of fat are deposited and her muscles grow. She's starting a period of major weight gain—she'll put on as much as 2½ ounces this week, and during the next month her weight will nearly double.

Your baby's brain also expands quite a bit in the coming week, gaining the folds and wrinkles necessary for cell-to-cell communication. Also this week your baby begins to have the rapid eye movements associated with the dreaming phase of sleep.

You

Your care provider should be monitoring your expanding uterus and weight. You should be feeling movement at this point. If you haven't, talk to your care provider. No feeling of movement could be a sign that your placenta is in front of the baby. It may also take more time to feel movement if you're overweight.

As your size expands, you may want to keep an eye on your sodium intake, which can make you swell and bloat. Care providers recommend a limit of 3 grams of sodium per day. If you experience rapid bloating, call your care provider.

As your baby gains weight, so do you. You've probably gained at least 15 pounds by now. Some women enjoy the fact that pregnancy is a chance to gain weight without worry. For others, weight gain can inflame existing body-image issues.

As you expand, you may begin to feel itchy as your skin stretches and your skin cells are infused with pregnancy hormones. You even have fetal DNA cells circulating in your own blood, which some researchers theorize can trigger an *immune system* reaction leading to itchy pregnancy-related skin conditions. (For more on itchy pregnancy skin conditions, see "Itching" in Chapter 2).

There's no need to buy moisturizers made especially for pregnancy. Any product that absorbs well will do, though do opt for moisturizers with simple ingredient lists that don't contain fragrance.

What you can do: Are you thinking of decorating? Now is a good time, while you have the energy. If you live in a house built in the 1970s or earlier, you need to have a professional painter get rid of any chipping, flaking, or peeling paint as soon as possible. Lead paint chips and dust are poisonous to humans and especially dangerous to small children and infants. If you plan to paint the baby's room or refinish the floors, wear an industrial-quality mask, and open plenty of doors and windows for ventilation. The same goes for laying new carpeting, putting up vinyl-coated wallpapers, or sanding down windowsills and doors. Try to have your project completed by the end of this month, so there will be enough time for the paint's chemical fumes to air out. Wall-paint fumes aren't dangerous, but their intense odor can make you feel dizzy and sick. You may want to consider using only low-VOC (volatile organic compounds) paint. Don't climb up more than a few rungs on a ladder—your balance has shifted, putting you at risk for falls. (See "Painting" in Chapter 2.)

> *"It's so exciting to feel real movement! It started as little flutters, and now I feel it several times a day."*

24 WEEKS

Fetal Age: 22 weeks (155 to 161 days)

16 to 15 weeks, 111 to 105 days until your due date

Baby

Size: Your baby weighs a little over a pound and is about 8½ inches long—the length of a banana.

Development: Your baby's skin becomes less translucent as pigment is deposited, and it looks wrinkly because her body is making her skin more quickly than it makes the fat to pad underneath it. Her circulation system continues to expand.

Your baby's unique hand- and footprints are forming. You may feel jumps as she has bouts of hiccups. In fact, it may seem like the baby is in perpetual motion. Some babies now kick in response to sounds and touch from outside the womb. Encourage your partner to talk to the baby, and you may be able to feel her move in response.

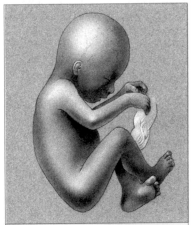

Fetus, 22 weeks post-conception

You

Your uterus is about 1½ to 2 inches above your belly button, and your bump is definitely apparent and hard to disguise! You may be suffering from heartburn, muscle aches, sore feet, fatigue, and dizziness.

Call your care provider if you feel dizzy often or if you faint; it may be a sign of anemia. Dizziness is often caused by low blood sugar or by standing up too fast. Rise slowly, and eat regularly.

What you can do: Iron levels are usually checked in the first trimester, but if you feel tired and/or dizzy often it's not a bad idea to ask to have them checked again, given how much your blood volume has increased over the past few months. As many as 20 percent of pregnant women are anemic, and the condition can cause serious complications.

Have you picked out a name yet? Bestowing a name is so much fun— and so much responsibility! You could name your child anything— even a one-letter initial or a symbol. Whatever it is, remember that the baby inside your stomach will be burdened or blessed with it for life (or until she's 18 and can legally change it). So pick wisely!

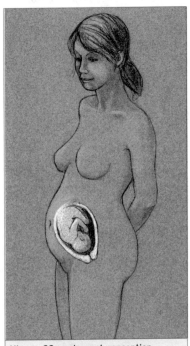

Uterus, 22 weeks post-conception

Tips:

- **Avoid deliberate misspellings of traditional names.** Your child will spend much of her life spelling out the name and correcting those who are confused. Plus, studies have shown that kids with a "misspelled" name are often perceived as being less intelligent and are less likely to land job interviews when they grow up.

- **Remember nicknames.** If you can't stand "Liz" (and rumor has it Elizabeth Taylor couldn't), then don't name your daughter Elizabeth. Nicknames are bestowed on the playground, and you'll have no control over them. Try to think of any unflattering variations that 6-year-olds could come up with.

- **Check the popularity.** Your kid might like finding a key chain or pencil with her name on it every so often, and not having to spell her name for every teacher and camp counselor, but she would probably feel a little generic if five other kids in her class share her name. Still, name popularity can be tough to predict and can fluctuate like the stock market (whoever would have foreseen the rapid rise and decline of "Madison" in the early 2000s?).

- **Consider the initials.** If your last name is Smith, think twice before naming your daughter Ann Susan. Also traditional monograms have the last name in the middle, so if your son's name is Dan Garrett O'Brien, his traditionally monogrammed tote bag of the future will spell "dog."

- **Search the Internet.** It's not a bad idea to verify that your child's name is not also that of, say, a notorious criminal. Speaking of online searches, note that if your child has a unique name he or she will be more easily found on the Internet, for better or worse.

WEEK 25

Fetal Age: 23 weeks (162 to 168 days)

15 to 14 weeks, 104 to 98 days until your due date

Baby

Size: Your baby weighs 1¼ pounds and is a little more than 11 inches long, about the size of a small bag of sugar. In the last third of pregnancy, she'll double and triple her weight.

Development: Her hands are completely developed. Your dexterous baby can touch and hold her feet and make a fist. You may be able to hear your baby's heartbeat with a simple stethoscope, and your partner may be able to hear it by pressing his ear against your belly. Your baby has a regular sleep schedule now and active and inactive periods. You may or may not be able to discern when these periods are. Her nostrils, which have been plugged, open up.

You

Your belly can't be disguised. Your uterus is the size of a soccer ball, and your ribs, diaphragm, and stomach are becoming compressed. This compression forces acid back up into your esophagus, which can give you heartburn and make you feel full after eating only a little food. Antacids (see Chapter 2) are safe to take while you're pregnant, though you don't want to take them on a daily basis because they can prevent the absorption of some nutrients.

As your weight gain increases, you may become one of the 20 to 50 percent of pregnant women who develop hemorrhoids.

> *"I really recommend the hospital tour. As a first-time mom who has only ever been in a hospital three times (when I was born, when one of my siblings was born, and to visit a relative), I didn't really know what to expect. I'm scared of hospitals, so seeing everything before I went into labor helped a lot."*

Taking a Hospital Tour

If you'll be delivering in a hospital, taking a tour of the maternity wing before the big day is standard. Here are some suggestions for ways you can make the trip more helpful and questions you might want to ask:

• Call ahead, since most hospitals have regularly scheduled tours once or twice a week.
• Time your trip to the hospital, including parking. Take notes on the quickest route to get there, and note any alternate routes in case of traffic jams or construction. (But remember that there's usually no need to panic when you're in labor: most first-time babies take 14 hours or more to arrive).
• Find out where you and visitors can park, during regular and late hours.
• Ask where to go to be admitted when you arrive and if there is a different entrance or procedures if you arrive after hours.
• Ask if there are any pre-admission forms you can complete while you're there that will let you be admitted more quickly when you're in labor.
• Ask what the ratio is of certified labor and delivery nurses to patients, and if there's an upper limit to how many patients a nurse may be assigned to care for at one time.
• Ask if there's a limit to how many visitors you can have in the delivery room, waiting room, or recovery room and if there are special rules for visits from siblings or other children.
• Ask if there are any restrictions on taking photos or filming in the delivery room.
• Check out both the birthing suites and also the recovery rooms. Lots of hospitals offer a few palatial birthing suites to entice new customers, but tiny and considerably less-deluxe postpartum rooms, which is where you'll be spending most of your in-hospital time.
• Inquire about the level of the NICU (**neonatal intensive care unit**). A level III NICU is

the highest, able to care for the earliest-born preemies and babies with the most serious problems.

- Ask what kind of services the hospital offers for moms who plan to breastfeed. Are there lactation consultants on staff? Will they visit you in your recovery room after the baby is born? Will you be able to call with questions or get other support services should you have questions or problems after you check out of the hospital?
- Locate the hospital cafeteria, and scope out the closest convenience stores, delis, and restaurants offering takeout, in case hospital food turns out to be unappealing.
- Ask about what kind of security procedures are in place to keep unauthorized visitors out of the maternity ward, and to make sure babies aren't accidently swapped.
- If your hospital is a teaching hospital, find out if medical students and/or *resident*s might be involved in your care, observe procedures, or deliver your baby and what the procedure is for requesting second opinions from physicians in case of complications.
- Ask what happens if you need a cesarean. Will your partner be permitted in the operating room with you? What will happen with the baby after your c-section?
- If you know you want an epidural, ask if the birthing wing has its own anesthesiologist and if women need to be dilated a certain amount to have one. If you have special conditions that might make your epidural more complicated (you're taking certain medications such as blood thinners, you are obese,

or you have a spinal condition like scoliosis) ask if it's possible to meet the anesthesiologist to discuss them before you go into labor.

- If you're having a boy and plan to have him circumcised, ask where the hospital performs circumcisions, who performs them, and what kind of pain medication they use. (For more on this, see our discussion on page 216.)

What you can do: Now is a good time to get into the habit of doing back stretches, which can help with your aches and pains throughout the day. It's also a good time to be walking, swimming, and practicing yoga. Now is not a good time for weightlifting or kickboxing—exercises that might injure your softened ligaments.

You may have cramps in your calves, back, tailbone, and even arms, as your ligaments soften. Calcium and magnesium, found in cow's milk and vitamin supplements, may help. (For more on your vitamin and mineral requirements, see Chapter 3.)

If you're considering breastfeeding, this is a good time to start attending *La Leche League* meetings. These informal sessions will supply you with solid, practical information on how to breastfeed and tips on good nutrition and the process of childbirth. La Leche League groups often are listed in the white pages of the telephone book, and you can also find a local group by calling the organization's national number or by visiting their Web site. (See the Resources.) Most groups offer a leader on call for support 24/7 if you're having problems after your baby is born.

WEEK 26

Fetal Age: 24 weeks (169 to 175 days)

14 to 13 weeks, 97 to 91 days until your due date

Baby

Size: Your baby weighs about 1⅓ pounds and has undergone a growth spurt in the past few weeks. From weeks 20 to 28, she almost doubles in height and now would be about a foot tall if she could stand and is about 9 inches long curled up.

Development: This week marks a major milestone in your baby's hearing and sight.

Your baby's hearing system (cochlea and peripheral sensory end organs), which began connecting during week 18, is now completely formed, and starting now and over the next few weeks, she'll become increasingly sensitive to sound. In about a month, you may feel her jump if she hears a sudden loud noise, especially if you're in the bathtub, where sound waves are amplified through the water.

Her eyes are almost fully formed. All babies have blue eyes in the womb, no matter what their genetic inheritance is, and a baby's eyes don't get their final color until a few months after they are born. The air sacs of the lungs, called *alveoli*, will be developed by the end of this week and will begin to secrete a substance called *surfactant* that will keep the lung tissue from sticking together.

About half of your baby's energy is spent developing her brain.

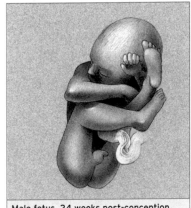

Male fetus, 24 weeks post-conception

You

Sleeping is definitely getting uncomfortable. Lying on your back is now too uncomfortable: Your baby will be pressing into your backbone and your uterus will put pressure on a major *artery*, restricting blood flow. Lying on the right side also puts the weight of the baby on a major vein. Sleeping on the left side has been associated with a lower risk of stillbirth than right-side or back sleeping, so try to sleep left-sided if you can.

Between now and the next 3 weeks, you may be tested for *gestational diabetes* with a *glucose tolerance test*. This test requires you to drink a glucose-rich liquid, usually in the form of a syrupy orange-flavored drink. After an hour, a blood sample is taken. If you have a positive test, you'll be given another, longer, 3-hour diagnostic test. If you do have gestational diabetes, you'll be advised to adopt a low-carbohydrate diet.

Gestational diabetes is a temporary condition that usually

goes away after the baby's born, though in some cases what looks like gestational diabetes is type II diabetes that continues after the baby's born.

How you may feel: You may feel like your body has been taken over: It's weird to have another person sharing your body with you, especially one who kicks so much. Nature has taken over, and there's not a whole lot you can do about it but cope, rest, relax, and marvel. You probably wish that you could take a vacation from your pregnancy sometimes. Floating in a swimming pool with your eyes closed may be as close as you can get.

Pregnancy-related *carpal tunnel syndrome* affects one in four pregnant women. It's most common for women who type on keyboards or otherwise work with their hands and wrists all day. What happens is the extra fluid in your body can accumulate in your wrists and cause sharp pains that can run up your arm, or numbness in your fingers and hands. Take as many typing breaks as you can, use a wrist rest at the computer, and consider wearing a plastic splint at night and sleeping with your wrists elevated.

What you can do: If you're planning a home or hospital birth, now is a good time to look into hiring a labor assistant or doula if you are planning to do so. Your care provider, hospital, or childbirth educator can help you locate one, or you can find an assistant yourself by contacting DONA (Doulas of North America, *www.dona.org*) or the International Childbirth Education Association (ICEA, at *www.icea.org*).

The *birth assistant* you call will set up a meeting with you and your partner prior to labor to talk about your birth philosophy and what kind of services you may find helpful. Are you preparing for a home birth? Your attending midwife will certainly give you detailed lists of what you'll need.

If you've decided on a home birth, be sure to do your research— read every home-birthing book and watch every video you can get your hands on. Now is a good time to pack your clean linens, nightgowns, plastic sheeting, and so on into a large box that you can keep in a safe place until you need them. Make sure you know what your midwife's plan is should there be a medical emergency. (See page 198 for more about home birth.)

Support During Labor

Having continuous support during labor can make a big difference. Support can be from a partner, a chosen friend, a midwife, a doula, or others. Studies on the effects of support during labor have found that mothers having continuous support:

• **Need less medication.** Mothers with adequate human support are less likely to require an epidural or need other pain medication.
• **Have more effective labors.** Supported mothers are less likely to need a forceps or vacuum extraction during birth.
• **Are less likely to have surgical deliveries.** Supported mothers are less likely to need cesarean sections.
• **Have a better birth experience.** Supported mothers give higher ratings for overall

satisfaction with their births and had a feeling of having more personal control over their labors.

- **Have the best outcomes.** Starting support early in labor and relying on someone other than hospital staff members is associated with better outcomes for both mother and baby.

Things to Ask a Doula (Labor Assistant)

- Will you be available on my due date?
- How many births have you attended?
- Are you certified by Doulas of North America or do you hold any other certifications?
- Do you have someone who works as your backup in case you can't make it, and will I have a chance to meet that person?
- What type of childbirth classes do you recommend? (Some doulas may require that you take certain classes.)
- Will you still work with me if I plan to have an epidural or a c-section?
- At what point should I call you when I go into labor?
- Have you worked with my care provider before? If so, what were your impressions of him or her?
- What kind of relaxation techniques do you know?
- What do you think about women eating, drinking, and getting out of bed during labor?
- Do you usually bring accessories for labor, like a birth ball, massaging foot roller, aromatherapy oils, or other relaxation devices?
- Are you also a licensed massage therapist?

WEEK 27

Fetal Age: 25 weeks (176 to 182 days)

13 to 12 weeks, 90 to 84 days until your due date

Baby

Size: Your baby weighs about 2 pounds and is about 12 to 15 inches long, about the size of a small pot roast.

Development: If your baby were born now, he would have an excellent chance of surviving, though he still isn't fully developed and would probably not be able to breathe by himself. He would need to stay in an *incubator* to keep his body temperature regulated, and he would have a weak liver and immune system.

You

The weight of your baby is putting pressure on your back, which can cause shooting pains (*sciatica*) in your lower back and legs. Lifting, bending, and walking can make the pain worse. Warm baths, ice packs, and changing positions may help.

Your cholesterol levels may rise. Cholesterol is used by you and your baby's placenta to help make progesterone, a hormone with wide-ranging effects, such as preventing preterm birth, helping maintain cells' oxygen levels, and regulating metabolism.

The volume of your amniotic fluid is now reduced by about half of what it was earlier in pregnancy. With less cushioning to block the view, you'll be able to see bony knees and elbows poking out of your stomach when the baby kicks and turns. His kicks may be vigorous—others will be able to see them if they stare at your stomach.

As you grow, you may start to see stretch marks on your breasts and abdomen. You may also have a hard time bending over and tying your shoes. Your heart rate may have increased, causing you to feel flush and winded with less exertion.

What you can do: Have you thought about getting a pregnancy massage? It can be the most comfortable hour of your month! Massages may even be covered by your health insurance. You may be able to find a doula who also certified in pregnancy massage.

Here are some other safe indulgences:

- A manicure. Your nails are long and strong, so take advantage. Get them polished at a salon that's hygienic and well-ventilated.
- A pedicure and foot massage (but don't get a leg massage if you have *varicose veins*). Your poor feet will be subjected to 500 pounds of pressure or more every time you take a step, so treat them well!
- A warm bath in a dim room with soft music playing. Treat yourself to new sponges, loofahs, a waterproof bath pillow, gently scented glycerin soaps, and bath oils.
- A home facial. If you have dry skin, mix up papaya, avocado, and a few teaspoons of oatmeal. Leave the mask on for 15 to 20 minutes, then massage your face and rinse. The fruits are rich in natural oils, and the oatmeal will slough off dead skin.

If you have oily skin, substitute cornmeal for oatmeal; the gritty grain will help you exfoliate.

The Third Trimester

Weeks 28 through 41

Welcome to the third trimester! You'll be two-thirds of the way through your pregnancy when your fetus is 177 days old.

While reaching the third trimester feels like great progress, with it comes a return to fatigue, dizziness, and constant trips to the bathroom.

WEEK 28

Fetal Age: 26 weeks (183 to 189 days)

12 to 11 weeks, 83 to 77 days until your due date

Baby

Size: Your baby has doubled her weight in the past month and is the size of a bag of flour. She now weighs about 2¼ pounds. Her total length is nearly 15 inches.

Development: Were your baby born now, there's an 80 percent chance she will survive, but she will still be at risk for complications and will probably need a stay in the hospital's Neonatal Intensive Care Unit (NICU). About one in four babies who arrive this early develop serious, lasting disabilities, and about one in two have milder problems with learning or behavior later on.

Your baby's main job right now is to put the finishing touches on major organ systems, such as her brain, lungs, and liver. As you can probably tell, she's also working on gaining layers of fat. Her body fat is about 2 to 3 percent.

Your baby's eyes, which were covered by her eyelid folds at the sixth week of development, are capable of opening this week, and her retinas have rods and cones, which are the specialized nerve cells that make vision possible. Cone cells detect color, and rod cells are used for vision in low-light conditions. Her sucking and swallowing skills are also improving.

You

At some point in the third trimester, if it hasn't already happened, you will cross the line from pleasantly round to verging on uncomfortable. Your legs may ache or cramp, it's hard to get a good sleeping position, and the baby is big enough to give you some sharp kicks to the ribs! Your perspiration can get trapped in the folds of your skin, which can be irritating and make you feel grubby. Try applying talcum powder under your breasts before you put your bra on, and in any other nooks and crannies you may have developed. If you're going to get stretch marks, you probably have them by now.

Remember that hot weather, standing for long periods of time, or low blood sugar can make you prone to dizziness and fainting. Drink water, and stay in the shade if you're pregnant in the summer.

With 12 weeks to go until your baby is officially due, you may start having more regular visits to your care provider. If you're Rh-negative, you should get the RhoGAM shot this week to prevent complications at delivery.

Between now and the next few weeks, you'll be given blood tests for your iron levels and offered a glucose tolerance test if you haven't already had one.

What you can do: Feel your belly to see if you can find the baby's head, bottom, knees, and elbows. Try mapping your belly by lying in a semi-upright position on your back. Your baby's head will feel like a hard mass with a distinctive round, smooth texture. Put your palms on either side of your belly, and try gently pushing back and forth—the side where your baby's backbone is will feel firmer and offer more resistance to moving. Walk your fingertips across your abdomen—your baby's back will be firm, and the arms and legs will be knobby.

Once your baby moves into the head-down position, you may start to feel your baby's heel kicking around your ribs; the heel will be a small, mobile knob the size of a large bubblegum ball pressing out just below your rib cage. If you're not sure what parts of the baby you're feeling, ask your physician or midwife to show you where the baby's head, back, and bottom are at your next visit.

Once you figure out where the baby is, it can be fun to use makeup or body paint to sketch out where the baby is on your belly (you don't need special belly paint, any non-toxic body paint will do).

Your Partner's Role in Childbirth

In the old days, numerous cartoons were drawn of anxious husbands pacing in the waiting room while their wives gave birth behind closed doors. Today, most fathers-to-be want to play an active role in the birth process. Most dads who have been able to be present during birth report afterwards that it was an important and unforgettable transition for them, too.

It's up to you to decide how involved you'd like your life

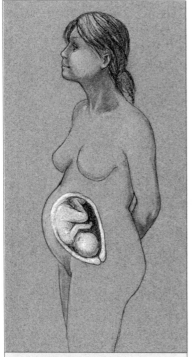

At 26 weeks post-conception, your belly announces your condition to the world.

partner to be in your birth experience. And, some fathers-to-be are so intimidated by the whole birthing process that they may want to opt out.

It's critical to have support from at least one other familiar person during your labor to help you stay relaxed and to assist you with important decisions, but there's no hard-and-fast rule that says the person you choose has to be your husband or boyfriend.

If your baby's dad is skittish about blood or medical procedures, there are other ways he can still help, like driving you to the hospital, alerting family members, and making sure your other children and pets are taken care of while you are hospitalized.

So, talk to your chosen birth partner about what kind of labor support you would like from him or her. Do you want him at your head whispering encouragement, or supporting you for walks in the hall? Or would you rather your partner stayed out of the way and let your mother or labor assistant do those jobs?

WEEK 29

Fetal Age: 27 weeks (190 to 196 days)

11 to 10 weeks, 76 to 70 days until your due date

Baby

Size: Your baby is about 2½ pounds and would be between 15 and 17 inches tall if she could stand.

Development: Your baby's adrenal glands are producing a chemical that will be made into *estriol* (a form of estrogen) by the placenta. This estriol is thought to stimulate the production of *prolactin* by your body, and the prolactin makes you produce milk.

So even if your baby comes early, you'll still be able to breastfeed. Each passing week improves the likelihood that your baby will be born strong and healthy. Her brain can direct rhythmic breathing and control body temperature, so she's less likely to need breathing assistance should she be born early.

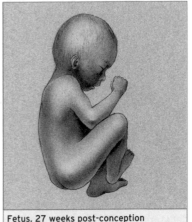

Fetus, 27 weeks post-conception

She's growing eyelashes, adding fat, and developing her brain.

Because of brain wave activity, researchers have speculated that babies can even dream at this time!

Between now and your due date, she will double her weight. This week her bones are also fully formed, though they remain soft and pliable.

You

How you're feeling physically: As the levels of prolactin increase in your body, your breasts may start to leak a little bit of colostrum, sometimes enough to dampen your bra. Prolactin also has a sedating effect, and you may feel the need to take naps the way you did in the first trimester. Your uterus is now in a position where it exerts pressure on your bladder, requiring frequent bathroom visits day and night.

Things to organize: Your closet. Now is a good time to shop for versatile clothes that you can wear in both the next months and for a few months postpartum. You'll most likely be the size you are now for about the first 2 months after the baby's born.

Good clothing buys include:
• Jeans or pants with elastic in the sides. If you buy pants now, make sure you have at least 2 inches of room in the hips to allow for second-trimester pelvic spread. As you get larger, pants with a tummy panel may become more comfortable.
• Comfortable cotton bras with a flap that converts them into nursing bras. If you're large-breasted, look for supportive wide straps. Only buy one or two bras at a time, because your breasts will continue to grow.
• Button-down shirts long enough to cover your pants' elastic and panels. (You can unbutton bottom buttons if the shirt gets tight.) These shirts can also be used for nursing later.
• Maternity dresses with drawstrings in the back to loosen or tighten the fit.
• Bikini-style maternity underwear.
• A bra that fits well. It's better to pay a bit more for a quality bra at a store that offers personalized fittings and specialized maternity and nursing bras than to play hit-or-miss with the selection at a discount store. Or, try on bras at a full-service boutique, then see if

you can find a better deal online for the brands and sizes that fit you best.

- Maternity hose or an adjustable garter belt with stockings.
- Small hats and sunglasses to protect your face from the sun.
- Flat-soled, slip-on shoes.

  Bad buys include:
- Non-maternity plus sizes—they'll fit your stomach, but will drape badly everywhere else.
- Thong-style and/or synthetic-fabric underwear; both can enable urinary tract infections.
- Over-the-stomach underwear, which tends to be too big for postpartum use.
- Bras made of synthetic fabrics, which can cause skin problems such as *eczema* and nipple irritation.
- Normal, non-pregnant panty hose or tights, which are sure to roll down at the waist and/or bag at your ankles.
- Shirts too short to cover expandable panels on maternity pants.
- Wide-legged pants, which will make you look wide all over.
- A-line tops, which will start to look like tents as months go on.
- Finger and toe rings, anklets, and cuff bracelets—if they fit now, they'll be too small in a few months and too big after the baby's born.
- New piercings or tattoos—they'll bleed more and be more prone to infection.

WEEK 30

Fetal Age: 28 weeks (197 to 203 days)

10 to 9 weeks, 69 to 63 days until your due date

Baby

Size: Her length is about 16 inches—about as long as a laptop computer—and she measures about 10½ inches from crown to rump and weighs approximately 2½ to 3 pounds. From now until delivery, every baby will gain weight at a more individual rate, at an average rate of about half a pound a week.

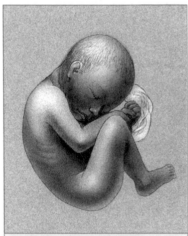

Fetus, 28 weeks post-conception

Development: Your baby's most important organ, her brain, continues to develop at a rapid pace. Her eyes are able to track light, and some researchers have theorized that exposing your belly to light may stimulate development. Try moving the beam of a flashlight slowly over your belly in a dim room to see if she reacts.

You

If you can, keep up your swimming, walking, yoga, or other non-weight-bearing exercise, though you're not feeling as energetic (and as comfortable) as you did last trimester. Exercise can help relieve your back, hip, and leg pain and help you have a speedier physical recovery after childbirth. If you've been lifting free weights or using weight machines, you don't have to stop, but keep the weight level and the repetitions and range of motion at maintenance level. Don't try to add muscle mass or increase your range of motion, because your ligaments are relaxed and more prone to injury.

As the weight of the baby puts pressure on your bladder, you'll find yourself running to the bathroom, only to pee a tiny amount. The tubes that link your kidneys, bladder, and **urethra** are also compressed, which means you can't empty your bladder as efficiently. You may also leak urine when you laugh or cough. One exercise you don't want to slack off on is the Kegel, especially if laughing or coughing is already making you leak urine.

If you have light skin, you may notice enlarged veins on your legs or elsewhere.

You can help prevent aches and pains by not staying in one position for very long. Take walks, and move around to improve circulation. If you work at a computer, put your laptop on a box on top of your desk so you can work standing up.

Wear loose clothes, including loose socks, to keep your circulation from being restricted, though if you have varicose or enlarged leg veins, many care providers recommend support hose that you put on before you even get out of bed to keep your veins from bulging.

You've now been officially pregnant for 7 months, and the home stretch is in sight. You're big now, no doubt about it! Your belly is about the size of a watermelon. Tying your shoes is a challenge, and you may have adopted a pregnant "waddle," which is caused by loosening of pelvic ligaments.

> *"I've started to get out of breath just from walking up a flight of stairs or up a little hill! It really makes me sympathetic to people who are out of shape."*

You may feel your heart pounding and have shortness of breath as you exert yourself. If you've been exercising and are in good shape, you will experience less breathlessness. Hormonal changes make your lung capacity expand so you can breathe more frequently and deeply.

If you feel short of breath, take slow, relaxed, and deep breaths.

The damage that can be done by continuing to smoke increases as you get closer to term. If you haven't quit, give it another try.

Things to organize: Your birth plan: You can't anticipate everything that's going to happen during labor and delivery, but a birth plan is a tool that can facilitate a conversation between you and your care provider. Don't expect that the labor and delivery nurses at your birthing center will have an opportunity to read it (depending on the time of day and the hospital, they may have to be tending to as many as seven other laboring women at a time).

Instead, view your birth plan as a way for you to figure out for yourself what kind of birthing environment you'd like, how you want to manage your pain, what kind of interventions you want (and which to avoid), and what your friends and family's roles will be. Then use your plan as the start of a discussion with your care provider about what you can expect during labor. Also be sure to involve your partner in the plan, so he or she will be prepared to express your wishes if you're otherwise occupied.

There are also lots of Web sites that offer interactive programs that let you generate your own birth plan to print out.

What to Include in Your Birth Plan

Your strategy for comfort and pain management. Do you want to be offered:
• An epidural?
• *Narcotics*, sedatives, and/or opiates?
• The use of a birthing tub or the shower?
• The opportunity to walk around?
• The services of a labor assistant or doula?
• Low lights, soft music, or a specific ambience? (Candles and incense will not be allowed.)

• Labor accessories, such as a birth ball or birthing stool?
• Acupressure, *acupuncture*, or guided relaxation techniques?

If you know you want an epidural, ask your care provider at what point during your labor you can get it. If you have qualms about getting one, set up a consultation with one of the hospital's anesthesiologists assigned to the obstetrical unit to learn more about the procedure.

Your Hospital Experience

What levels of intervention are you comfortable with?
• Do you mind having a routine IV in your arm or on the back of your hand for fluids or a *heparin lock* (hep-lock) a sealed needle unit placed on the back of your hand or in your arm to allow ready access to a vein? Hospitals have different policies on IVs—some will routinely insert a hep-lock as soon as you're admitted, making it easier to administer intravenous medication or fluids. Others will only insert an IV needle if you have an epidural or a need for extra fluids. As a patient, you can request to postpone the hep-lock until there's actually a need for it.
• Are there interventions you want to avoid for religious reasons, such as blood transfusions?
• If you've previously had a cesarean delivery, do you want the opportunity to deliver vaginally this time? (See "Vaginal Birth after a Cesarean" in Chapter 2).
• What circumstances would make labor induction or augmentation necessary? Ask how many days past term you can go before

your care provider will consider induction, and how many hours the hospital will give you to go into labor after your water breaks. (For more on labor inductions and augmentation, see pages 98–99.)

- Can you eat and drink in labor? Some hospitals forbid eating and drinking during labor—it's ice chips only. You probably won't feel like eating, but you may appreciate being allowed to drink when you're thirsty.
- Whom do you want to have in the room with you? Tell your care provider if you want to have extra people in your room, such as your labor assistant or children.
- Are there certain individuals you *don't* want in the room?
- What's the policy on fetal monitoring? Some hospitals require that your contractions and both your and your baby's heart rates be electronically monitored at certain intervals (such as once an hour). Having to stand still or lie down to be monitored when you're in labor can be aggravating.

Delivery

How do you want to participate in the birth? Do you want to:
- Be told when to push, or to push as you feel the urge?
- Touch the baby's head as it crowns?
- Watch the birth in a mirror?
- Have your partner catch the baby or cut the umbilical cord?
- Have the baby be placed on your chest immediately after delivery?
- Have newborn procedures such as weighing and fingerprinting be

performed in the room, or in the nursery?

If a cesarean is necessary:
- Will your partner be allowed in the room?
- Can you have the drape removed when it's time for the baby to be lifted out?
- Can you be given some time to get acquainted with the baby before she's cleaned and whisked away?
- Will your partner be allowed to take pictures or videos in the operating room?
- How long can you expect to be in the hospital afterwards?

Recovery

- How soon after delivery will your care provider check up on you?
- Will the baby be in your room around the clock, only when you're awake, or just for feedings?
- If you're planning to breastfeed, ask how the hospital supports breastfeeding. Will the baby be placed on your chest for feeding immediately after birth? Is there a lactation consultant on staff? If the baby has to go to the NICU, will the hospital help you pump milk?
- How long are you likely to stay in the hospital?

WEEK 31

Fetal Age: 29 weeks (204 to 210 days)

9 to 8 weeks, 62 to 56 days until your due date

Baby

Size: She weighs between 2½ and 3½ pounds. She continues to gain weight at a faster pace than she lengthens, which will give her those cute chubby cheeks. She's about 14 to 16 inches tall, although individual growth rates vary.

Development: Your baby begins to run out of room as she puts on weight. You should feel about 10 kicks an hour. Some care providers suggest keeping a record of kicks by taking time daily to write down how many kicks you can feel in an hour so that you are aware if there's a decrease in activity. Other care providers may advise that as long as it feels like the baby's active, there's no need to keep notes. If you do sense a decrease in activity, try drinking a large glass of juice. If that doesn't make the baby energized, or makes her less energized than she usually would be, call your care provider.

You

How you're feeling:
- **Bloated.** If your blood pressure is normal, and you don't have protein in your urine, your puffy face, hands, legs, and feet are probably normal.
- **Tired.** If you are working, you probably keep a secret calendar in your desk that counts the days, hours, and minutes until your maternity leave starts.
- **Clumsy.** Extra inches and a shift in your center of gravity can make you bump into furniture, knock things over, and be more prone to accidental falls.

TIP

Get plenty of calcium and magnesium this week and for the rest of your pregnancy. They help harden your baby's bones, and will also help prevent your late-night leg twitches and muscle cramps.

Things to do this week:
- Add to your baby registry.
- Baby showers are traditionally held around week 36, though if you are expecting multiples, earlier might be better. Guests want to see you in all of your pregnant glory, and you want to be spry enough to enjoy your own party!

Here are some registry tips:
- Refer to the Baby Gear Primer, Chapter 6, and take stock of what you have and what you'll need.
- Pick at least one national or online store to register in, so friends and family from out of state will also be able to send gifts.
- Select items from every guest's price range.
- Test out items in the store, and choose carefully. You can always return stuff, but it's better to get what you want the first time.
- Venture out of the baby department. Consider adding towels, washcloths, clothes hampers, unscented detergent, or an extra trash can or two. You'll need that stuff too.

> *"I think the baby's running out of room. I used to feel more kicks, but now it feels more like squirmy knots in there."*

WEEK 32

Fetal Age: 30 weeks (211 to 217 days)

8 to 7 weeks, 55 to 49 days until your due date

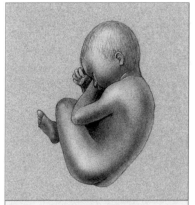

Fetus, 30 weeks post-conception

Baby

Size: She weighs about 4 pounds and is about 15 to 17 inches tall.

Development: Hair is growing on her head, and lanugo, the fine hairs on her body, is beginning to be shed. She also has toenails.

Photographs of babies in utero at this stage show their skin becoming less translucent and pinker, as layers of fat are deposited under the skin. Her skeleton is rapidly ossifying (turning from cartilage into solid bone), which means that kicks will feel stronger and more intense. Kicks may even become visible through your shirt as the trimester progresses. Well-placed kicks under your ribs can take your breath away!

You

From now until delivery, you'll be gaining about a pound a week. About half of that gain is the baby's, the rest is all kinds of fluid—amniotic fluid, blood, mucus, and so on—which you'll lose soon after delivery or in the weeks following. To avoid fluid pooling in your bottom and ankles, try to keep moving all day. Work standing up as much as possible, take 15-minute breaks to walk around the block or the building, and if you have to drive for work, get out of the car at least every half-hour for a stretch.

What you can do: Admission procedures vary among hospitals, so it's an excellent idea to take a tour of the hospital prior to going into labor to get a general lay of the land, if you haven't already. Say hello to the nurses in labor and delivery, take in the sights, and if you have any questions about your health insurance coverage, get those straightened out with the hospital's billing office before you go into labor.

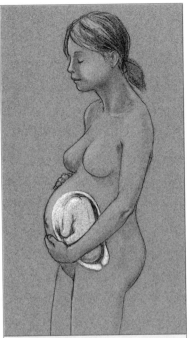

With two months to go, you may wonder how much bigger you can possibly get!

WEEK 33

Fetal Age: 31 weeks (218 to 224 days)

7 to 6 weeks, 48 to 42 days until your due date

Baby

Size: Your baby's crown-to-rump length is about 11½ inches (and about 17 inches crown to heel). She weighs about 4½ pounds and gains an average of 7 to 8 ounces every week.

Development: Your baby has probably moved to the head-down position and may descend into your pelvis at any time in the next 6 weeks and begin to press into your cervix. This position not only prepares her for birth but allows blood to flow to her developing brain. The dark quiet of your womb is perfect for this activity. Right now, your baby is also in the process of receiving your antibodies. If she were born right now, her immune system would be immature, and extra care would need to be taken to keep her in a sterile environment.

You

You continue gaining weight at the rate of a pound a week, and it probably seems impossible that your body will find somewhere to fit 6 more pounds. Your amniotic fluid has reached its maximum volume of 2 to 6 cups.

Anyone who says, "Wow, you *only* have 6 weeks to go!" doesn't understand how time slows down during the last weeks of pregnancy.

If you're still working, you're probably already counting the minutes until your maternity leave starts. During the next 6 weeks, you may be trying to decide if you'll be one of the 66 percent of moms who will return to the workforce in the year after having a baby, or if you'll be among the 34 percent who stay home.

Call your care provider if you suddenly feel puffy in your face or hands; this is a sign of preeclampsia, sometimes called toxemia, which can be life-threatening for you.

What you can do:
• If you know that you don't want to go back to work after the baby's born, or you're undecided, now is a good time to update your résumé. Collect a copy of your job description and samples of your work, and download any useful contact names and addresses

onto a flash drive in case they'll come in handy later.

- Write down all of your duties and accomplishments now, while they're fresh in your mind. Copy down important phone numbers from your address book and files, and save a list of the e-mail addresses stored on your work computer.
- Save a list of the e-mail addresses stored on your work computer and delete any personal e-mails or correspondence that may have found their way onto your work computer.

WEEK 34

Fetal Age: 32 weeks (225 to 231 days)

6 to 5 weeks, 41 to 35 days until your due date

Baby

Size: Your baby weighs about 5 pounds or more, like a bag of flour. She will continue to gain about 2 or more pounds in the next 6 weeks.

Development: Now that your baby's brain has formed billions of neurons, it must accomplish the even more complex feat of hooking the neurons and synapses together. Your baby's brain is forming trillions of connections, making it possible for her to learn in the womb.

All of this brain development may be the reason that your baby sleeps frequently at this stage. She may even be dreaming—her eyes dart around rapidly just as an adult's might in REM sleep. And your child's brain development is in no way complete at birth. In the

first year after birth, a baby's brain triples in size and becomes three-quarters of its adult size.

You

The volume of your uterus is five hundred to a thousand times larger than before you got pregnant, so it's safe to say you're feeling huge and slow. If your partner wonders what it feels like to be pregnant, try filling a backpack with as many pounds as you've gained (dried beans or bags of sugar make good weights) and have him wear it around the front of his torso.

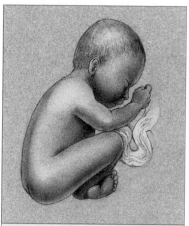

Fetus, 32 weeks post-conception

You're still running to the bathroom frequently and probably will be from here on out. Try to drink a lot of water early in the day, so you don't get thirsty at night and have to get up that much more.

What you can do: Install that car seat. If you haven't purchased your baby's car seat and installed it facing rearward in the backseat of your car yet, do it now. Your baby might come early, and the hospital staff won't let you drive your baby home without one. And there's nothing worse than watching from a hospital wheelchair as your partner goes nuts trying to install it while parked in the fire lane. To get the most value from your car seat purchase, get one that holds a baby weighing at least up to 30 pounds.

> **TIP**
>
> Contact your care provider if you experience blurred vision, severe headaches, severe swelling, or sudden weight gain. These symptoms can be a sign of preeclampsia.

WEEK 35

Fetal Age: 33 weeks (232 to 238 days)

5 to 4 weeks, 34 to 28 days until your due date

Baby

Size: At more than 5 pounds and between 16 and 20 inches, your baby is becoming more ready for birth with every passing hour. She's the size of a roasting chicken.

Development: Her nervous system and immune system are still maturing, and she's adding the fat that she'll need to regulate her body temperature. But everything else, from her toenails to the hair on her head, is fully formed.

If she were born now, she'd have higher than 99 percent odds of surviving.

You

You're carrying so much extra weight and fluid that even simple tasks can be tiring.

If your job requires sitting all day, it's probably getting hard to work.

You should take frequent breaks to walk around and stretch your legs (if you have the privacy to lie down for a few minutes or do stretches on your hands and knees, even better). Change your sitting position frequently, and bring in pillows to support your back. You'll be seeing your care provider once every 1 to 2 weeks now.

If your initial group B strep (GBS) screening was negative, another screening will usually be performed between now and week 37. This involves taking a vaginal/rectal swab and then culturing it to detect the presence of GBS bacteria. GBS is a fairly common bacterium that usually doesn't cause symptoms in a mother but can potentially cause a serious infection in the newborn. If you're found to have GBS you'll need an IV of antibiotics during labor to protect the baby.

What you can do: If you have other children, this can be a poignant time, because it is the last few weeks of being a family in the way that you're used to. It can seem hard to imagine that there will be enough of you to go around, and you may wonder if it will ever be possible for you to love a new baby as much. You may feel guilty about the sacrifices your other children will have to make to accommodate the new baby. No matter how many children you have, each new baby is a leap of faith that the sacrifices will be worth it.

Don't forget to arrange care for any children or pets for the 2 to 3 days you'll be in the hospital. Ask a neighbor to collect your newspapers and mail. You probably will send your partner home to check on things at some point, but you don't want to have to worry, especially if the hospital or birthing center is far from your home.

And have you figured out who you're going to tell about your new baby, when and how? A special e-mail mailing list allocated to "baby news" could save a lot of time in getting the word out.

WEEK 36

Fetal Age: 34 weeks (239 to 245 days)

4 to 3 weeks, 27 to 21 days until your due date

Baby

Size: With 1 month to go, she weighs about 5 to 6 pounds and is fattening. Her full length from crown to feet is about 20½ inches.

Development: Has your baby's movement slowed down? If so, you shouldn't worry.

Five to 10 percent of all mothers report that babies start to slow down as they grow larger and get more cramped for space. Still, you should be able to feel your baby move more at least 10 times in 2 hours. If you're concerned, try drinking a sweet beverage, such as orange juice, and then lying on your side for a while. Most babies will wake up and start to move. If you're still concerned, contact your healthcare provider.

You

As women in the grocery store may have already told you, you look like you could go into labor at any minute. And they might be right—your due date just suggests a time when the baby's likely to be born. In reality, you could go into labor any time between now and 6 weeks from now!

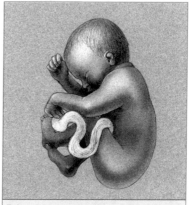

Fetus, 34 weeks post-conception

Your belly button is becoming flattened or may even stick out like a wine cork. You may feel a *lightening* sensation on your ribs and organs as your baby descends into your pelvis.

Breathing and eating will be easier, but the tradeoff is you'll be running to the bathroom more often than ever, and the change in pressure may cause shooting pains in your groin and leg.

If you're aching (and we don't see how you couldn't be), indulge in a pregnancy massage from a professional prenatal-massage therapist, or find a pool and take a swim. At home, try sitting on an exercise ball (also known as a birth ball). This will take pressure off your back because it forces you to sit straight and with good balance, using your legs to support and stabilize you. This is good practice for labor.

If you'll be breastfeeding, you'll want to stock up on nursing bras and shirts that button down the front (or are specifically made for breastfeeding). This is a particularly good time to buy nursing bras, since your breasts are about the size they'll stay for the duration of your nursing experience. Make sure that your bras fit well, don't itch, don't have armpit-jabbing underwires or tight straps that could bind around your breasts, and are made of natural, breathable materials (synthetics may cause a rash!).

Some women report going into an intense and obsessive nesting phase in the weeks, days, and hours before labor begins—cleaning out closets, sorting clothes and drawers, mopping and vacuuming with intensity. (Who knows, maybe early labor hormones wake up the primitive part of the brain that makes birds fluff their nests and prairie dogs clean out their dens.) Go with it—moving around will feel better than staying in one position. Just be sure to mind your form as you kneel, lift objects, and stretch upwards so you don't fall over or pull a muscle.

WEEK 37

Fetal Age: 35 weeks (246 to 252 days)

3 to 2 weeks, 20 to 14 days until your due date

Baby

Size: An average of about 7 pounds, with an average length from crown to heel of about 19 inches.

Development: Your baby is practicing her breathing with amniotic fluid, but she has increasingly less space to practice stretching and kicking. Your baby's intestines are also building up *meconium*, a greenish-black substance made of baby by-products such as dead cells, shed lanugo, and amniotic fluid.

This meconium, sticky and thick, will become your little darling's first bowel movement, to be passed soon after she is born. Her body fat has increased to about 8 percent. By birth, it'll be about 15 percent.

If your baby is a boy, his testes will have descended into his scrotum.

While your baby could be born at any time, the longer she stays in, the more time she has to develop the connections in her brain in the pleasant peace and quiet of your womb. At this point, she can do all the things a newborn can, with the exception of breathing air, crying, and pooping in a diaper. Just as you're feeling stretched, your baby is being squeezed on all sides. Some of your antibodies are crossing the placenta, giving your baby's immune system some support for her first days in the world.

You

You're carrying around 15 to 25 or more pounds: extra stores of fat will account for 7 pounds or so, add 4 pounds for extra fluid, 2 pounds (or more) for your breasts, about 1 to 1½ pounds for the placenta and umbilical cord, and about 5 to 7½ pounds for the baby.

After 37 weeks most healthcare providers will want to see you once a week, and twice a week from week 40 on, to check cervical changes and the baby's position and to monitor your blood pressure and urine for signs of preeclampsia (for more on this, see "Preeclampsia" in the Pregnancy Dictionary).

The hormone *relaxin* is causing all of the smooth muscle in your body to unclench. You'll feel like you have loose "rag-doll" joints. Even tall, fit women will start to get a waddling gait as ligaments soften. Inside, the smooth muscle layer of your uterus is flattening and relaxing to accommodate your baby's weight gain. You may have round ligament pains (sharp muscle cramps around the place where your bathing suit's leg holes would be) as these ligaments are softening and being pulled by the weight of the baby.

You're probably having Braxton-Hicks contractions, periodic hardening of your belly, which you may or may not notice. How can you tell these contractions from the real thing? If you have to ask, they probably aren't. Real contractions grow progressively stronger, more intense, and more regular. They may start and stop in a series over a day or night before they get down to business. Use a timer to see how far apart they are and how long they last. If they start to come at regular intervals, let your care provider know. You may expel bloody *show*, also known as your *mucus plug*, at any time. This is a blood-tinged mass of mucus that has been covering your cervix for the past 9 months. It doesn't mean that you'll go into labor right away—it can take as long as 2 to 3 weeks after bloody show before labor begins. (For more about this, see page 87.)

As you approach your due date, you'll start to get frantic calls from well-meaning friends and relatives who just want to check and see if you're in labor yet. Of course, only 5 percent of moms deliver on their due date. Any care provider who can tell you when you're going to go into labor is lying or planning to induce you. Waiting for labor can make you feel discouraged. Make plans every day, go to the movies, walk outside, and enjoy the last few days of quiet.

Keep your car filled with gas, and make sure you can always get in touch with whoever is designated to drive you to the hospital. Write down the phone number of a local taxi or ambulance service in case you go into labor when you're home alone. If you're impatient, take plenty of walks and keep swimming. The activity may or may not move things along, but you'll feel better.

> *"I asked my midwife when she thought the baby would be born, and she said, 'If I could tell that, I wouldn't be a midwife, I'd be down betting at the track.'"*

Stay rested, nourished, and hydrated to prepare for labor. In addition to waiting for serious contractions to start, be on the alert for the **rupture of membranes** (water breaking). You'll have a lot of discharge now as the birth canal cleans and prepares itself for the big event, but your water breaking is usually (but not always) hard to miss. It'll be a gush or a rapid trickle that smells like the ocean. Sometimes, but rarely, the fluid can leak out and seem like a heavy, watery discharge. Only one in ten moms experiences her water breaking before labor begins. If this happens to you, call your care provider right away.

You may or may not go into labor immediately. If you don't, your care provider may wait for 24 hours for labor to start naturally, but then will probably induce you out of concern for the possibility of infection. You may also be given intravenous antibiotics to reduce the possibility of infection.

You continue to add a pound a week and may have an increasingly hard time getting around gracefully. To get out of bed, roll to your side, then push yourself up with your arms.

WEEK 38

Fetal Age: 36 weeks (253 to 259 days)

2 to 1 weeks, 13 to 7 days until your due date

Baby

Size: An average of 7½ pounds and 20 inches, though due to individual variation, your healthy baby's size could vary by 1 or 2 pounds on either side.

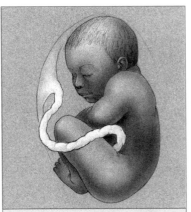

At week 38, your baby could be born healthy at any time.

Development: She is fully developed, though still adding connections between neurons in the brain (this continues well after birth).

Extra large! Your baby is likely to have hit the 6-pound mark by now, and the total weight of your uterus is about twice of that. At this point, you can try to make a guesstimate of her height yourself: try to find her head and rump, then measure your hands' distance with a tape measure or a string and ruler. Your baby's back will feel smooth and hard, while the front area will be soft with hard bumps that move when pressed. Your baby's head will feel hard and round and will move in response to a gentle nudge. The baby's forehead and brow will also feel hard, and the rump will feel larger and bulkier than the head and won't move as readily as other body parts. Don't worry too much if you baby seems sideways sometimes, some babies wait until labor starts to get into the proper position.

At week 38, your baby could be born at any time, though the odds are against it, with pregnancy for first-time moms lasting an average of 41 weeks and a day.

If you have had previous late-term stillbirths, though, or your baby seems dangerously *small for gestational age*, your doctor may recommend induction between now and week 39.

If you are not being induced or delivering with a scheduled c-section, the uncertainty of when labor will begin is the hardest part of the third trimester. Your due date may very well come and go, especially if you're a first-time mom, and the current recommendation is that doctors wait at least 2 weeks after a due date passes before considering induction unless there's a medical problem.

Don't be tempted to try to induce labor with herbs or castor oil, no matter what it says on the Internet. Herbal supplements are unregulated by the FDA and can contain highly variable concentrations and unlisted ingredients. Their effects can be nonexistent, unpredictable, or even dangerous, and no herbal

supplements are tested for safety for pregnant women by the FDA.

Keep eating frequent small, nutritious meals, and if you think that your contractions may be the real thing, eat something. The calories will help fortify you for what could be a long labor. Also keep yourself hydrated with water, tea, milk, or juice. Avoid carbonated beverages, which can increase bloating.

What you can do: Finalize arrangements for someone who can cook and do chores to live in or drop in for several hours a day. For 2 to 4 weeks postpartum, you'll need more help than just your partner can provide, especially if he'll be going back to work soon after the baby's born. If you have other children, you may also need additional babysitting help.

Also consider the possibility that you might be away from home for longer than the typical labor-plus-48-hours. If you have a c-section you may be away for as long as 4 days, or even longer should you or the baby experience complications.

Are you still working? We understand that starting your leave early means less time with the baby, and that you may not have paid maternity leave, but even so, you may want to seriously consider starting your leave soon. If you sit all day, you could be plagued with back pain, hemorrhoids, varicose veins, swollen ankles, carpal tunnel syndrome, or all of the above. If you do a lot of standing or walking at work, your muscles will be easily and seriously fatigued as they strain to keep supporting your frame.

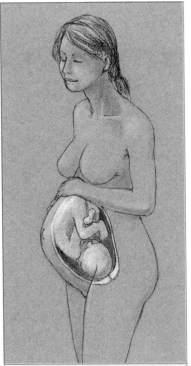

Waiting is the hardest part of the third trimester.

What's a Mucus Plug?

Soon after you conceive, a barrier of thick cervical fluid will form a seal that keeps bacteria out of the uterus. During pregnancy the fluid is cloudy, sticky, and jelly-like, then as labor nears the cervix begins to soften and stretch, which can tinge the barrier with blood and skin cells. In the weeks before pregnancy you may shed the barrier little by little, in the form of mucous-y and sometimes pink-streaked discharge, like what you might see on a tissue if you had a head cold and blew your nose too hard. Or you may shed it in larger parts, in the form of bloody mucus on your underwear or toilet tissue, in what's called show (see below) or bloody show. Sometimes vaginal intercourse or a cervical exam can also dislodge a little show. Or you may see no snotty or bloody discharge at all until you are about the deliver the baby. If you do pass bloody show, though, let your healthcare provider know at your next appointment.

How Big Is the Baby Going to Be?

Be skeptical of any weight estimates that you hear. It's really hard to tell a baby's size from the outside, even for experienced healthcare providers equipped with ultrasound. To you the baby will feel huge no matter what: After 37 weeks you will be carrying around 15 to 25 or more pounds: extra stores of fat will account for 7 pounds or so, add 4 pounds for extra fluid, 2 pounds (or more) for your breasts, about 1 to 1½ pounds for the placenta and umbilical cord, and about 5 to 7½ pounds for the baby.

In any case, a baby's weight doesn't affect the birth experience as much as you might suppose. Your baby's head is the largest part to be delivered, and a baby's skull size doesn't vary much between a 5 or a 10 pound baby. What matters more is how the baby's skull is positioned as he or she descends into to your "pelvic outlet"—the ring of your pelvic bones and tailbone.

Baby's heads are also joined together by moveable plates of bone connected by membrane-covered spaces. This allows the plates to slide over one another, making the baby's head more compact for birth, called **molding**. In the best case your baby's head descends from forehead to tailbone; less optimal is if you and baby are back-to-back or the baby is rump down (**breech presentation**). Also, your pelvis will expand before and during birth, with the lower rim widening by as much as one-third for your baby's descent.

Can't They Just Knock Me Out?

There are women who claim to have had painless or even "orgasmic" deliveries, but they're the exception. Nine out of 10 women agree that some, most, or all of labor is best described as painful.

When it comes to the pain of labor and birth, it can be tempting to take a "just give me the epidural" mindset. But there are drawbacks to a head-in-the-sand approach to labor pain.

The reality is, you will have to learn to handle pain in some capacity because there is no such thing as just being knocked out for the entire birth and recovery process. Every birth will involve *some* amount of physical discomfort. Even women who have 10-minute pushing stages will have to cope with uterine cramps afterward. A scheduled c-section may keep you from feeling discomfort during delivery itself, but the recovery will involve many more hours of recovery discomfort, disability, IV pokes, and catheterization, which can be more painful overall. Drips and **catheter**s also confine you to bed for the rest of labor and much of recovery and can interfere with breastfeeding, all of which can make you feel vulnerable.

The pain of labor itself is also not like the pain of a needle, broken ankle, or cavity. It comes and goes in waves, never the same from one moment to the next. Thrashing, demonic laboring women are only in the movies. Most women are able to ride the waves, find a part of their minds where it doesn't hurt, and breathe, squat, and adjust through contractions.

Yes, epidurals are magic, but they also have drawbacks (see page 189 for more about epidurals).

When it comes up epidurals our advice is to not decide you will or won't get one. Focus on getting yourself through the first stage of labor with whatever pain management technique works for you—breathing deeply, finding comfortable positions, walking, visualization—and tell yourself that you can do this. You can always request an epidural if you feel you need one.

WEEK 39

Fetal Age: 37 weeks (260 to 266 days)

6 to 0 days left until your due date

Baby

Size: Anywhere from 5½ to 9½ pounds. Don't be too worried if your care provider says that your baby is large. It's extremely difficult to judge a baby's weight from the outside, and baby seeming big from the outside should not be considered evidence that labor should be induced before 40 weeks or that a c-section will be necessary.

Development: Your baby is adding neural connections and growing hair and still gaining weight. Researchers have found that labor begins when the fetal lungs emit a protein that signals their development is complete. If so, it's proof of the old saying that "only a baby knows when it's ready to be born."

You

How you may be feeling:
- "Like a dump truck."
- "Like I'm doing nothing but waiting."
- "I wish people would quit calling to ask if I'm in labor."
- "One minute I want labor to start, the next I'm worried about labor and what I'll do with her when she gets here."

To get some relief from your weight and aches, do plenty of hands-and-knees cat stretches and pelvic tilts. Soak in a warm bath, swim, or just float in the pool to take a break from gravity.

Things to organize: People want to help, but they need to be told what to do (and sometimes how to do it).

Is your partner prepared to take over your household duties? Help prepare him by writing a list of any phone numbers he may need and posting it somewhere visible:
- Numbers for your doctor, midwife, and/or labor support person or doula
- The pediatrician
- Household repair providers
- Your mechanic
- Grocery delivery service
- Cleaning service
- Veterinarian
- Dentist
- Any other medical specialists you use (dermatologist, psychiatrist, podiatrist, etc.)

Make a to-do list of anything that you think he should take care of for the next several months: routine car maintenance, household repairs, changing the sheets in the guest room for your mother, and so on.

Make a file of important documents:
- Receipts for products and services
- Vehicle maintenance records
- Contact information and policy numbers for any insurance policies you have
- Mortgage or rental contract documents for your home
- Create a mail area in your house, if you don't already have one. Get a box to put bills in that's furnished with stamps, envelopes, and pens that work. Put a trash can nearby to keep junk mail from accumulating and a place to keep magazines until you can get to them.
- Get a calendar with lots of room to write, if you don't already have one, and record trash days, recycling days, upcoming appointments, birthdays, and other occasions that you'd usually keep track of in your head.

Stock up on nonperishable goods so you'll have less shopping to do later:
- Paper towels and napkins
- Canned, jarred, and frozen foods
- Extra-absorbent maxi pads
- Paper plates and cups and plastic flatware (so you'll have fewer dishes to wash)
- Trash and recycling bags
- Batteries
- Local carryout and delivery menus, with foods you like circled

Yes, we know, it sounds like you're hunkering down for a hurricane. But you'll want (and deserve) to spend any spare time relaxing, not on chores and getting the car fixed!

Call Your Care Provider If You Experience Any of These Symptoms

- Vaginal bleeding
- Pain or burning when you urinate
- Very bad or frequent headaches
- Severe vomiting
- Pelvic pain or cramps
- Increasing pelvic pressure
- Decreased fetal movement
- Intense bloating of your face, hands, and/or feet

What Makes Real Labor Start?

Most moms can't precisely answer the question "What time did your labor start?" Unless your water breaks spontaneously (which happens less than 10 percent of the time), the start of labor is usually pretty subtle. You might have a series of strong contractions every 15 minutes for an hour that disappear for hours or days, only to come back and then fade again. Your doctor or midwife might tell you that you've lost your mucus plug and are a centimeter dilated, but you might not feel contractions for a week or more after that.

Labor starting is much more like a snowball gaining momentum as it rolls down a hill than a horse leaping out of the gate when the starter pistol fires. Researchers believe that a hormone secreted by the baby's lungs and **pituitary gland** initiate a complex cascade of hormonal interactions—a chemical conversation, if you will—between baby and mother that starts to relax her smooth muscle tissue and ligaments (this is why diarrhea and sometimes vomiting can be an early sign of labor). Then uterine muscle fibers to start contracting and releasing, to push the baby out in a gradual way that lowers the risk of injury the baby or mother.

When Your Water Breaks

All during pregnancy, your baby has floated inside a tough, watery balloon called the amniotic sac. Usually the amniotic sac breaks sometime after labor is well established, called rupture of the membranes. It's not clear what makes about 10 percent of women's sacs break before labor, but recent research appears to show that 1 out of 3 mothers whose waters break early have mild infections.

A ruptured sac is painless—you'll simply feel gushing, warm fluid coming out.

Typically, it will break while a woman is at home in bed, or while she's sitting on the toilet. (Nothing special about these places, they're just where third-trimester moms spend most of their time.)

If your membranes rupture, you may see the mucus plug and white flecks of vernix, the sloughed-off waxy covering for your baby's skin.

If you're walking around, the

Coping with Nighttime Contractions

Sometimes Braxton-Hicks contractions feel more intense and bothersome at night, especially as they begin to shift into *prodromal labor*. If you're awakened by discomfort in the middle of the night and are having trouble sleeping, try to conserve your energy for the big work ahead. Drink water, eat something, and try to relax around your contractions as best you can. Here's a handy list of coping strategies:

- **Don't watch the clock.** While you do want to check your contractions once in a while to see if they're changing, you don't need to record every contraction over the many long hours of early labor—you could wind up staring at the clock for days. Trust your contractions to let you know in no uncertain terms when it's time to take them more seriously.
- **Take a shower or bath.** Nothing soothes like warm water. Dunk a full-size bath towel in warm water, and use it as a blanket for your back or belly, or roll it up to make a warm compress to drape across your neck and shoulders. (Not too hot, or it will make your baby's heart rate speed up.)
- **Drink a soothing beverage.** Try non-caffeinated liquids, such as warm milk with honey or an instant breakfast beverage, to make you sleepy.
- **Urinate frequently.** It will make you more comfortable, and an empty bladder will make more room for your baby to move down in preparation for birth.
- **Eat a snack.** Try eating cereal, a banana, or a turkey sandwich. Turkey contains an amino acid called tryptophan that may make you drowsy.
- **Turn on some music.** Listen to a relaxing CD of surf or nature sounds, or pull out your self-hypnosis birthing tapes.
- **Change beds.** Try sleeping on the couch wrapped in a cozy comforter and propped up with piles of pillows.
- **Ask about medication.** It's okay to take sleep medications with diphenhydramine (such as Tylenol PM or Benadryl) as directed if your healthcare provider has already given you the go ahead.

fluid may dribble out and dampen your underpants, or it could gush out and run down your leg—a shoe-soaker.

If your water breaks, put on a maxi pad, call your care provider and partner regardless of what time it is, and pack your bag with last-minute items and catch a ride to the hospital (or if you're having a home birth, make yourself comfortable and time any contractions while you wait for the midwife).

If the fluid is greenish, has green or brown spots or is foul smelling, this could be caused by meconium (baby stool), which is a sign that your baby may be in trouble. If you see meconium, do not attempt a home birth—call your midwife and proceed to the closest hospital.

Packing a Hospital Bag

Think about what you want to bring with you to the hospital. Perhaps find a corner of your closet to start piling things in. Don't forget a newborn- size and photogenic outfit for the baby to wear home, and a blanket to swaddle her with.

(The nurses can show you how to swaddle.)

Hospitals are usually pretty good at providing everything you'll need while you're there. Some even give you disposable underpants. Still, it's nice to have things from home.

Here are some things you may want to include when packing for the hospital:

- Health insurance card
- Baby car seat already installed firmly in the backseat of your car in the rear-facing position
- An outfit for the baby to wear home
- Address book with phone numbers of relatives and friends to be notified
- Cell phone and charger cord, though you may have to have to keep your phone off until you are in a recovery room—cell phones may interfere with hospital monitoring equipment
- Deodorant, brush, comb, toothbrush, and toothpaste
- Maternity underwear (hospital may supply, but just in case)
  Optional items:
- Birth plan
- Music player and earphones or speakers
- Snacks for you, your partner, and guests
- Bottles of juice or sports drinks
- Legal pad and pen for taking notes for recording things you want to remember
- Folder for carrying home discharge papers, copies of your medical records, and the baby's footprints
- Bathrobe and slippers
- Lightweight blanket for your partner
- Moisturizer, face wash, and/or makeup (if you wear it)

- Lip balm
- Hair clips, elastics, and/or a headband
- Maternity outfit to wear home (you'll only be about 10 pounds lighter, so bring what was comfortable last month)
- Camera
- Change for snack and soda machines
- Natural childbirth pain relief supplies
- Birthing ball
- Two-level footstool for supporting your feet as you sit in a chair or on the toilet
- Back massage supplies, such as a tennis ball

The following are usually supplied by the hospital (but bring if you prefer your own):
- Socks with non-slip soles
- Pillow with a colored pillowcase (so it doesn't get lost)
- Nightgown with front openings for nursing (something that you don't mind getting stained)
- Box of disposable breast pads
- Heavy-flow sanitary napkins

WEEK 40

Fetal Age: 38 weeks, days 267 and beyond

Baby

Size: Your baby is newborn size—the average newborn weighs 7½ pounds and has a length of 21½ inches.

Development: The baby is fully formed. Her brain is about one quarter of its eventual size, and contains about 100 billion neurons. The placenta is providing her with antibodies that will last until about 6 months after birth.

Before birth, circulating blood bypasses the lungs completely. Then, when she takes her first breath, her brain cues the muscle of the diaphragm to contract and the rib cage to expand, and blood pressure drops in the lungs and air begins to flow into them. The passage in the heart that lets blood bypass the lungs begin to close and will be permanently shut in 12 to 24 hours after birth.

You

If your due date has come and gone, your pregnancy is officially post-date. But don't panic, staying pregnant past 40 weeks is really common, even normal, especially if you're a first-time mom and/or of European genetic descent.

If your care provider starts talking about scheduling an induction, first make sure your due date is as accurate as possible. You may also want to ask for a second opinion from a *maternal-fetal medicine* specialist—a specially trained obstetrician—if you're concerned that your healthcare provider is suggesting an intervention that seems risky.

At the same time, after 41 weeks (39 gestational weeks) other potential risks of continuing the pregnancy need to be taken into account, like the potential for placental problems and low amniotic fluid. Women and babies of Asian and African genetic heritage appear to be particularly vulnerable to post-date risks. (Note it doesn't matter what the baby's father's genes are, it's apparently mom's genes that appear to affect

how long an average pregnancy lasts.)

So, before you talk induction, discuss with your healthcare provider to make sure that your estimated due date (EDD) has taken into account the length of your cycle, your genetic makeup, and whether or not this is your first baby.

In the meantime, your care provider will check your *dilation* (how open your cervix is, if it all) and *effacement* (how thick your cervix is) to see if changes are occurring that may predict the onset of *active labor* using a grading system called a Bishop (or Bishop's) Score.

There are plenty of methods of attempting to induce labor, such as stripping the membranes (page 96), herbs, and cervical massage, but unless your care provider has a real concern that you or your baby's health is compromised, you shouldn't try any of them. Any attempts to induce labor should only happen in a well-equipped medical facility.

You are bigger and more uncomfortable than you ever thought possible, and probably can't sleep well or do much more than watch television, read, and make trips to the bathroom.

These are tedious times, but do try to enjoy the peace and quiet. As the saying goes, babies are easier to take care of in there than out here. Don't feel guilty about just sitting around. Do try to stretch your legs and encourage labor with daily walks.

Your care provider may use ultrasound to see if your baby has enough amniotic fluid. If the baby seems fine, you and your

Bishop's Score

The **Bishop's Score** is a grading system used to assess if active labor is near and which moms-to-be are most likely to have a successful induction of labor.

Each of the conditions on the assessment is assigned ratings from 0 to 3, with 3 being the most favorable. If the mother's score is 0, then she's nowhere near active labor and it's unlikely labor can be successfully induced. But if her score is greater than 8, then the conditions for using labor-inducing medications are favorable, though note that someone could have a high score and still not go into labor for many days, or have an attempted induction not work (which happens to about 1 in 6 moms). Each one of these points is given a score of 0–2 (for position and consistency) or 0–3, with the highest score being 13:

- Cervical dilation: No dilation gets a score of 0, 1-2 centimeters is a 1, 3-4 centimeters is a score of 2, and more than 4 centimeters scores a 3.
- Cervical effacement: This is how thin the cervix is, expressed as a percentage. Zero to 30 percent effacement gets a score of 0; 80 percent or more gets a score of 3.
- Cervical consistency (as in how soft or firm it is): Firm gets a score of 0, soft is a 2.
- Cervical position: The more anterior the position, the better aligned for delivery. Add 0-2 points: 0 for posterior, 2 for anterior, and 1 point for somewhere in the middle.
- Fetal station: How far down the baby's head is. Three points for way down, 0 or up to -3 points for way up.

care provider can discuss when to schedule induction of labor. No matter what, one way or another, somehow, that baby is getting out!

All About Contractions

Some women who have never given birth mistakenly believe that labor is just one long pain. Actually, the uterus contracts in rhythmical waves of hardening and softening throughout labor with time to rest in between. The pain of a contraction builds and then peaks for a few seconds in the middle of the wave, and then it slowly disappears. No contraction lasts more than 90 seconds, and the time between contractions can be 10 minutes, 5 minutes, or 1½ minutes, depending upon what stage of labor you are in.

By now, you've experienced plenty of contractions during your pregnancy, but most of them were so painless and mild, you probably weren't aware of them. A simple test for whether you're having a contraction or not is to press down on the top of your uterus—the ridge at the top of your belly below your rib cage. If the ridge feels soft like the tip of your nose, then you're not having a contraction. If the ridge feels hard like your forehead, then you are.

Unless your contractions are getting stronger, longer, and closer together, then you're probably not in labor, but having Braxton-Hicks contractions, which are the painless tensing of the smooth muscle fibers of your uterus as it stretches and adapts to your baby. You can usually make these practice contractions go away by drinking water, changing positions, or lying down for a while.

Prodromal labor involves contractions that lead up to labor, but start and stop in the weeks and days before active labor gets under way.

Prodromal labor helps the mouth of your cervix start to soften, thin, and stretch open. If you aren't certain whether your contractions are prodromal or real, get a watch with a second hand, a pen, and a piece of paper, and write down the time when each contraction starts, when it ends, and when the next one begins for about an hour.

"Real" Contractions

It's not always easy to tell which contractions are causing dilation and effacement and which are Braxton-Hicks contractions or prodromal labor, but you can generally assume your contractions are going to lead to birth in the near future if:

- The contractions don't go away if you drink water or change position.
- Contractions are unmistakably getting stronger and closer together.
- Contractions are coming at regular intervals, like every 15 or 10 minutes, for at least an hour.

Most of the time "real" contractions are unmistakably stronger than the Braxton-Hicks kind—they may be actually painful and take your breath away, and it's difficult to talk through them. But not always. If you're not sure, call your healthcare provider.

When You're Overdue

It's not uncommon for a baby to seem overdue based on confusion about when conception actually happened, since many women don't keep accurate records of their periods. A baby may appear to be abnormally late even though he's right on schedule according to his mother's cycles.

About 18 out of every 100 pregnancies go beyond 41 weeks; and approximately one out of every six mothers has a pregnancy that lasts beyond 42 weeks.

In rare instances, an overdue pregnancy can signal a medical problem. A mother's placenta may lose efficiency in supporting the baby. Her amniotic fluid may begin to dry up; a baby's growth may be halted; or he may keep on growing larger, making his trip through a narrow pelvis more challenging. Babies who are more than a week overdue are more vulnerable to not getting enough oxygen during labor and birth.

If you've gotten to 41 weeks of pregnancy with no signs of going into labor, you may be asked to take tests to evaluate your baby's activity levels and heart rate and to measure the volume of fluid in your amniotic sac to make sure it is adequate to support your baby.

WEEK 41

Fetal Age: 39 weeks

Size: About a half-pound more than last week.

Your due date's come and gone, your healthcare provider may be requiring biweekly fetal testing, and the "you haven't had that baby yet?" remarks are getting you down. If you were hoping for a home birth but your midwife won't do homebirths after 41 weeks, you may be in a slight panic.

A few things to try, in order of effectiveness:

- **Stripping or sweeping the membranes.** This is when a healthcare provider, using a gloved hand, takes a finger and sweeps around the inside of the cervix to loosen it from the amniotic sac. This can stimulate contractions or cause your water to break and should only be done by an experienced medical professional; don't try it at home.

  The procedure involves inserting a gloved finger up into the rim of your cervix and rotating it between your baby's amniotic sac and the rim of the cervix. This detaches the amniotic membranes from the lower part of the uterine cavity in order to encourage the start of labor. The sweeping is used to help stimulate the hormones that start labor, but can sometimes be painful and lead to minor bleeding afterward.

  A series of studies have found that sweeping the membranes increases the chances of going into labor within a week. Women who've had sweeping done are less likely to have their labor artificially induced. There appears to be no increased incidence in adverse outcomes for mothers who had the procedure or higher levels of infection, although the procedure may cause temporary bleeding and discomfort.

- **Nipple stimulation.** Nipple stimulation can bring on contractions, but your cervix has to be ready in order for it to work, and it can't be just a few twiddles or honks: you need to simulate the actions of a breastfeeding baby for at a solid 20 to 30 minutes at minimum. Use a breast pump, preferably a double-horned one, for 2 minutes, then rest for 3 minutes, then stimulate for 2 minutes again. Or use your hands, milking both breasts with vigor (you'll know you're doing it right when you see fluid on your nipples). If you get no contraction action at all after 20 minutes, give up. If you feel contractions, keep it up for 60 to 90 minutes, or until your contractions are coming at a rhythmic pace on their own.

- **Long walks and staying upright.** Keeping the baby's weight on your cervix will help gravity encourage effacement, and moving around will help your circulation. At home, sit on a birth ball to read or watch TV.

- **Intercourse.** Sperm contain *prostaglandins*, which can encourage *cervical ripening* (in fact, prostaglandin gels applied to the cervix for hospital inductions are made with pig or bull *semen*). For maximum effectiveness, have sex in the missionary position (or as close to it as you can manage), make sure your partner ejaculates, and it's a bonus if you can have an orgasm too (orgasm causes a uterine contraction). Then prop your hips up with a pillow and stay lying down for at least 2 minutes to keep the sperm at your uterus. It's often repeated on the Internet that prostaglandins are more effective if ingested, but we have yet to find any studies that confirm this.

- **A belly band.** Sometimes, particularly with women who have had more than one child, the baby's head can move on and off of the cervix, causing prodromal labor that can seem like honest-to-goodness strong and real contractions for hours, that then stop when the baby changes position. Using a belly band or even a baby sling wrapped around your lower belly can help keep the baby's head positioned on the cervix to encourage dilation and effacement.
- **Spicy food.** Lots of women swear by super-spicy Indian or Thai food, though there's no evidence that it works.
- **Fresh pineapple or papaya.** Fresh pineapple contains an enzyme called bromelian, which can break down protein, which could theoretically help kick-start labor. Fresh papaya also has a similar enzyme. These fruit enzymes are quickly destroyed by exposure, though, so canned or heated fruit won't do, you must cut and/or juice your own (or get fresh-squeezed juice at your local juice bar, if you happen to have one in your town). Pineapple and

papaya enzyme supplements are also available in grocery-store vitamin aisles, though note that as with almost every dietary supplement, they have not been tested for safety or effectiveness for use during pregnancy (or any other time).

- **Acupuncture.** Results of studies have been mixed as to whether or not acupuncture can induce labor, and most studies done to date have been on relatively small groups of women. One 2001 study found that women who had acupuncture delivered 2 days sooner than women who didn't,[2] in 2006 a study of first-time pregnant women at 38 weeks' *gestation*, found no difference in the rates of *spontaneous labor*,[3] then in 2008 a study found that women who had acupuncture were actually pregnant even longer than the control group.[4] So to make a long story short, no one really knows if acupuncture works to induce labor or not, but the evidence seems to lean toward the direction of it not making a difference.

What's a Non-Stress Test?

If you're past your due date, or if you have certain high-risk conditions like hypertenstion, intrauterine growth restriction, or gestational diabetes, your healthcare provider will probably demand (or at least strongly encourage) one or more non-stress tests, *biophysical profiles*, or *contraction stress tests* a week. When you're post-term there is a risk that the placenta will begin to break down, depriving the baby of nutrients and oxygen. This can happen with no warning or symptoms, and needless to say, it's not good.

Non-stress tests, biophysical profiles, and contraction stress tests are basically the same thing: your belly is hooked up to monitors for 20 minutes to an hour (be sure to use the bathroom first!) while a technician monitors the fetus for certain signs. A non-stress or contraction stress test checks the baby's movement and heart rate in response to your contractions (which in this late stage of pregnancy you will have a lot of, even if you're not always aware of them).

The technician will be checking to make sure that the baby's heart rate is normal, then slows a little during contractions and speeds up after. A biophysical profile is the same as the above, but includes more detailed observations such as the condition of your placenta, the flow through the umbilical cord, the amount of your amniotic fluid, and your baby's body and breathing movements. If your baby's heart rate doesn't respond to contractions, fluctuates when there isn't a contraction, or doesn't recover quickly after a contraction, these are all signs that the fetus is could be having circulation problems, and you will probably be admitted right away to the hospital for an emergency c-section. If all is well, then you'll be sent home and may be directed to make an appointment for another test in a few days.

Medical Induction

If you have certain medical issues, or labor starts and stops over and

over, or you've gone well beyond your delivery date, then your physician or midwife may suggest an induction. Augmentation of labor is making your contractions stronger once your labor has already started. Both augmentation and induction use medications to make your uterus contract or employ special devices that artificially stretch the mouth of the uterus, your cervix, as a way of jumpstarting labor.

An induction can be potentially lifesaving if the placenta isn't supporting your baby any longer; your baby has stopped growing normally; you have started having preeclampsia, affecting your blood pressure and other body functions; you've got poorly controlled diabetes mellitus; you have an infection in your uterus; your baby's blood type is incompatible with yours (*isoimmunization*); your amniotic sac has broken prematurely (rupture of the membranes), exposing your baby to the danger of an infection; or your baby has died inside you (stillbirth).

Your doctor or midwife may also suggest that you have an induction if your baby is weeks overdue, especially if tests indicate that your placenta may be starting to decline in function. Placentas work most efficiently up to about 40 weeks, and 42 weeks is about the longest most clinicians are comfortable letting a pregnancy continue.

Some mothers opt to have labor induced when there's no medical necessity, which is called having an elective induction. Some healthcare providers will gladly let you schedule an induction after 39 weeks or sometimes sooner, even if there's no specific medical reason for it. Other healthcare providers will only let you schedule one if you're past your due date.

The Risks of Inducing Labor

- **Heightened cesarean risk.** An induction nearly doubles your risk of having a c-section. A survey of the induction experiences of 14,409 women found that having an induction was associated with an 11 percent higher risk of having a cesarean section for first-time mothers. (See our list of c-section risks on page 197.)
- **Immature baby.** Your baby's lungs are one of the final organs to mature during the last weeks of pregnancy, and dating a pregnancy is not an exact science. If your provider wants to schedule an induction because you're past-date, make sure the length of your cycle and other factors are taken into account first.
- **Uterine hyperstimulation.** Overmedication can make the uterus cramp up and cut off the baby's supply of oxygen and blood, which can slow down the baby's heart rate.
- **Uterine rupture.** Having an induction after you've previously had a cesarean section is associated with an increased risk of *uterine rupture*, so you shouldn't have an induction if you have previously had a cesarean.

Other mothers at risk for rupture during induction are older mothers, women who have given birth to a large number of children, women carrying larger-than-normal babies, and women with an enlarged uterus.

Induction for a "too-large" baby?

An extra large baby is thought to have trouble fitting through a mother's pelvis and to cause a mother's contractions to be ineffective.

Current studies show that a doctor's or midwife's suspicions about the baby's size shouldn't be the only reason to opt for an induction. If your healthcare provider wants to schedule you for an induction only because the baby looks large from the outside, consider seeking a second opinion from a specialist in maternal-fetal medicine.

When to Leave for the Hospital

The first and most protective thing you can do in preparation for going to the hospital is to ensure that your contractions are well under way before you take off. Waiting also makes it less likely that you'll be sent back home from the hospital once you get there. First-time parents often panic and convince themselves (as in the movies) that they should race off at the first sign that contractions mean business.

But rather than speeding off to the hospital, before you go into labor ask your healthcare provider at what point you should call her. Write down the time that a contraction begins and how long it lasts.

Relax. Take cat naps. Eat a high-protein meal if you have the urge. Take a shower (or a bath if your water has not broken yet). Drink plenty of fluids to prepare yourself for the hard work ahead. Once contractions are strong, so much so that you're having trouble talking while they're going on, you can let your doctor or midwife know and finalize packing your hospital bag.

Getting Admitted

When you're admitted to the hospital, you'll be asked to submit your insurance card, your birth date, your social security number, and other identifying information. You may be given waivers and other paperwork to sign, stating that you'll allow the hospital to perform emergency surgery if necessary, and promising you'll pay your medical bills if your insurance company won't.

Note that even if you've filled out reams of paperwork before you arrived, there will likely still be yet more forms to fill out before you get to "relax" in triage or a delivery suite.

You will then be rolled in a wheelchair with your patient record to the labor and delivery area of your hospital. A labor and delivery (L&D) nurse will assess your general health, and she will try to determine how far along you are in labor. Here are some questions that you will likely be asked:
• When did your contractions start?
• How often they are coming?
• How strong are they?

• Has your water broken yet?
• If so, when did that happen, and what color was the fluid?
• Is your baby moving as much as usual?
• Have you had any problems during your pregnancy?
• Do you have any ongoing medical problems, such as diabetes or heart problems?
• When did you eat last?

You'll also be asked about any medications you may be taking (bring along your bottles); and if you have any allergies.

If you have a birth plan that you've discussed with your healthcare provider, this would be a good time for you, or your partner, to ask that a copy be put in your medical folder (keep a copy for yourself).

After the admitting staff has gotten all of the information they need, you'll be walked or wheeled into a room. Depending on the procedures at your hospital you may be wheeled to a delivery suite right away, or you may be waylaid in a triage area for fetal monitoring until your provider arrives and/or a delivery suite becomes available.

And off we go! For what happens next, see the "Birth" chapter on page 171.

What (and What *Not*) to Worry About

Pregnancy is a stressful time: who wouldn't fret about growing a human being who you're completely responsible for, but can't see or communicate with? Then there are so many warnings directed at you, combined with vague information. Don't take a hot bath or eat a ham sandwich; don't eat this kind of cheese; be sure to exercise—but not this way or that way. It can seem like the world is a dangerous place full of accidents waiting to happen. It's not just your imagination—on one hand we find out more every day about how important the fetal stage is for lifelong health, yet at the same time, solid, definitive studies about exactly what is safe during pregnancy are tough to find.

The lack of good pregnancy-safety information is in large part because it's considered unethical to use pregnant women in randomized clinical trials, so studies of food ingredients, drugs, or activities either are based on animal studies with pregnant rodents, or are after-the-fact studies of things that pregnant women were doing anyway, like taking aspirin, lifting weights, or drinking coffee. While studies like those can give you a little information—you don't want to take any drug that makes rats grow extra limbs—it won't give you the more precise information that a controlled, randomized double-blind study might. Even if controlled studies were performed on every drug, 9½ months is a long time, and pregnant women come into contact with thousands of things, and babies and mothers have millions of traits. So was it the drug that made the child become hyperactive later in life, or was it the sugar in all the cream puffs mom ate in the third trimester?

That's not to say you should ignore warnings based on solid information, but when it comes to headline-making stories about one scary study or another, always remember that your local news, a

Web site, or somebody's blog may not be the best filter for helping you assess real risk or telling which studies are weak or misleading. With studies, generally you can assume the more subjects the better (a study of 1,000 moms or babies is better than a study of 20), but on the other hand, the more subjects, the more other factors can come into play. For instance, one study of caffeine users find a very small increase in the rate of miscarriage for women who consume more than 200 mg per day, and it was immediately a lead story on every local news channel and morning show with a health report. But was it the caffeine causing that increase, or was it that pregnant women who drink a lot of caffeine are also exposed to other things, like coffeemaker germs or coffee pesticides? Or maybe the increase was a side effect of side effects: maybe women who drink more caffeine tend to be more dehydrated, and that's what was increasing the miscarriage rate. As it turned out, we'll probably never know—that study was quickly contradicted by another study, but not before pregnant women nationwide were wracked with guilt over drinking a few mochas.

And then there's all that darned-if-you-do-or-don't information, like leafy greens and fish are some of the most nutritious things you can eat, but by the way, also the foods most likely to be contaminated with bacteria or mercury or worse.

So while it's a good idea to lower whatever risks you can, it's also important to practice the art of accepting the reality that there's a certain amount of risk involved with everything in life. There is nothing anyone can do to make pregnancy (or life) completely risk-free. It's also human nature to worry about the things we can't control more than the things we can: we'll stay up all night worrying about the possible harm from some cough medicine we took before we knew we were pregnant, but not spend a second worrying about, say, driving a car. It helps to put things in perspective: you probably should not worry any more about the 3-in-100 risk of birth defects any more than you would fantasize about how you'll spend the money you might win from a raffle ticket with those odds.

Also keep in mind that once you hear a heartbeat on Doppler, you have about an 88 percent chance of carrying your pregnancy to term and giving birth to a healthy baby, even if you're over 35, take hot baths, and drink coffee. (And odds are if something goes wrong, it won't be the thing you stayed up all night worrying about).

But avoiding worry is easier said than done. Of course you'll worry, no matter what some book says. So without further ado, following is an alphabetical list of the things most pregnant women worry about, and the current available evidence on what is safe and what isn't, what tests you'll encounter, and common fears.

The following topics of most concern during pregnancy are listed in alphabetical order.

Age Over 35

If your due date is past your thirty-fifth birthday, most hospitals will consider you to be a "high risk" patient, which can be startling to hear, especially if you're otherwise in good health. While it's true that as we age the risks of birth defects, miscarriage, and stillbirth go up, remember that 35 is by no means a magic number. Fertility peaks between 20 and 25, and after that risks begin to increase little by little, week by week. At 25 your risk of having a baby with Down syndrome is 1 in 1,250; at 30 it's 1 in 1,000; at 35 it's 1 in 400; at age 40 it's 1 in 100. You're also statistically at higher risk for gestational diabetes, pregnancy-induced high blood pressure, and cesarean delivery. It all can sound scary, but remember that the vast majority of women who are 35 and even 40 have healthy and otherwise unremarkable pregnancies. If you're over 35 most healthcare providers will offer you even more opportunities and varieties of genetic testing: the option of CVS or amnio, instead of the quad screen. Some hospitals and healthcare providers will also offer genetic screening and counseling to help put risks in perspective.

Air Travel

Air travel is generally safe when you're pregnant, as long as you're in a pressurized cabin. If you fly your own small plane, though, stay below 7,000 feet to avoid oxygen deprivation and pressure.

There is a slightly higher risk of first-trimester miscarriage for pregnant professional flight attendants and pilots, which may or may not be related to radiation exposure.

If you're traveling on a commercial airline in the third trimester, note that every airline will have its own policy as to how close to your due date you can be when you travel. If you're obviously in advanced pregnancy, some airlines will require a dated doctor's note or medical information form with your due date and a statement that you're free of complications.

Airline requirement or not, it's a good idea to take a sheet from your healthcare provider with a quick rundown of your medical history, including your blood type, any chronic health problems, a listing all medications you are currently taking, any medical or food allergies, your healthcare provider's name, and your due date. Most airlines won't let you travel after 36 weeks, or 32 weeks if you're expecting multiples, because they don't want to have you go into labor en route, and some airlines won't let you on the plane at all after week 34.

Pregnancy, combined with sitting still for 4 hours or more, also increases the risk for deep-vein thrombosis, or DVT, a rare but serious blood clotting disorder. DVT isn't specific to air travel—your risk goes up whenever you sit for 4 hours or more. To prevent DVT, stay hydrated and stretch your calves (get up for a walk or a leg stretch) at least once an hour. Studies have found no benefit to wearing special compression stockings.

When you travel:

• Opt for an aisle seat or a bulkhead seat, which will make it easier for you to get up to take a walk or use the bathroom.

• Fasten the seat belt across your hips and below your belly.

• Don't worry about radiation from the metal detectors used at airport security gates; the level of radiation is very low.

• Stay hydrated: drink plenty of water before, during, and after your flight.

• If you're traveling alone and have heavy bags, spring for curbside check-in instead of risking muscle strain or injury.

• If your pregnancy is high risk or you are within a month of your due date, ask your healthcare provider to recommend a provider at your destination. If you experience spotting, your water breaking, or signs of premature labor while you're away from home, your best bet is to proceed to the closest emergency room.

Alcohol

Drinking alcohol can severely damage a fetus. Some research has found that one drink a week is okay (as in one 5-ounce glass of wine, one 8-ounce glass of malt liquor, one 12-ounce beer, or a 1.5-ounce shot of hard liquor), but any more than that—as few as two drinks a week—has been linked with brain damage and/or other birth defects.

Don't worry about any alcohol that you drank before you found out you were pregnant, though—before 6 weeks or so, basic structures are developing and if anything damages fetal DNA, it will also cause a miscarriage. So if you had a few before you knew you were pregnant and you're still pregnant, everything is probably okay. It is also safe to eat dishes that have cooked alcohol in them: beef burgundy, chicken marsala, beer-battered shrimp, and so on. But avoid more than a few bites of flambéed dishes, such as bananas foster, crepes suzette, cherries jubilee, and the like. These are made with high-alcohol spirits and the brief flambé action is not usually enough to burn off all of the alcohol.

Allergy Shots and Asthma Medications

If you're taking allergy shots for asthma or other chronic allergic conditions, it's okay to keep taking them in the lowest dose possible, according to the American Congress of Obstetricians and Gynecologists (ACOG). Says their statement: "It is safer for pregnant women with asthma to be treated with asthma medications than it is for them to have asthma symptoms." If you do have

asthma, it's important to keep your symptoms under control and have your lung function checked periodically throughout pregnancy, because the oxygen deprivation can cause growth restriction and increase the risk of preterm birth.

Amniocentesis

Amniocentesis, also known as amnio, AFT, or an amniotic fluid test, is a genetic test that takes a sample of amniotic fluid, which contains fetal DNA. With this DNA sample, geneticists can determine if your baby carries the genes for Down syndrome, trisomy 13 or 18, Fragile X, *neural tube defect*s, or other genetic abnormalities. It can also determine fetal blood type and gender. An amnio in late pregnancy can help predict fetal lung maturity, Rh incompatibility, or signs of inflammation. Healthcare providers usually offer the option of amnio if you are over 35 or have a family history of genetic disorders, or if a triple screen, quad screen, or AFP test result is abnormal, though increasingly the test is being offered to all women.

Amnio is usually performed between weeks 15 and 20. While in the 1970s the risk of amnio-induced miscarriage was about 1 in 200, more recent studies have found the risk to be closer to 1 in 769.

The test is performed by numbing an area on your belly with a local *anesthetic* (though not all providers do this), and ultrasound is used to guide a larger needle through the abdominal wall and

uterus and into the amniotic sac. About 2 tablespoons of fluid is extracted, then the fetal cells are separated out and cultured, fixed, and stained so the chromosomes can be examined. While the test itself just takes a few minutes, it usually takes about 7 to 10 days before complete results are available, because it takes time for the cells to be cultured, and sometimes the sample has to be sent to a specialized laboratory.

While tests such as the triple screen, quad screen, and AFP can reveal a potential risk of an abnormality, an amnio is a diagnostic test that can determine with certainty if an abnormality is present. An amnio can't detect every type of abnormality, though, only the specific gene disorders that are being tested for.

As with other kinds of tests, the important thing to consider is what you will do with the result. Some women opt to test even if they are sure they would not terminate the pregnancy no matter what, so that they will know what to expect at delivery and work toward being prepared emotionally and practically for a child with special needs.

Antacids

Antacids in the form of calcium carbonate, magnesium hydroxide, or magnesium oxide are safe to take during pregnancy, though long-term use (as in daily use for more than 2 days in a row) can prevent the absorption of nutrients. If you do take antacids, avoid using them within a half-hour of eating or taking your prenatal vitamin, and avoid antacids that contain aspirin (which may be listed on a label as salicylate or acetylsalicylic acid). Talk to your healthcare provider before trying acid blockers (such as rantidine, cimetidine, or famotidine). There is scant evidence about the safety of their use during pregnancy, though a large study found no increase in birth defects, fetal death, premature delivery, or low *APGAR scores*.[1]

Antibiotics

Some antibiotics appear to be safe to take during pregnancy, and others aren't. Considered safe are amoxicillin, ampicillin, clindamycin, erythromycin, and penicillin, but antibiotics in the tetracycline family should all be avoided as they've been linked to birth defects. A recent study has also found a possible link between rare birth defects and nitrofuran derivatives and sulfonamides (which are commonly used to treat urinary tract infections). So before you take antibiotics for an infection, make sure that the prescribing healthcare provider knows that you're pregnant.

Artificial Sweeteners

Stevia, sucralose, and acesulfame potassium are all considered safe for moderate use during pregnancy. Aspartame is considered safe as long as you don't have liver disease, *phenylketonuria* (PKU, a rare metabolic disorder), or high levels of the amino acid phenylalanine in your blood. When it comes to saccharin, after all of these years it's still not a settled question if it is safe for use during pregnancy. Saccharin does cross the placenta and is stored in fetal tissue, though, so if that bothers you, skip the Sweet 'N Low.

Aspirin

Because of its blood-thinning qualities, aspirin isn't recommended for regular use as a painkiller during pregnancy. But if you have certain specific conditions, like high blood pressure or a blood clotting disorder, your healthcare provider may recommend a low-dose (81 milligram per day) aspirin regimen, which appears to be safe, though most recommend stopping low-dose aspirin treatment after 32 weeks of pregnancy to reduce the potential risk of fetal blood flow issues and excessive blood loss during delivery.

Baths

See Hot Tubs.

Bed Rest

Many pregnant women are sent to bed by their doctors at some point in their pregnancy, for conditions such as preterm labor, pregnancy-related hypertension, slow fetal growth, carrying multiples, *placenta previa*, and *incompetent cervix*. But for all of these conditions, there is no evidence that bed rest works. There's also no standard protocol for prescribing bed rest, and much evidence that the side effects of the bed rest may be as bad or worse than the complications it's supposed to prevent.

Being put on bed rest and the extent of how restricted your activities will depend more on your care provider's style than on your physical symptoms. Many healthcare providers readily admit that they prescribe bed rest for problem pregnancies because they want a patient to feel like they're doing everything they can, even if the complications are out of anyone's control.

While lying in bed seems like a harmless activity, side effects can include headaches, blood clots in the legs, muscle *atrophy*, weight loss, depression, and anxiety. Often, even after delivery, the effects of passive immobility can continue, such as difficulty walking up and down stairs and deep soreness in your back and leg muscles.

The bed rest prescription also usually means you have to stop work, certainly a shock to your employer or anyone else who relies on you.

If you've been advised to go on bed rest, ask your healthcare provider the following questions:

- **Predicted outcome.** How and why will bed rest help my condition?
- **The details.** Make sure you know what he means by the concept of bed rest. Are you going to be allowed to sit up? Or, should you lie on your left side all the time? Can you get up to go to the kitchen or bathroom? Can you work from home? Should you limit your sexual activities?
- **Side effects.** Are you aware of the side effects of bed rest, and do you think that the benefits will outweigh them?
- **Second opinion.** Consider getting a second opinion, particularly if you begin to experience the side effects listed above.

Birth and Genetic Defects

A birth defect is any type of abnormality that affects the way a baby's body looks or functions. They can be caused by genetic or environmental factors, infections in early pregnancy, or a combination of factors. For about 60 percent of defects the cause can't be identified.

Every mom-to-be worries about birth defects. Fortunately, they're rare, with only about 3 in 100 babies born having any of 4,000 identified birth defects. Of those 3 percent, most are minor and easily treated (e.g., an extra toe). The other good news is that prenatal screening tests can identify 95 percent of abnormalities before birth.

Heart defects are the most commonly identified birth defect, affecting about 1 in 150 pregnancies. Some heart defects may resolve on their own; others may require surgery. Orofacial clefts, such as *cleft lip* or *cleft palate*, are the second-most common type of birth defect, affecting about 1 in 700 babies. Neural tube defects, which are defects of the spine or brain, affect about 1 in 1,000 pregnancies.

Cystic fibrosis, a genetic glandular disorder, affects about 1 in 2,500 to 3,500 Caucasian newborns, about 1 in 17,000 African Americans and 1 in 31,000 Asian Americans. (For more on CF screening, see page 118.)

If your baby is found to have a birth defect, you'll be referred to a genetic counselor who will help you determine the severity of the defect, what to expect, and what your next steps should be.

Birth Control During Pregnancy

If you became pregnant while using some method of birth control, you have a lot of company. One-fourth of all pregnancies in America are due to contraceptive failure—that's more than a million pregnancies every year! If your pregnancy is one of the "lucky" ones, you may have extra concerns about birth defects or pregnancy problems. Most often, there's nothing to worry about in terms of the baby's safety.

BIRTH CONTROL PILLS AND CONTRACEPTIVE PATCHES

Birth control pills can fail if a dose is skipped, when there's a chemical interaction with certain antibiotics or antacids that block their absorption, or if anything prevents them from getting digested, like a stomach virus or food poisoning. Birth control patches and rings, which eliminate these problems, are therefore theoretically more reliable. But all three methods, even when used absolutely correctly, do fail on rare occasions.

If you became pregnant while taking the pill or while wearing a contraceptive patch, there's no need to worry. There appears to be no increased risk of problems with the pregnancy or fetus. Just stop taking the pills or remove the patch as soon as you know you're pregnant.

SPERMICIDES

The majority of birth-control-failure pregnancies are from the failure of spermicidal methods, like a diaphragm with spermicide, contraceptive foam, the sponge, or contraceptive film. The failures of these methods result in more babies every year than there are residents of the city of Baltimore. Fortunately, studies have found no link between spermicides and birth defects or pregnancy complications.

IUD (INTRAUTERINE DEVICE)

The IUD is very effective, with an average annual failure rate of less than 1 percent. Still, failures do occur, usually if the IUD has fallen out unnoticed. If you become pregnant with an IUD, call your gynecologist right away, and check to see if you can still feel the IUD string. If you can't find the string, the device has either fallen out or has gotten out of position. Your care provider will probably order an ultrasound to see which is the case. If the IUD is still there, the current recommendation is to remove it because of the increased risk of infection.

Though no one knows for sure, researchers believe that an IUD works by causing a chain reaction of chemical messages that disorient sperm. You're about 5 percent more likely to miscarry if you

become pregnant with an IUD, and pregnancies conceived with an IUD in place also have a greater risk of being an ectopic pregnancy than those conceived without.

SHOTS

Depo-Provera is a contraceptive shot which contains a medication similar to the hormones in birth control pills, but in doses high enough to prevent pregnancy for 3 months.

It's extremely effective: You're as likely to get pregnant in the 3 months after getting a Depo-Provera injection as you would be if you had an operation to be sterilized.

Before you got the shot, your care provider should have tested you for pregnancy or administered the shot during your period, because some studies have shown the drug to be statistically associated with an increase in the incidences of low birth weight, stillbirth, and infant death, particularly in women who become pregnant in the 1 to 2 months after the shot. If this happens to you, discuss the risks with your care provider.

If you've decided to stop taking the shots and want to conceive, many practitioners recommend using a non-hormonal birth control method (such as **condom**s) for at least 6 months before you start trying.

TUBAL STERILIZATION (TUBAL LIGATION)

Hard to believe, but women do sometimes become pregnant

even after their fallopian tubes are "tied," sometimes many years after the operation. Often, these are ectopic pregnancies—meaning that a sperm has somehow managed to cross the divide and fertilize the egg, but the zygote can't descend into the uterus and implant and instead grows in the tube and must be removed.

On the other hand, it's quite possible to get pregnant after you or your partner has had the sterilization operation reversed. How likely and easy it is to get pregnant afterward depends on the type of sterilization procedure. The pregnancy rate after a male vasectomy is reversed can be as high as 90 percent. For reversed female sterilization, the rate can vary between 55 and 85 percent depending on individual circumstances like which sterilization procedure was employed, and how well the reversal operation went. If you do become pregnant after a reversal, however, there's no reason why your pregnancy shouldn't proceed as usual.

Bisphenol A (BPA)

BPA is an industrial chemical that acts like estrogen on the body. It's used to make lightweight plastics and is in a wide variety of products, from water bottles to DVDs, cash register receipts and food-can liners, and even some baby bottles and liners of baby-formula cans.

While BPA has been linked to cancer, obesity, and infertility in lab animals, it's currently controversial just how much BPA exposure is safe for humans. So, bottom line: avoid it whenever possible, without making yourself crazy in the process.

Some tips:
- When possible, opt for fresh food over canned. One study of pregnant women's urine found that women who ate canned vegetables daily had 44 percent higher concentrations of BPA.
- Wash your hands after you handle money and cash register receipts, and if you handle both regularly as part of your job, wear gloves. One study found that 50 percent of cash register receipts and 95 percent of dollar bills are contaminated with BPA (BPA is used in the thermal printing process of receipts, then is transferred to the money it comes into contact with). If you save receipts, keep them in a zippered plastic bag, not in your wallet.
- Buy water bottles, baby bottles, and sippy cups specifically labeled "BPA-free."

Black Cohosh and Blue Cohosh

Black cohosh is an herb with estrogen-like properties and can trigger labor; Pitocin is a synthetic counterpart. Because of these labor-stimulating properties, you should only take it if you are in post-term pregnancy (after 42 weeks) and only under the supervision and advice of an experienced medical professional.

Blue cohosh is another story. In spite of the similar names, the two herbs are not related. Blue cohosh can cause heart and organ failure and should be completely avoided during pregnancy and lactation.

Botox

Botox (onabotulinumtoxinA) is an injected neurotoxin primarily used to paralyze certain facial muscles to give a more youthful appearance. There are no adequate and well-controlled studies to show the effects of onabotulinumtoxinA on human fetuses, so don't get Botox while you're pregnant. But if you had injections before you conceived or knew you were pregnant, though, there's no need to worry.

Breastfeeding During Pregnancy

It's safe to breastfeed while you're pregnant; just be aware of a few things:

- **Breastfeeding burns a lot of calories.** In addition to the extra 100 calories per trimester you should add to your diet, also consume an additional 300 or so to replace the ones you burn breastfeeding.
- **Breastfeeding requires a lot of nutrients, too.** Don't skip your prenatal vitamin, and maintain your calcium intake at at least 1,300 mg per day.
- **Keep up your fluids.** Dehydration can be dangerous during pregnancy, so keep a bottle of water at hand at all times.
- **Nipple stimulation can cause contractions.** If you have a history of preterm labor consider weaning by the third trimester, or sooner if you experience lower back pain or painful or strong contractions.
- **Keep an eye on your baby's weight.** Your body will direct calories and nutrients to the fetus first, your breastmilk second, and your own body last of all. Supplement with formula at the first sign your baby is not gaining according to age guidelines in the chart below, if you find yourself feeling listless and run-down, or if you lose weight or don't gain at least a pound a week after the first trimester.

Baby Weight-Gain Guidelines

AGE	WEIGHT GAIN PER WEEK
0-4 months	5.5-8.5 ounces
4-6 months	3.25-4.5 ounces
6-12 months	2-4 ounces

Caffeine

Caffeine, also known as mateine and guaranine on ingredients labels, is the world's most popular psychoactive drug, and 90 percent of people in North America consume it every day.

Caffeine definitely has been linked to certain pregnancy unpleasantnesses, including:

- Higher rates of urinary tract infections (UTIs).
- Lower absorption of essential minerals, including calcium, iron, and copper.
- *Diuretic* effects (in other words, it makes you pee a lot), which can contribute to dehydration.
- An increase in nausea, heartburn, stomach pains, and diarrhea.
- An increase in sleep difficulties.
- Heart arrhythmias in fetuses who have a caffeine sensitivity.

If you have a UTI, severe nausea, and/or vomiting, or other digestive issues or anemia, it's a good idea to cut the caffeine out totally and as soon as possible. Also note caffeine is an MAOI (monoamine oxidase inhibitor), so you should avoid it completely if you are taking antidepressants or certain other drugs with warnings against possible interactions with MAOIs.

There are conflicting reports on

How Much Caffeine?

Black Tea: 8 ounces, 40-70 mg
Coffee: 6 ounces, 80-130 mg
Coca-Cola: 12 ounces, 34.5 mg
Dark chocolate bar: 1.5 ounce, 25 mg
Diet Coke: 12 ounces, 46.5 mg
Espresso: one 1.5-ounce shot, about 70 mg
Excedrin (headache medicine): 1 tablet, 65 mg
Green Tea: 8 ounces, 25-40 mg
Milk chocolate bar: 1.5 ounce, 12 mg
Pepsi: 12 ounces, 37.5 mg
Red Bull: 8.3 ounces, 80 mg

whether or not caffeine contributes to the risk of first-trimester miscarriage, with one study finding a "small but statistically significant" increased risk of miscarriage with amounts as small as 150 mg per day (the amount in about three 6-ounce cups of coffee), and other studies finding no increased risk. One 2008 study found a doubled risk of miscarriage for women who consumed 200 mg of caffeine or more, yet in the very same year a different study came out showing no correlation between caffeine and miscarriage at all.

In better news, caffeine has not been linked with birth defects, preterm labor, or low birth weight. Trying to break a caffeine addiction can be rough: the body becomes tolerant of caffeine after just a few days, and cutting back or trying to go cold turkey can cause headaches, nausea, irritability, and even depression, because caffeine stimulates the brain's production of seratonin (aka the "happiness hormone"), so stopping abruptly can cause a sharp mood crash. Your best bet is to step back your intake slowly, over the course of a week or so. Every serving mix a little more decaf and/or milk into your morning coffee, and replace soda with seltzer or decaf tea.

Carnival Rides

You go to an amusement park, a water park, or the fair, and on every ride there's that silhouette of a stork with a big red slash through it. What gives?

The worry with rides is that often a ride's restraints, such as a lap bar or over-the-shoulder bar, are positioned right at below-belly-button level, and this can risk dangerous impact on your lower abdomen. If you're still in the first trimester (early enough that no one can tell you're pregnant anyway) you don't need to worry: your baby is well protected by your hips and abdominal muscles and the amniotic sac, and it would take a serious and near-fatal impact to cause fetal harm—much more than what even the most extreme roller coaster or water slide could dish out. But once your uterus starts growing out of the pelvis in the second trimester, your baby loses the extra protection of your hip bones, making it a good idea to avoid anything that potentially risks a direct blow to your abdomen, including any ride with restraints, bouncy houses, fast-moving water slides, high dives, jousting with lances, and/or vigorous wrestling in an inflatable sumo suit.

Castor Oil

A dose of castor oil is sometimes mentioned as a way to stimulate labor in a post-term pregnancy. What it does is cue stomach cramps, which lead to diarrhea and vomiting, which can lead to dehydration and muscle cramps, which may (or may not) trigger labor. So, probably needless to say, it's not a great idea. If you're desperate enough to consider such a drastic measure, at least first try sex (see Week 41), nipple stimulation with a breast pump, or if you've been pregnant for at least 41 weeks or longer, asking your healthcare provider about stripping your membranes and/or medical induction methods.

Cat Litter Boxes

If you have a cat and can't convince anyone else to change the litter box, get your cat a new box, wear gloves when scooping and disposing of litter, and scoop the box daily to avoid risking exposure to the parasite *Toxoplasma gondii*. Cats can pick up the parasite from contact with an infected rodent and shed it in their poop, which can become infectious after a few days. You don't need to worry about exposure if you scoop daily, or if you don't have mice and your cat never goes outside, or from just petting or brushing a cat. The parasite can stay active for as long as a year, though, which is why it's a good idea to gift your cat with a new box when you find out you're pregnant.

About a third of people are immune to infection from previous exposure, and a blood test, which some care providers perform at the first prenatal visit, can determine if you have been exposed and are immune. Exposure to the parasite doesn't usually cause any symptoms or complications in healthy adults, but being exposed for the first time during pregnancy can be dangerous and serious because pregnancy compromises your immune system. Symptoms of toxoplasmosis are similar to flu symptoms—swollen glands, aches and pains, a headache, sore throat or fever—but can go on for a month or more, so if you are not immune to the infection and experience these symptoms and they don't go away in a day or so, let your healthcare provider know. The most common source of exposure to toxoplasmosis during pregnancy is actually not cats or soil, but raw or undercooked meat, so cook meats thoroughly, keep food-prep surfaces clean, and consider wearing disposable gloves while handling raw meats.

Cell Phones

Research seems to suggest that children who were exposed to cell phones during pregnancy are at a greater risk of developing behavioral issues later in life. We know that electromagnetic radiation emitted by a nearby turned-on phone affects the way adult brain cells metabolize glucose, and it stands to reason that fetal brain cells are even more vulnerable, because they divide at a much quicker pace than adult cells, plus fetuses lack a thick skull for protection.

So when it comes to cell phones, play better safe than sorry. Use a headset with a long cord and keep the phone away from your abdomen (and skull). Consider keeping your phone with you for emergencies but turned off (finally, a valid excuse to be unreachable!).

Chorionic Villus Sampling (CVS)

CVS is a diagnostic test that can identify 99 percent of major genetic abnormalities using a sample of specific cells from the placenta (but bear in that they don't routinely test for the hundreds of genetic diseases that they can test for—only the ones you are most at risk for—not the really rare ones). While CVS was once only offered to women who had certain risk factors, the new standard of care is to offer the testing to all women.

The big advantage of CVS testing over amniocentesis is that CVS can be performed much earlier than amnio (11 to 13 weeks as opposed to 15 to 20 weeks). This gives you the option to terminate the pregnancy at a point where abortion is relatively safer and before the pregnancy is apparent.

And while not long ago CVS used to be considered a considerably riskier procedure than amnio, the so-called loss rate has much improved in the past decade to about 1 in 360. (Individual doctors and labs may have lower or higher loss rates.) The loss rate from amnio is estimated at about 1 in 769, which sounds like a big difference, but keep in mind that amnio is performed later when the risk of miscarriage is already statistically much lower, and that 1 in 360 is already less than one-third of a percentage point. If you have a choice, it's best to opt for a lab and doctor that perform the procedure frequently.

There has also concern that CVS testing has been associated with limb defects in babies (as in missing fingers or toes), but this appears to be just for testing done before 10 weeks, and there does not appear to be an increased risk at 11 weeks or later.

One major difference between amnio and CVS, though, is that CVS can't detect neural tube defects such as *spina bifida*, and amnio can. If you opt for CVS testing, you'll be offered the option of a blood test between weeks 15 to 20 to screen for these. CVS testing and amnio also allow prenatal paternity testing to be performed, too, though that's not usually covered by health insurance.

If you do opt for CVS, you will need to make an appointment at a specialized lab. You'll be advised to come with a full bladder, usually with instructions on how much to drink and when.

The CVS test aims to take a sample of the chorionic villi, which are tiny, hair-like projections on the edge of the placenta that contain fetal DNA. There are two ways of obtaining this sample: through the cervix (transcervically) or through your belly (transabdominally). Which one you have will depend on the position and location of the placenta. The loss rate for transcervical and transabdominal sampling appears to be statistically similar.

For either method of obtaining a sample, an abdominal ultrasound will be used to determine the location of the placenta. For the transcervical procedure your vagina and cervix will be cleaned with antiseptic, then a thin plastic tube will be inserted into the cervix to guide the needle that will take the sample. For the transabdominal version, your abdomen will be swabbed with antiseptic, a local anesthetic cream is usually applied to the abdomen, then the needle is guided in. You should be able to watch all of this on ultrasound, which can be reassuring.

If you are Rh-negative, you'll need a shot of Rh immunoglobulin after the procedure, just in case you and your baby's blood are incompatible.

While most labs advise that you can drive yourself home after CVS testing, it might not be a bad idea to have someone else with you at the test for moral support.

You'll be told if you need to limit your activities after CVS testing; most labs advise that you avoid strenuous activity, heavy lifting, air travel, and intercourse for 72 hours after the test.

Some cramping and spotting is normal after the test, but if you experience severe cramping, bleeding that doesn't stop, clear watery discharge, or a fever of 100.4 degrees or above, call your healthcare provider right away.

Test results are usually available about a week later, depending on the lab.

Occasionally a sample won't collect enough cells for testing, in which case you'll have to repeat the test. Also in about 1 to 2 percent of samples there are both normal and abnormal cells, or the results can be inconclusive if maternal cells somehow contaminate the sample.

In the unlikely event that CVS testing triggers a miscarriage, this typically happens within 3 days.

Cocaine

Cocaine has not been associated with birth defects, but it is very dangerous to fetuses, tripling the risk of fetal death. It crosses the placenta in about 5 minutes after exposure and constricts blood vessels, restricting blood flow and oxygen to the fetus. Users have a high risk of **placental abruption** (see the Pregnancy Dictionary at the back of this book). Babies born to habitual users will also experience painful withdrawal after birth.

Cold Medicines

With 9½ months of pregnancy, odds are you'll catch a cold at least once. When it comes to cold-symptom medications, some are considered safe, some are not, and for many there is not much information at all. If you aren't sure if a medicine is safe or not, ask your healthcare provider or a pharmacist.

Considered safe:
• Acetaminophen (Tylenol) has

been used safely by pregnant women for decades now. If you use it, be careful to follow dosing instructions and don't take more than 1,000 mg at one time, or 4,000 mg within 24 hours, to avoid potentially dangerous liver damage.
• Saline nasal sprays, rinses, facial steamers, and room vaporizers are all safe to use, and for nasal congestion may be even more

effective than medication. Warm salt water gargles are also safe and effective for a sore throat; dissolve ¼ teaspoon of salt in warm water, then lean back and gargle a mouthful. Adding a tablespoon of honey can also contribute to the soothing effect.
- Sleeping with your head propped up with pillows can also help congestion.
- Peppermint tea is safe and effective—try warm green tea with mint for extra decongestant effects.
- Sugar- or honey-based lozenges or candies, such as cherry Ludens, can help soothe a cough or scratchy throat.

Not sure:

The following medications are classified as a pregnancy category C, meaning that there is not enough data to determine conclusively if they are safe or not.
- Oxymetazoline hydrochloride (Afrin) nasal spray: Studies have found no effect on fetal growth or pregnancy outcome, but there just has not been enough research to draw a conclusion.
- Pseudoephedrine (Sudafed) narrows blood vessels, which can help ease nasal congestion. Many studies have found no link between pseudoephedrine and birth defects, but some studies found an association between the use of pseudoephedrine in the first trimester and increase in the risk of gastroschisis, an opening in the baby's abdominal wall. Because this birth defect is so rare, though, with only about 2 cases in every 10,000 births, there is not enough evidence to show a clear connection. If you're in your first trimester and can't breathe out of your nose, try some other things first, like a steamy shower, saline nasal spray, or nasal rinse. But if nothing else works and you can't sleep, a dose or two of pseudoephedrine is unlikely to cause harm. Ask your healthcare provider and do not use it if you have high blood pressure.
- Guaifenesin (Mucinex, Robotussin): Guaifenesin thins mucus and lubricates the respiratory tract. Some studies have suggested a possible link between guaifenesin exposure and the incidence of inguinal *hernia*s and neural tube defects, but the number of babies affected was too small for the results to be conclusive. Because of these concerns, though, some care providers recommend avoiding guaifenesin during the first trimester. A safe—and possibly more effective—alternative is warm lemonade or hot caffeine-free tea with lemon juice. Grape juice and limeade and other citrus juices are also effective at cutting phlegm, and drinking lots of fluids of any kind will help thin mucus and make coughs more productive.

Not safe:
- Aspirin: Not recommended because of its blood-thinning qualities.
- Ibuprofen: Ibuprofen or other nonsteroidal anti-inflammatory medications like naproxen should be avoided, especially in the third trimester, because they have been associated with low amniotic fluid levels, delayed labor, and a specific heart defect. Ibuprofen should also be avoided while breastfeeding.

Cystic Fibrosis Screening

Cystic fibrosis is a genetic disorder caused by an abnormal recessive gene, which means both parents must carry a copy of the abnormal gene for it to be passed on to the child. If both parents are carriers, each of their children has a 25 percent chance of having the disorder. You can be screened for the CF gene at any point, and if tests determine that you are a carrier then your partner should be tested also.

More than 10 million Americans are carriers of one *mutation* of the CF gene, including one in twenty-nine people of Caucasian descent. In other races or ethnicities, one in forty-six people of Hispanic descent, one in sixty-five people of African descent, and one in ninety people of Asian descent carry a mutation of the CF gene.

CVS can sample fetal genes and diagnose CF with a 99 percent degree of accuracy.

Deli Meats

Pregnant women are advised to avoid prepackaged cold cuts because of the small but serious risk of contamination with listeria bacteria. Deli meats (and raw hot dogs) are suspect because of the possibility of contamination after cooking and before packaging. While listeria infection is very rare, with only about 2,500 cases a year in the U.S., the infection can be serious for pregnant women and cause fetal death. Also frightening is that food contaminated with listeria won't smell or look spoiled,

and symptoms can be mild. You can greatly reduce or eliminate your risk by heating your deli meats to steaming hot (160°F), making your own cold cuts at home, or, if you must eat at a deli, substituting a sandwich not made with lunchmeat, like meatball or steak subs or tuna salad. The CDC also recommends avoiding soft cheeses like brie, camembert, and queso fresco. But processed cheese spreads like cream cheese, cheese balls, and cottage cheese are all safe.

Depression and Antidepressants

It was once believed that pregnancy made women immune to depression, but research has found the opposite to be true: hormonal changes and the stress of pregnancy seem to actually increase the risk. Depression appears to be a combination of

genetics and situation, and your risk is higher if your mom, dad, or siblings have struggled with it, and also if there are other stressful situations in your life, such as if you're having problems with the baby's father and/or your pregnancy was unplanned, you're having financial problems, or you have a history of pregnancy loss. Making matters worse, when you're depressed you're not up to taking care of yourself, which makes it hard to ask for help or believe that anything actually will help.

So how can you tell depression from plain-old sadness or pregnancy hormones? The symptoms:

- You dislike yourself and feel hopeless, like life isn't worth living, or you imagine killing yourself. If you experience these feelings, let your healthcare provider know right away, even if you have no other symptoms.
- You feel irritable and short-tempered most of the time and/or have constant negative, guilty, or anxious thoughts.
- Things that you used to like don't make you happy any more.
- You can't sleep or you sleep too much, or you can't eat or eat too much. These symptoms can also be due to other causes, though: hormonal effects can make you lose appetite or feel ravenous, baby kicks and discomfort can disturb your sleep, and anemia can make you listless and tired.

If you are depressed, you face the decision of how to treat it. Your health plan or finances may or may not make talk therapy an option, or you may be offered the choice to take antidepressant medication or to try to manage your symptoms without it.

Starting, stopping, or changing antidepressant medications during pregnancy means that you and your healthcare provider will need to weigh the risks of depression,

such as self-destructive behavior, possibly not being able to take care of yourself, and/or self-medicating and the risk of suicide, versus any potential harm of medication.

Some antidepressant medications are riskier than others: the ACOG has specifically stated that pregnant women should avoid paroxetine (Paxil), which has been linked with heart defects when taken in the first trimester. If you are taking paroxetine, you will need to work with your prescribing doctor to step down your dose gradually to avoid withdrawal symptoms. Fluoxetine (Prozac, Sarafem), Citalopram (Celexa), Phenelzine (Nardil), Sertraline (Zoloft), and Tranylcypromine (Parnate) have all been associated with an increase in rare but serious septal heart defects. Of those drugs, about 2 percent of babies were born with the heart defect, versus about 1 percent of babies who were not exposed to antidepressants. Bupropion (Wellbutrin) has not been associated with birth defects as of now, but may not work for everyone's depressive symptoms.

Any risk of side effects needs to also be balanced against the very real risks of depression. Stopping SSRIs is linked to a 70 percent risk of the recurrence of depression and can cause other symptoms, such as nausea, irritability, anxiety, and insomnia, and untreated depression is associated with an estimated 5 percent risk of suicide.

If you decide to continue treatment with antidepressants, also note that your dosage should be re-evaluated as your pregnancy progresses, because your metabolism goes up, especially in the second half of pregnancy. Let your healthcare provider know right away if you suspect that your symptoms are coming back.

For the most up-to-date and detailed information on the safety of specific antidepressants, talk to your healthcare provider or call the Infant Risk Center at Texas Tech University Health Sciences Center, which publishes the manuals on the safety of medications during pregnancy and breastfeeding used by healthcare providers.

> **TIP**
>
> The Infant Risk Center takes calls from the public Monday to Friday, 8 a.m. to 5 p.m. Central time, at (806) 352-2519.

Diarrhea

When you're pregnant, your body is more reactive to toxins in foods, in the form of bacteria or chemical additives. At the slightest suggestion, your body will probably expel food as quickly as possible to keep out harmful foodstuffs. Your bowels may naturally loosen as labor nears, in response to hormonal surges.

Mild diarrhea is nothing to worry about, but if you're having severe abdominal cramps, feel light-headed and/or have a temperature, call your healthcare provider. Also call if your diarrhea doesn't go away in 24 hours.

Discharge

It's normal to have increased vaginal discharge during pregnancy; only worry if you experience itching, an unpleasant odor, bleeding, a gush of fluid, or discharge any color but white. (For more on symptoms and treatment of vaginitis and yeast infections, see those entries in this chapter.)

Dogs

While cat poop can carry toxoplasmosis, there are no such concerns with dog waste. Dog poop can carry bacteria and parasites, though, so you don't want to be handling it with your bare hands. But there's no danger in picking up after your dog using a bag to cover your hands, or with a scooper. (If you do come into accidental contact with dog poop, just wash your hands thoroughly with warm water and soap.) There's also no danger in petting a dog or letting your dog lick your face or, later, the baby's high chair tray.

Dogs can pose a threat of injury to babies and toddlers, though.

While most dogs instinctively respect the offspring of the alpha female of their pack, any dog will nip if it feels threatened. And you can't tell which dogs will be dangerously aggressive by breed or size—babies have been killed by golden retrievers, cocker spaniels, and in one instance a 4-pound Pomeranian.

Before your baby is born, you'll need to make sure your dog has some basic training to not to jump up on people, to follow basic commands like "sit," and to walk at heel (a very important skill if you plan to walk the dog and push a stroller at the same time). It can also be helpful to train your dog not to share the stairs with you, but to stay at the top or bottom until you're up or down so he won't bowl you over when you have the baby in your arms. If you're going to train your dog or introduce new rules, e.g., no dogs on the couch, it's a good idea to do this training before the baby comes home, so the dog won't associate banishment with the baby.

While you're pregnant it can also help to expose your dog to babies and young children, while keeping him leashed and under control. Praise him and offer a treat if he stays calm and friendly and lets himself be petted, so he'll associate babies and kids with positive rewards.

Get your dog used to what the routine will be after baby: if your partner is going to take over walking the dog, get the dog used to that while you're pregnant. Also get your dog used to being fed regular meals, rather than having his food left out all day, because

when your baby gets to the "chew on everything" phase, it will help keep your child out of the dog dish if you store the food off of the floor and feed the dog his meals during naps and after bed.

Also accustom him to being in a crate sometimes, like when you're not at home or are cleaning house.

After baby is born, some trainers suggest having your partner or a friend bring a blanket and a dirty diaper with baby's scents home from the hospital (transport them in a plastic bag), and introducing your dog to the baby's smell so the arrival of the actual baby won't be so shocking.

When baby does come home, first go in, greet your dog warmly, then leash him. When baby is walked in, stay calm and keep the leash slack, and if your dog remains calm and respectful, let your dog sniff the baby, and reward him with a treat if he's good. It's normal for your dog to be inquisitive and want to sniff the baby, but don't let your dog paw, jump up on or lick the baby. If your dog is hyper, jumps up, or barks, don't shout or strike him, just put him directly in his crate and try again later.

No matter how sweet your dog, never leave your baby and dog together out of arm's reach. Don't let your dog chew baby toys (and don't let your baby chew dog toys), and keep your baby away from the dog's feeding area. Once your baby gets mobile, make sure your dog always has somewhere to escape to when he's had enough baby time, like to his crate with a dog bed in it.

If you find you just can't train your dog, for instance, he doesn't respect your leadership or nips at you or others, keep him confined and ask your vet for advice. If your dog is out of control after a decent effort, don't risk bringing your baby home to a dangerous dog; instead find your dog another home.

Dreams

As the third trimester progresses, your sleep becomes lighter, and your dreams may seem more intense or weird. More often than not, a pregnant woman's dreams are more vivid, more emotional, and more memorable than ordinary dreams. During your pregnancy, odds are you'll probably have at least one or two dreams that you remember for a long time, because they were so strange, scary, marvelous, or symbolic. Why?

One reason dreams are so memorable is that in late pregnancy, baby kicks, bathroom trips, and pregnancy discomforts can wake you up while you're dreaming, so you're better able to remember the dreams you have. Why the dreams themselves are so weird is more of a mystery.

There are countless theories about the causes and meanings of dreams. One of the more plausible theories about dreaming is that it helps your subconscious mind sort the information it received during the day, kind of like a secretary filing a pile of the boss's random message slips. Information from the recent past is being added in with older memories, and the mingling of the old and new information creates a strange story, a sort of mental Mad Lib. Add to this mix all of the extra hormonal messages and physical changes your body and brain are going through, and the result can be some deeply strange images.

The strange dreams of pregnancy may also serve as a way for your mind to rehearse for future events. It's critical to your baby's survival that your subconscious mind, the part that has you swerve before your car hits a tree, is ready to react to new potential threats and surprises. Perhaps this is why pregnant women often report having dreams about things like giving birth to a litter of kittens, or dreams where their babies are demonic. It doesn't mean that your baby will actually have a tail, but it could be that your brain is rehearsing so that if your baby is born, and he doesn't look like you expected, or there are surprises while you're giving birth, you'll be able to react appropriately to keep you and your baby safe.

Echinacea

Studies have found no link between echinacea and birth defects or pregnancy complications. Unfortunately, studies have also found echinacea no more effective for treating a cold than a placebo.

Ecstasy Pills

Ecstasy, also known as MDMA or methylenedioxymethamphetamine, has not been tested in pregnant women, but it has been shown to cause lasting damage in the areas of rats' brains that control planning, impulse control, and attention span. Rats exposed to ecstasy in utero appear to show evidence of lasting learning and behavioral problems. If you've taken ecstasy during your pregnancy, inform your care provider.

Electric and Magnetic Fields (EMF)

Power lines and every kind of electronic device produces an electric and magnetic field of what's called non-ionizing electromagnetic radiation. The kind that comes out of household appliances is known as ELF, or extremely low-frequency radiation. The kind that comes out of cell phones and makes food cook in a microwave is radiofrequency and microwave radiation (RF/MW radiation). There have been about 25,000 scholarly articles published about the potential effects of non-ionizing radiation from power lines, electric blankets, home appliances, and so forth, and while there's evidence that high doses of it isn't good and does have biological effects—heating up tissues, disturbing nerve responses, and raising blood pressure—not much clear evidence has emerged on how much exposure is harmful.

One 2002 study may be worth paying attention to, though. The study equipped 1,063 pregnant women with magnetic-field measuring monitors on their bellies for 24 hours, and went on to find a two- to six fold increase in risk of early miscarriage for those who had an average continual dose of 16mG of electromagnetic radiation a day (a level that 75 percent of the women in the study were exposed to).

Magnetic fields are measured in milliGauss, or mG. A modern cell phone emits about 2 mG as you use it, an electric blanket emits about 4.5 mG, and a hair dryer emits about 500mG. But the amount of radiation goes way down with distance from a source. For instance, your average computer monitor will emit about 8 mG at a distance of 1 inch, but less than 1 mG at 8 inches away. Simply putting your cell phone in your purse instead of your pants pocket, putting your laptop on a desk instead of in your literal lap, or holding your hair dryer at arm's length can reduce exposure considerably.

Or, if you're really worried about EMFs, you can buy a handheld home sensor (called an EMF meter) for about $20 and walk through your house, Ghostbuster-style, to detect them.

Electric Blankets

There are two things that are potential causes for concern when it comes to electric blankets: the potential of the blanket to raise your body temperature and the electromagnetic field (EMF) created by the blankets. The good news is that studies so far have found that there's no reason to be concerned with either. As long as you keep the temperature set to low enough that it doesn't make you sweat or burn your skin, there's no risk of the blanket raising your internal body temperature. Electromagnetic fields are still a relatively new area of study, but research so far has found no connection between electric-blanket use and preterm or low-birthweight babies, childhood cancers, or neural tube defects. Blankets made after 1992 also have much weaker electromagnetic fields than earlier models. If you're still worried, though, an easy way to eliminate any potential risk is to turn on the blanket to let it heat up your bed, then turn it off when you get in.

Femur Length

Ultrasound technicians sometimes measure the length of the fetal femur (upper leg bone) between weeks 14 and 20, and sometimes the humerus (upper arm bone) as well; a shorter-than-average arm or leg bone is a considered a potential indication of Down syndrome. But if your doctor or a technician says that your baby has a relatively short femur or humerus, do not panic. By itself, with no other indicators, this is nothing to worry about. Genetics, fetal age, and simply the angle of the ultrasound picture can all make a bone appear abnormally short when everything is fine.

Fibroids

Uterine *fibroids* are growths in the muscle of the uterus, and they are really common—most women will have at least one in their lifetimes, and most will experience no complications or other problems with their pregnancies. About one-fifth of women with fibroids will experience issues, though: if you have a lot of fibroids it can become more difficult to become pregnant, and once you are pregnant the extra estrogen of pregnancy can cause the fibroids to grow larger. A large fibroid in the uterus can obstruct labor or force the baby into an unusual position, and/or cause excess bleeding after birth. If you have fibroids your healthcare provider will keep tabs on their growth and position during your pregnancy. Fibroids can't be treated or removed during pregnancy, but may be removed afterward.

Fish

Fish is packed with nutrients that build the fetal brain and body, is high in protein and vitamin D, and is full of healthy fats. Research has found that moms who eat 12 ounces or more of fish have higher verbal IQs, better motor coordination, and better social skills later in life.

But, as you've probably heard, many species of fish come with the risk of contamination from mercury and other pollutants, like PCBs, petrochemicals, and pesticides. These pollutants can do all sorts of terrible things to a developing fetus, like increasing the risk of birth defects, impaired cognitive development, and certain cancers. Further muddying the waters, genetic testing has found that fish is often mislabeled: consumers think they're buying one species may actually be buying another. One FDA study found that 37 percent of seafood they tested was mislabeled, so it's possible that when you think you're eating trout, it's tilefish. The FDA also does not routinely test domestically caught fish for mercury or other pollutants.

What can you do?

• Skip the fish and take purified fish-oil supplements or cod-liver oil. While you don't get protein this way, you do get the omega-3s and usually some vitamin D as well. The downside: some supplements can cause unsavory "fish burps."

• Avoid the big fish. The higher up in the food chain a fish is, the more likely it is to be contaminated. Shark, pike, albacore and yellowfin tuna, tilefish, marlin, king mackerel, swordfish, and halibut are all very likely to be contaminated with mercury. Mercury levels in salmon can vary a lot, with FDA salmon samples finding some with very low levels and other samples with dangerously high levels.

The Web site www.gotmercury.org features a calculator that uses your body weight and how much of what species of fish you plan to eat to determine safe mercury levels.

• Avoid farmed salmon. Farm-raised salmon have been found to have high levels of PCBs and dioxins.

• Avoid rockfish. Also known as black bass or striped bass, there have been numerous reports of rockfish with high levels of contaminants.

• Be wary of catfish and tilapia. While American farmed catfish and tilapia are safe, any catfish over 2 pounds and wild-caught or Asian farmed tilapia and catfish have a high risk of being contaminated with pollutants. If you're not sure where your catfish or tilapia is from, avoid it.

• Small fish and shellfish generally contain very low levels of mercury: anchovies, herring, sardines, shrimp, clams, oysters, and crabs. Avoid raw oysters or clams due to the risk of food poisoning.

Flu Shots

Flu shots, which are manufactured with killed virus, are totally safe during pregnancy and recommended: not only can they prevent you from getting the flu, but it will also protect your baby from the flu for 6 months or so after birth. You should not take the seasonal-flu nasal-spray *vaccine* if you're pregnant, though, because the spray is made with live virus. You should also get vaccinated against the H1N1 flu virus, because the H1N1 flu, while very rare, can be fatally serious for pregnant women and their babies. As with the seasonal flu vaccine, you should not take the H1N1 flu mist if you're pregnant.

Gardening

There's no harm in gardening, as long as you wear gloves to avoid possible contact with parasites in the soil (and bend at the knees to avoid back strain).

Gas and Bloating

Your digestive tract has slowed down to allow your body to get maximum nutrition from your food and bacteria, and enzymes in your stomach now have more time to process whatever you eat. A side effect of this change is burping, a bloated feeling, and passing more gas than you usually would.

Keeping a food journal can come in handy. If you find yourself unusually gassy, you can look back and see what you ate a few hours ago. You may discover that certain vegetables cause more gas than others.

If milk products are causing your problem, you may suffer from *lactose intolerance* (which means you're allergic to some of the sugars in cow's milk).

In later pregnancy, your growing uterus will crowd your abdominal cavity and put pressure on your stomach, which can further slow digestion, making you feel even more bloated after eating, and more gassy.

Over-the-counter products containing simethicone, such as Gas-X, Phazyme, Mylanta Gas Relief, and Maalox Anti-Gas, are considered safe to take during pregnancy, but activated charcoal tablets are not.

Ask your practitioner for advice, and call right away if your gas discomfort ever feels more like abdominal pain or cramping or is accompanied by blood in your stool, severe diarrhea or constipation, or more vomiting than usual.

Gingko Biloba

Supplements containing gingko biloba should be avoided during pregnancy, because there is evidence that, like aspirin, gingko has blood-thinning qualities.

Glycolic Acid

Glycolic acid is a common ingredient in women's skin care products. It's safe to use skin care products containing glycolic acid as directed while you're pregnant and breastfeeding.

Group B Strep

GBS is a fairly common bacterium, found in about 25 percent of all moms. It usually doesn't cause symptoms in a mother, but can potentially cause a serious infection in the newborn—today, untreated Group B step infection is a leading cause of infant death in the United States. Most pregnant women are screened with a urine test at the first prenatal visit, and if that test is negative, again between weeks 35 and 37. If you're found to have GBS at the first or second screening, or if you have not been screened, you'll need IV of antibiotics during labor, which will prevent infection in the baby.

Hair Products

It's considered safe to dye, perm, or relax your hair during pregnancy. Very few of the chemicals in hair dye are absorbed through the scalp. If you dye your own hair, though, be sure to keep the room well-ventilated to avoid inhaling the chemicals, and don't leave the dye on any longer than necessary, to minimize exposure. Do note that the hormonal changes of pregnancy may cause hair dye to take unevenly or cause unusual color results, and changes in the protein bonds in hair can mean that perms won't work or will work unevenly.

If you work as a hairstylist, take precautions: make sure your work area is well ventilated and always wear gloves.

Hairs, Strange and More

Thanks to your pregnancy hormones, you'll have more hair from head to toe, and your hair will have a different texture. You may notice that your hair is different as soon as you find out you're pregnant, or changes may take a few weeks. Some women have such extreme changes that their curly hair straightens, or their straight hair gets waves!

Normally, the hair on your head grows for about 7 years, stays on the scalp for about 6 months, and then falls out. But during pregnancy, this growth pattern is interrupted, and the old hair isn't shed as easily. Your hair will feel thicker and stronger and may be easier to style. For most women, the second trimester begins the best hair days of their lives, when the "no-shed" effect becomes noticeable.

Your body hair undergoes the same change of cycle. Even leg and toe hair will appear to grow longer and more quickly. In the months after birth as your hormone levels return to normal, you'll lose the extra hair, though, thankfully, not all at once.

Your scalp condition may also change while you're pregnant. Depending on your genetic makeup, your oil-producing glands may either speed up or slow down production in response to hormonal changes, so your hair may be drier or oilier than normal.

Change your shampoos and conditioners for the next 9 months to suit your new hair texture. If your hair is dry, shampoo once only every few days. Use deep-conditioning packs or hot oil treatments once a week. If it's oily, wash once per day, applying conditioner only when needed to detangle.

With oily or dry hair, get a trim every 6 to 8 weeks to get rid of split ends or breakage, and brush your hair gently and only when necessary. For body hair, shave, or trim with scissors. Waxing or depilatory creams may irritate your skin and follicles.

Headaches

Pregnancy headaches are common, and dehydration, low blood pressure, and/or sinus congestion are usually to blame. Some women also have their first migraine headaches, or worse migraine headaches, possibly because of hormonal shifts. Fatigue and/or nausea can also make headaches worse.

If you get a headache, first try drinking a large glass of water and lying down. If that doesn't help,

acetaminophen (Tylenol) is the *analgesic* of choice for pregnancy. If taking a dose of acetaminophen doesn't help and you have a sharp headache behind your eyes, ask your healthcare provider to recommend an over-the-counter sinus medication.

If you get migraines, note that not all medications are safe to take during pregnancy, so work with your healthcare provider to develop a safe treatment plan.

Heart Rate

Conventional wisdom once held that when you're pregnant you should keep your heart rate below 140 BPM. While you're pregnant you don't want to work out to the point of dehydration, muscle pulls, or light-headedness, but there's no evidence that you need to keep your heart rate below a certain specific level.

Heated Car Seats

Because heated car seats, a common feature in newer vehicles, only warm your back and backside and don't raise your internal body temperature, they're safe to use while you're pregnant.

Heating Pads

Excess heat in the first trimester has been linked to neural tube defects, so you don't want to put a heating pad directly on your stomach. But it is fine to use a heating pad anywhere else.

Heavy Lifting

The concern with heavy lifting is that your muscles and connective tissues are softer during pregnancy, which makes muscle pulls more dangerous. Pregnancy also changes your center of gravity, making you more prone to falls. So it's okay to lift anything that you were able to lift before pregnancy, just take care to stabilize yourself first and not strain or extend beyond your usual range of motion.

Hemorrhoids

Hemorrhoids are swollen veins around the anus that can cause itching or pain. Sometimes they may even bleed a little. They can look like a bump or a small cluster of grapes. Sometimes they protrude after a hard bowel movement. They often appear when a woman becomes constipated because of the slowing down of her digestive system.

Treating constipation can help, and so can gentle witch hazel compresses or wipes, pain killing ointments, rinsing off your bottom with warm water after each bowel movement, and sitting in a warm bath.

Hemorrhoids are made worse by the pressure of birth, but they usually shrink or even mostly disappear as you recover postpartum.

Herbal Tea

Most herb teas are safe to drink during pregnancy, but do avoid teas that contain yerba mate, which contains high levels of caffeine. Some extractions of yerba mate also contain high levels of carcinogenic polycyclic aromatic hydrocarbons (PAH). High amounts of yerba mate have also been linked to liver disease.

High Altitudes

If you live in a high-altitude town, your body is already used to functioning with less oxygen. If you don't, then it makes sense to avoid traveling anywhere with an altitude of higher than 7,000 feet—the Swiss Alps or Aspen, for example—or flying in an unpressurized cabin above this level. The decreased oxygen will put a strain on your system and may even cause altitude sickness: nausea, headaches, and vomiting.

High Heels

The risk of high heels in pregnancy has to do with balance: pregnancy changes your center of gravity, making you more likely to lose your balance even in flat shoes. Pregnancy also increases the amount of weight and pressure your feet are subjected to. Wearing heels, especially in the second half of pregnancy, can cause even more pressure on the balls, arches, and joints of your feet, and can cause lower back pain. Lots of women go up a half a shoe size (or more) after pregnancy anyway, and the added pressure of wearing heels can increase this effect because of the extra pressure on the foot joints between your arch and toes. So while you're pregnant flats are a better bet.

Horseback Riding

Like water slides and amusement park rides, horseback riding is safe in the first trimester, because your fetus is surrounded by not just the amniotic sac but three layers of uterine muscle, your abs, and also the bones of your pelvis. After the first trimester, though, your uterus grows up past your pelvic girdle and the fetus loses that extra protection, making horseback riding no longer safe because of the danger of being kicked by, or falling off of, the horse.

Hot Tubs

There a couple of good reasons to avoid hot tubs while you're pregnant. One is that heat exposure in the first trimester has been linked to an increase in the risk of birth defects, with one study finding that women who soaked in hot tubs in the first trimester had double the rate of neural tube defects than women who didn't. This doesn't mean you have to take tepid baths throughout your pregnancy, but it's a good idea to avoid soaking in any bathwater that's hot enough to raise your body temperature, particularly during that very delicate 8- to 12-week developmental period.

Another good reason to avoid hot tubs, especially public ones, is bacteria that can grow in them that can cause or encourage yeast infections or vaginitis, even if the tub is cleaned regularly. If you have a hot tub at home and want to use it, set the temperature to 102°F or less, don't soak for more than 15 minutes at a time, and make sure the tub gets cleaned at least once a week with the filter changed at least once a month.

Insect Bites

Pregnancy makes you more appealing to mosquitoes and other biting insects, because your blood vessels are more dilated, and you're giving off more body heat and carbon dioxide. Mosquitoes also are attracted to carbon dioxide, and pregnant women take larger and more frequent breaths. Use insect repellants that are labeled as being okay for children, and avoid products containing DEET—they've been associated with neurological and dermal reactions in humans. Also avoid natural repellants that contain oil of pennyroyal—though you probably won't absorb enough through the skin to make a difference, pennyroyal is known to induce abortion.

If you're unlucky enough to get an ant, roach, termite, or flea infestation while you're pregnant, investigate what measures you can take to avoid bombing the house. No one knows whether the bug sprays used by exterminators are safe for pregnant women or not, but the lists of warnings are certainly scary and extensive. If you must bomb, we suggest staying somewhere else for a week, and letting someone else go in and air out the house and wipe down the surfaces before you move back in.

If your neighborhood is being sprayed, stay inside with your windows closed. Again, no one knows whether the sprays are safe for pregnant women or not, but if they can kill all those bugs, it makes sense to avoid them.

Itching

Feeling itchy? There are at least seven different skin afflictions specific to pregnancy, including in early pregnancy, pregnancy-aggravated eczema, pruritic folliculitis of pregnancy, and prurigo gestationis. Or, if you're in later pregnancy, your itching may be from PUPPP (pruritic urticarial papules and plaques of pregnancy), impetigo, gestational pemphigoid, or intrahepatic cholestasis of pregnancy. It all sounds very complicated, but bottom line, about half of women experience itchy, rashy areas and/or zit-like bumps and/or discolorations somewhere (usually on the belly, arms or legs) to some degree at least once during pregnancy.

Let your healthcare provider know about any rashes you experience (he or she will likely recommend a mild steroid cream) and do your best to not scratch or pick. If the area is intensely itchy it can help to apply an ice pack, and many women report success with oatmeal, applied in a cream or as a paste made with colloidal oatmeal bath and water.

Do note that being infected with chicken pox for the first time during pregnancy is potentially serious, though. If you've never had chicken pox and get a fever and an itchy rash at the same time, call your healthcare provider right away or go to a clinic so you can start treatment with oral antiviral drugs as soon as possible.

Manicures and Pedicures

There is evidence that some chemicals in some brands of nail polish, dibutyl phthalate, toluene, and formaldehyde, can cause fetal harm at high levels of exposure, but there's no evidence that painting your fingernails or toenails is unsafe. Many brands have now eliminated these chemicals, and even if your polish contains them they won't be absorbed into your body so long as you don't bite your painted nails. To play it safe, use polish that claims to be free of these chemicals and only get your nails done in a well-ventilated room. The same goes for acrylic nail chemicals, nail polish remover, and acrylic-fingernail remover: you certainly don't want to ingest it or

breathe it in in a small, enclosed space, but brief exposure in a well-ventilated salon is nothing to worry about.

When it comes to pedicures there are a couple of additional concerns: the leg massage and the cleanliness of the foot bath. If you're in advanced pregnancy, decline the calf massage that can come with some pedicures, because an aggressive leg rub can aggravate varicose veins. And pregnant or not, it's important to pick a place that always disinfects its whirlpool foot spas with bleach between every customer and keeps spa drains very clean. Don't be afraid to bring your own instruments or to ask to see the disinfectant used to clean the foot bath. Believe it or not, people have contracted fatal staph infections (and plenty of other less serious fungal rashes and skin infections) from foot-spa bacteria. Never get a pedicure if you have any broken skin, even if it's just a little scrape, hangnail, or insect bite. If you develop any bumps, boils, or fever in the days or weeks following a pedicure, let your healthcare provider know right away.

Marijuana

Marijuana is the fourth most-used recreational drug in America (after caffeine, *nicotine*, and alcohol) and has been studied fairly extensively. A link has not been found between moderate use (as in a few times a month) and pregnancy complications. Smoking anything deprives the fetus of oxygen, though, and daily smoking of has been linked to premature labor and low-birthweight babies.

The drug does pass through the placenta to the baby, and babies exposed to marijuana during pregnancy will test positive for the drug in their urine for 2 to 3 weeks after their mother's use. Some hospitals do drug-screen newborns (without the knowledge or consent of the mother) and will notify child protective services of a positive drug test.

Massage

Massage during pregnancy is a great thing, especially in the final weeks when pregnancy starts to strain your neck, back, and leg muscles. Studies have found that regular massage during pregnancy reduces stress and is associated with a lower rate of labor and delivery complications.

If you opt for a pregnancy massage, it's important for your comfort and safety to pick a therapist who is certified and has experience specifically with prenatal massage (if you're tempted to get a massage during a cruise or a foreign vacation, note that other countries may have different, or nonexistent, certification procedures for massage therapists).

Positioning during a massage is important—after about 20 weeks of pregnancy you should be on your side or in a semi-reclining position, not flat on your back. While a table with a hole for your belly is cute, it may cause lower back strain if you're in advanced pregnancy. Your therapist should also avoid massaging directly on your spine or on any area with varicose veins or a rash. You should never experience pain during massage—let the therapist know right away if anything hurts.

Microwaves

You may have heard some people express concern about microwave ovens leaking radiation that could harm a growing baby. Fortunately, this is just an urban legend—there's no evidence of any danger. Microwaves don't generate enough radiation for there to be a risk of exposure.

Mold

There are no human studies available that examine mold exposure during pregnancy, but if you find mold in your house you should have it removed, or remove it yourself from hard surfaces by scrubbing with a solution of ½ cup of bleach to a gallon of water.

Muscle Spasms

Pregnant women are prone to muscle spasms in their calves and feet at night. No one knows the exact cause, but some evidence points to a calcium and/or magnesium deficiency. Make sure to drink at least 2 pints of milk per day or some equivalent, such as calcium-enriched orange juice, almond milk, or soy milk, and check that your prenatal vitamin has at least 350 mg of magnesium. It may help prevent leg cramps to wear socks to bed at night to keep your feet and legs warm.

Nitrous Oxide

You might be surprised to know that nitrous oxide (aka "laughing gas") is commonly used for labor-pain relief by many women in other countries, including 48 percent of women in Finland and half of women in the UK in the past decade.[2] It's only available in a handful of hospitals in the United States, though, because it's thought to not be strong enough to wipe out labor pain the way an epidural does. It can cause numbness, visual impairment, and clumsiness, and over-sedation can lead to oxygen deprivation and nausea.

On the plus side, though, the effects of nitrous oxide wear off quickly—you could try it for 5 minutes, decide you don't like it or it doesn't work, then try another approach to pain relief, in contrast to an epidural, which calls for a total commitment.

Nitrous oxide is potentially a good alternative for women who can't or don't want to have an epidural, or just need something to take the edge off of a long labor, and it's too bad it is not at least an option for women here. Hopefully, as more women request it, it will become more widely available. **Note:** You shouldn't have nitrous oxide during the first trimesters of pregnancy. Continual use can lead to fetal death, birth defects, anemia and B12 deficiency.

Nosebleeds

A lot of pregnant women get nosebleeds, because pregnancy increases blood flow and thins your *mucous membranes*. Dry, hot air can also cause bleeding, so consider using a humidifier to moisten air in your office or bedroom, or moistening a dry, itchy nose with a saline nasal spray.

If you get a nosebleed, sit up straight and lean forward to lower blood pressure in your nose and keep you from swallowing blood. Gently pinch your nostrils shut for at least a full 5 minutes. If that doesn't stop the bleeding, gently pinch again for 10 more minutes. If you still can't stop the bleeding, contact your healthcare provider; you may have a broken blood vessel and need to have your nose packed with a spongy material to compress the vessels, or in an extreme case, have the vein cauterized. After you get the bleeding to stop, be careful to not blow your nose vigorously, and if you have to sneeze, open your mouth so the sneeze isn't forced through your nose.

Opiates

Maternal use of opiates like hydrocodone, morphine, oxycodone, methadone, and heroin has been associated with more than double the risk of delivering infants with conoventricular septal defects, atrioventricular septal defects, hypoplastic left heart syndrome, spina bifida, or gastroschisis. Opiates can also suppress appetite, which can lead to nutritional issues.

If you're taking opiate prescription pain relief (like codeine or hydrocodone), talk to your healthcare provider about switching to a non-opiate medication for pain relief.

If you are addicted to heroin or taking more opiate painkillers than prescribed you should not attempt detoxification without medical supervision; stopping abruptly can be dangerous or even fatal to the fetus. Studies have found that buprenorphine is a safer alternative than methadone, but if buprenorphine isn't available, note that methadone detoxification is still safer than continuing to use opiates or stopping opiate use abruptly.

Overweight or Obese

If you're overweight you're not alone: as of 2011, about 65 percent of American adult women were overweight with a *body mass index* (BMI) of 25 to 30, and about 36 percent were obese, with a BMI of more than 30. (Note that online BMI calculators can be inaccurate, though, especially if you have a lot of muscle mass—having one of those skin-caliper tests where your healthcare provider "pinches an inch" and measures it is a more accurate assessment of BMI.)

Being overweight does increase the risk of certain complications, such as gestational diabetes, pregnancy-induced high blood pressure, and certain birth defects. The weight of extra fat compresses blood vessels and restricts circulation, which makes it more difficult to get pregnant and harder for nutrients and oxygen to reach the baby. Fat cells also cause inflammation, which increases this effect. Being overweight can also make it more difficult for Doppler devices and *fetal monitor*s to detect fetal heartbeat and for ultrasound to get accurate images of the fetus, which can make it more difficult to diagnose health issues.

There is also evidence that conditions in the womb will affect a child for life, and babies born to overweight mothers are more likely to have higher levels of appetite-stimulating hormones and to become overweight themselves.

Ideally the best thing to do is get your BMI down to below 25 before you become pregnant. If that's not possible, the next-best thing is keep a close eye on your diet and increase your activity. You don't want to cut calories below about 2,200, but you do want to make extra-sure that every calorie is a nutritious one, and watch your carbohydrates closely, just as someone with gestational diabetes would. Physical activity is also really important for helping improve circulation, burning excess calories, and keeping your blood sugar in check.

It's also important to find a healthcare provider who understands the issues and is helpful, not judgmental. And if you are obese (as opposed to just a little overweight) you will need to deliver at a hospital that is properly equipped to handle your delivery.

Oysters

Because of the high risk of food poisoning, it's a good idea to avoid eating raw oysters while you're pregnant. (Note that if you're craving oysters, that may be a sign of a mineral deficiency. Make sure you're getting enough calcium, iron and zinc in your diet.) Cooked oysters, as in fried or in a stew, are relatively safe, though avoid eating any fresh oysters between June and October due to the rare but serious risk of marine toxins that can't be killed by cooking.

Pains, Shooting

Sharp or twinge-y pains in the joints of your hips, around your backbone, and in your shoulders, arms, and/or neck are to be expected, as your lower-belly weight puts strain on your connective tissues. Striving for good alignment can go far: Stand with your tailbone tucked under your pelvis and the weight of your hips stacked directly on top of your feet. If you work at a desk, try to work standing up barefoot or in flat shoes, or alternate between standing and sitting. Hip stretches, pelvic tilts on hands and knees, and very gentle seated twists can help work out kinks. If you drive a lot, consider using a lumbar roll cushion or a rolled-up towel on your lower back to support your hips.

Painting

There simply aren't any studies that document the effects of painting a room or a picture with oil paints or enamels during pregnancy. It's difficult to measure exposure, but household painting typically involves very low levels of harmful emissions. Intense inhalation of paint (as in, say, recreationally, or working in the paint department of an auto-body shop) is dangerous, though. Miscarriages, low birth weight, birth defects, developmental disabilities, and higher risk of cancer for children later in life have all been linked to high levels of exposure to solvents over long periods of time.

If you do paint at home, keep the space well ventilated with open windows and fans. Don't use paint manufactured before 1990, as it may contain dangerous levels of mercury. Don't try to renovate a house with pre-1978 paint in it; instead hire a lead-safe-certified firm, because the lead-laden dust and paint chips can be hazardous to you and your baby. If your house was built before 1978, also call your local health department or water supplier to ask to have your water tested for lead.

PCB

PCB, or polychlorinated biphenyl, is a chemical compound used in electronic manufacturing and hydraulics. In humans, exposure can cause hormonal changes and various cancers. Since 1973 it's been banned in the United States in paints, adhesives, and waterproofing materials, but there have still been several environmental contamination "events" in the United States, usually the result of electric or chemical companies illegally dumping in public waterways. Because of widespread contamination, while you're pregnant it's a good idea to avoid eating fish caught in local ponds or lakes, or wild waterfowl that may have been eating contaminated fish.

Peanuts

Avoiding peanuts (or wheat, milk, eggs, or shellfish) during pregnancy has not been found to help prevent food allergies in your future baby. It also doesn't help to prevent a child's allergies by purposefully eating potentially allergenic foods while you're pregnant. If food allergies run in your family, there is evidence that you may be able to help to prevent or delay the onset of allergies by breastfeeding exclusively for 4 to 6 months, and continuing to breastfeed as you introduce potentially allergenic foods. If you can't breastfeed and allergies run in your family, opt for hydrolyzed formula. Whether your child is consuming breastmilk, solids, or both, call your doctor or pediatrician if you or your baby experiences allergy symptoms, such as hives, itchy eyes or mouth, vomiting, pale skin, fainting, difficulty breathing, or swelling of the eyes, tongue or lips.

Phthalates

Phthalates are a group of chemicals added to plastics to make them more flexible and harder to break. They're also found in personal-care products like moisturizers, soap, and shampoo. Phthalates are known to change hormone levels and affect human and animal metabolic and reproductive systems. Some studies have suggested links between fetal exposure to phthalates and shorter pregnancy duration, and conditions including childhood asthma, insulin resistance, ADHD, and genital changes in boys. Perhaps most vexingly, we don't know what levels of phthalates are safe for humans, and it can be difficult to impossible to know what products contain them, since manufacturers are not legally required to list them on ingredient labels. (More than 10,000 ingredients are allowed for use in personal-care products, and we have toxicity data on only 7 percent of them.)

Here are some suggestions for limiting your exposure:
- Opt for soaps, shampoos, and body washes labeled as "phthalate-free" and don't contain "fragrance" as an ingredient if you can find them. If not, go for unscented products with fewer chemical ingredients on the label.
- Opt for a reusable metal water bottle over plastic disposable.
- Store and reheat leftovers in glass containers instead of plastic.

Piercings

Getting pierced (or tattooed, or doing anything that adds extra stress and pain to your life) while pregnant is probably not such a good idea. You'll bleed more and may be more prone to infection. If you're already pierced and any of your piercings hurt, swell, or smell bad, remove them immediately and call your doctor.

The major body changes of pregnancy can cause issues with your piercings, especially those in places that are tender and may stretch, such as your navel or nipples. Our advice is to remove any neck-down piercings to reduce the risk of infection and pain, especially if the site isn't completely healed yet.

Remember to wash your hands with a liquid antibacterial soap before removing the jewelry or touching the piercing, and be sure to keep your jewelry on a clean surface.

You almost certainly want to take out a navel piercing toward the end of your pregnancy or whenever it begins to annoy you. Your expanding stomach will make the hole stretch, which won't look so great.

Other piercings:

• Nipples. Nipple piercing does not prevent lactation, and having a piercing should not interfere with breastfeeding, provided you remove your jewelry first. Besides getting in your baby's way and increasing your discomfort, rings and beads can pose a choking hazard to infants if the jewelry comes loose with the motion of feeding. If you're pregnant, trying to conceive, or nursing and are interested in getting a nipple piercing, our suggestion is to wait until you are finished breastfeeding.

• Genital. Your care provider will most likely instruct you to remove any genital piercings because of the risk of tearing or stretching.

Raw Eggs

The USDA advises that pregnant women should not eat raw eggs due to the risk of salmonella contamination, and that all eggs should be cooked for at least 6 minutes to kill any bacteria, which means no real Caesar salad dressing, hollandaise sauce, or dipping your sukiyaki. But perhaps these warnings are overly cautious—scientists estimate that on average about 1 of every 20,000 eggs in the U.S. contain the bacteria. So, the likelihood that an egg might contain salmonella is extremely small—0.005 percent (five one-thousandths of 1 percent)—about the same odds as getting struck by lightning before you turn 35.

Reptiles

The majority of snakes, turtles, and lizards carry salmonella bacteria on their skin, but for you to become infected, you'd have to touch the reptile and then ingest the bacteria somehow. If you have reptiles as pets, always wash your hands thoroughly after handling them or cleaning out their tank and, probably needless to say, don't let them wander freely in your house or play on surfaces where you prepare food.

Rh Screening

Rh testing is usually performed as part of a first-trimester blood screening. If you're one of about 15 percent of moms who are Rh-negative, meaning you have a specific protein on the surface of your blood cells, you'll be given an intramuscular injection of RhoGAM at around 28 weeks of pregnancy and then again within 72 hours of delivery. This is because if an Rh-negative mom is carrying an Rh-positive baby, a mom's blood cells may attack the baby's if blood cells mingle during birth, causing anemia, *jaundice*, and/or enlarged abdominal organs in the baby. RhoGAM is a brand name of a solution of antibodies mixed with your own blood to prevent the **red blood cells** from attacking the baby's. If you're Rh-negative and experience spotting, miscarriage, or abortion, you'll be given a RhoGAM injection afterward.

Saunas

It's a good idea to avoid anything that could potentially raise your body temperature, especially during the first trimester. If you must sauna after that, stay hydrated, don't stay in for more than 5 minutes, and get out if you start to feel flushed or uncomfortable.

Screening Tests

A screening test is any kind of test that you take with no symptoms of a problem. A screening test doesn't diagnose an issue, but provides evidence that you might be at an increased risk. First-trimester blood and ultrasound tests and mammograms are all examples of screening tests.

A diagnostic test is one that can identify for certain if an abnormality is present; examples of diagnostic tests include CVS testing, amniocentesis, or blood count to detect anemia.

Self-Tanning Sprays

There's no research on the safety of long-term use of self-tanning sprays, but because they're basically dyes that stay on the surface of your skin, there's no reason to believe that they could hurt your baby. Because of hormonal changes, though, you may get an uneven result.

Sex

Sex is safe during pregnancy, unless your water has broken or your healthcare provider tells you to avoid it out of concern that it might trigger premature labor. If you clinician does tell you to abstain from sex, be sure to ask specifically what activities are off-limits.

Under normal circumstances, sexual activity won't harm the baby or induce miscarriage—in fact, there's evidence orgasms may be healthy for the baby, giving her a squeeze just like Braxton-Hicks contractions might. Don't worry that orgasmic contractions are premature labor: an orgasm always brings on minor contractions of the uterus, but now that your uterus is larger, you can feel them more. Only suspect that it might be labor if the contractions continue for more than an hour. Many positions may become impractical and uncomfortable in late pregnancy. Consider any position that keeps you off your back and is comfortable.

By the way, the famous Masters and Johnson study, which surveyed 101 women, reported that most women's interest in sex decreased or stayed the same during the first trimester. It was a different story by the second trimester though. Eighty-two of the women reported that their sex drives were in high gear, and the sex was the best of their lives. By the third trimester, however, interest had decreased again. For men, however, desire may slow over the course of your pregnancy. Men who live with pregnant partners produce less testosterone and more of other hormones such as *cortisol* and prolactin. While these hormonal changes make a man more relaxed and nurturing, they can also inhibit his sex drive.

Single Motherhood

If you're pregnant and not married, you're not alone. As of 2009, about 40 percent of births in the U.S. were to unmarried moms.

The good news for single moms-to-be is that studies have shown that marital status is not by itself an indicator of a child's well-being. Parental attention, access to social support, education, and financial resources are much more important to a child's mental and emotional health than a ring on your finger. Kids from amicably divorced couples do better than kids from high-conflict married couples, and financially stable, well-educated single moms have healthier children overall than impoverished married couples. In less-good news, being single can make it harder to become financially stable if you weren't already. You can't be two places at once, so you will need to find practical help—financial help, childcare, emotional support—to get through. Consider what options you have that can give you and your baby maximum stability: perhaps moving in with relatives or moving a relative or good friend in to your home to help. Take advantage of any social programs, scholarships, or food programs that you can.

The legal issues for single moms can also be stressful.

WHAT ABOUT CUSTODY?

If you are not married and the baby's father comes to the hospital with you, at some point you'll both be offered a form to sign that acknowledges his paternity (usually called an affidavit or acknowledgement of paternity, or AOP). (This form can't be signed while you are pregnant; you will need to wait until after the baby is born.) After both of you have signed, you will both have equal rights to the child, meaning that either of you can take the child anywhere as long as you don't deny the other parent access, until either of you files papers with the local family court and legally establish a specific custody and a visitation schedule.

Even if you don't have an official court-ordered visitation schedule, you are still required to allow the father to have "reasonable access" to the child. That doesn't mean you have to let the father and his new girlfriend drive off with your newborn for an unlimited amount of time, but at minimum you should agree on a few hours a week when he can come to your house and see the baby (for young babies, short and frequent visits are best). When the father comes to visit, make it easy and pleasant for him, because interfering with his access or making visits difficult may hurt your case if you have a custody dispute later. Also keep records of visits: dates, times, and anything notable that happened, such as if he was scheduled to show up for a visit but didn't.

If you don't put the father's name on the birth certificate or anywhere else, he will need to go to court to establish his paternity before he has any specific rights to visit the child or obligation to support him. If you know who your baby's father is but he won't sign a form acknowledging his paternity, you will need to contact a lawyer or your local family court to find out what steps you need to take in your state to establish paternity.

If you and your baby's father have a reasonably civil relationship but aren't living together, consider a session with a mediator (usually a family-law attorney) who can help you come to an agreement about custody, visitation, and support, which a judge can make official by signing. If you can't agree, or if your ex already has a lawyer, then it's important to contact a family lawyer or legal aid in your area to establish custody, a visitation schedule, and child support.

If you are married to someone other than the baby's biological father, or you have not been divorced for more than 300 days, your husband will be legally presumed to be the father of the baby. The biological father can only become a legal father if he fills out an AOP and your current or former husband also signs a denial of paternity. If the husband won't sign a denial of paternity, then either you or the biological father will have to take legal action to establish paternity.

WHAT ABOUT THE LAST NAME?

Think long and hard about giving your child his dad's last name if you aren't married to him. As far as the law is concerned, giving your child his dad's last name doesn't establish paternity or an obligation for child support, and having a different last name from your child can create all kinds of inconveniences, from confused receptionists at the doctor's office to suspicious ticket agents at the airport. Later in life, your child may be asked questions about his last name from people he doesn't want to share personal information with. And if your baby's father doesn't stay involved, the last name may serve as a constant reminder to your child and a point of resentment to you. It is not always simple to change the baby's name once it is put on the birth certificate; you will usually need permission from the child's father and a court order to change it. Alternatives are to hyphenate your and the father's last names, to make the father's last name the baby's first or middle name, or to wait to change your child's last name when and if you get married to the father.

Sit-ups

Avoid sit-ups and abdominal exercises after the first trimester, because the bump in your belly can train your abdominal muscles to go down and out instead of up and in, and increase the separation between your two vertical abdominal muscles.

Skiing

Skiing is fine exercise, but there are a few issues with skiing while pregnant: hormones soften your muscles and ligaments, making you more prone to pulls and sprains, and after the first trimester, the uterus loses the protection of your pelvic bones, so the baby could potentially also be injured if you suffer a serious fall. And pregnancy also throws off your balance, making falls and injuries more likely. So while slow cross-country skiing is safe if you're careful not to overstrain, downhill skiing and water skiing should be avoided.

Sleep Positioning and Problems

In the first half of pregnancy any position you can get into will be fine for you and the baby. But once you get to about 20 weeks, when the baby weighs a few pounds and the uterus and supporting structures weigh a few pounds more, sleeping on your stomach will start to feel like trying to sleep on a softball (then a football, then a basketball). Laying on your back will make the weight of your uterus compress your digestive system and major veins, and if you lie on your right side then the weight will squish your liver, though you won't be able to feel it. Healthcare providers have long recommended left-side sleeping in late pregnancy, and this recommendation was justified when a 2011 study found that women who slept on their back or right side had nearly double risk a late-term stillbirth than left-side sleepers.[3]

(Interestingly, the study also found that there was no connection between stillbirth and snoring, or stillbirth and the amount of daytime fatigue moms reported, and also that women who got up to use the bathroom more than once at night had a lower risk of stillbirth than women who didn't.)

Don't panic, though, if you wake up and find yourself on your back or the right side: the odds of stillbirth for wrong-side sleepers is still very low (a rate of 3.9 versus 1.9 of 1,000 pregnant women). Nevertheless, it makes sense to try to get into the habit of left-side sleeping as soon as your bump starts to pop.

And even with perfect positioning, most moms-to-be will find they have sleep problems in the last weeks of pregnancy. If it isn't baby kicks keeping you up, it might be muscle cramps, trips to the bathroom, Braxton-Hicks contractions, or even your own snoring or drooling. There's also evidence that hormonal shifts cause a mother's and baby's sleep cycles to synchronize in the last weeks of pregnancy, making a mom's sleep cycles shorter and deeper in the early part of the night and lighter in the early hours of the morning. You might find yourself getting in the habit of sleeping multiple places at night, like the first part of the night in bed, then a stint on the couch, sitting up in a chair, or even on the floor. (Whatever works, long as it's not flat on your back or your right side). It can also help to rest your right knee and elbow on a body pillow or a couple of regular pillows, with your left arm behind you.

Smoking

It's no secret that smoking during pregnancy is very dangerous, potentially causing miscarriage, stillbirth, placental abruption, childhood cancers, and lifelong learning and behavioral problems, among other issues. Smoking while pregnant is associated with a 60 percent higher rate of birth defects and a 200 percent increase in the risk of SIDS. There is no safe amount or safe kind of cigarette you can smoke—risk goes up the more you smoke, but even one or two cigarettes a day can cause harm. Quitting isn't easy, but it's a picnic in the park compared to having a baby that is stillborn or raising a child who is psychologically disturbed or has cancer, while always having to wonder if it was your fault.

When it comes to quitting, research shows that the safest, most effective method is old-fashioned cold turkey. Nicotine-replacement medications, switching to "light" cigarettes with lower levels of nicotine, or trying to gradually cut down all endanger the baby while making the process longer and more difficult.

If you're depressed or have a history of depression, talk to your healthcare provider about the potential benefits of taking antidepressant medication while you quit. Studies have found depression makes it more difficult to stop, because nicotine interferes with brain chemistry, essentially replacing your brain's own happy chemicals with itself. Quitting can also trigger depression, particularly in people who have been depressed in the past. Even people with no history of depression may be irritable and anxious in the first week, though it will get better every day as your brain adjusts.

Cravings actually pass quickly, but can make it seem like time has slowed down. If you have the urge to smoke, drink a glass of water to dilute those craving-causing chemicals and find a way to distract yourself (brush your teeth, take a shower, walk the dog, eat a carrot, do the dishes). If you can't think of anything to do, watch a clock, and you will find that within 3-5 minutes the craving will be gone.

St. John's Wort

St. John's Wort is an herb with active ingredients that some studies have found are as effective antidepressants for mild and moderate depression as Prozac. But the safety of St. John's Wort during pregnancy hasn't been studied, and there is some evidence that it may cause contractions or even induce spontaneous abortion in high doses. There's also the possibility that even if St. John's Wort helped ease your depression pre-pregnancy, it may not keep working while you're pregnant because of changes to your body chemistry and metabolism. If you are experiencing symptoms of depression it is safer and more effective to seek treatment from your healthcare provider or a psychiatrist.

Stillbirth

Stillbirth is the death of a fetus older than 20 weeks. Most pregnant women worry at least once (if not more often) about the horrifying reality that stillbirth does and can happen.

First know that stillbirth is rare: the odds are estimated at 4.9 in 1,000 pregnancies for Caucasian, Native American, Hispanic, and Asian women, and 11.5 per 1,000 pregnancies for black women.[4]

Unsettlingly, for most stillbirths a cause is never known, even after evaluation. Women who are pregnant for the first time after the age of 35 do seem to be at a higher risk, so if you're in this category it is a good idea to do daily kick counts. Some healthcare providers recommend monitoring how often your baby kicks for 30 to 60 minutes to get an idea of what a typical pattern is for your baby. An alternative method is to time once or twice a day how long it takes the baby to move ten times.

Fetal growth retardation is also a risk factor. If monthly uterine measurements are shorter than average you should have an ultrasound to monitor placental function and determine if the baby needs to be delivered early. Women who have had preterm stillbirths are also at risk for recurrence.

Cord accidents are often blamed for stillbirths in medical records, but it is difficult to know when or if the cord is to blame, as about 1 in 3 live babies are delivered with a cord around the neck, and it usually doesn't cause a problem.

While you may not be able to prevent stillbirth, avoid known risks like alcohol and cigarettes, wash your hands often, and employ safety precautions to prevent foodbourne infection.

Also be alert to warning signs: let your healthcare provider know immediately if the baby doesn't move 10 times over 2 hours or you experience unusual pain, bleeding, or discharge. Your clinician should make sure you are thoroughly evaluated with a non-stress test that checks placental and cord function (see page 97), a blood pressure check, and an ultrasound to measure the baby's growth. If you experience a notable decrease in baby movement, trust your instincts and insist on these tests, even if your doctor or midwife seeks to reassure you.

Sometimes, though, in spite of everyone's best efforts, babies simply die. A hundred years ago, and still today in some parts of the world, a mother might give birth to 5 or 12 children and expect to experience the loss of one or many through miscarriage, crib death, or accidents.

Today, most of us don't live under conditions where we reasonably expect fetal death; we usually have the fortune of seeing our fetus's heart light up on ultrasound and the luxury of very high odds of bringing a living baby home. A fetal death comes like a bolt out of the blue, and you cannot prepare for it.

Should the unthinkable happen, you can only trust that you have the strength inside of yourself to push through the worst. After the baby's born, it's important to see him and take all the time you need to let the whole family see, touch and hold him if they want to. The baby will still be yours and still beautiful.

Thanks to increasing awareness, hospital staffs are becoming most sensitive to the importance of letting parents express grief and create memories and providing support for patients' emotional pain. Baby loss is quite simply the most traumatic experience anyone could go through. It's not something one gets over, but a deep emotional and spiritual pain that will stay with you, just as your love for your baby does. While isolating in grief is normal, it's also crucial to reach out for support and understanding, available through groups of parents who have also experienced loss. For help locating these groups, see Resources on page 338.

Stress

Information about the effects of stress in pregnancy can be a little confusing. A little bit of stress is apparently good: one study found that women who reported moderate levels of anxiety and stress between weeks 24 and 32 of pregnancy had children who were somewhat more advanced in their mental and *motor development* at age 2.

But constant high levels of stress and anxiety may be harmful to your pregnancy. Stress hormones do cross the placenta, and in rare and extreme conditions can cause premature labor and, later, children who overreact to stressful situations. Interestingly, male and female fetuses respond to stress differently: boys by growing more; girls by growing less.

If you feel like you're under constant stress, first try to reduce or eliminate the stresses in your life: find a new job or work fewer hours, end high-conflict relationships, or treat your stress with moderate exercise. But, unfortunately, the kind of stress that's most harmful also comes with the kind of crisis situation that you can't foresee or avoid: war, natural disasters, the death or serious illness of someone close to you. If you're in an unavoidable high-stress situation you can only do your best to take care of yourself and seek and accept as much help and support as you can find.

Sushi

Conventional wisdom has it that sushi during pregnancy is a big no, due to the risks of food poisoning and mercury and other contaminants in fish. But sushi made fresh at a hygienic and sparkling-clean sushi bar is much less likely to be contaminated with bacteria than, say, cold cuts or salad at your local deli, and the servings of fish are so small that you're unlikely to exceed the recommended upper limits of mercury consumption, even if you have a few pieces of tuna. But if the element of risk bothers you, go for a roll that's cooked or vegetarian.

Swelling

In pregnancy, the changing levels of hormones affect the rate at which fluid enters and leaves the tissues, just like a massive case of PMS-related bloating. *Edema* is a fluid imbalance in your body, which can cause mild to severe swelling in one or more body parts.

Sometimes excessive swelling toward the end of pregnancy can be a sign of oncoming preeclampsia, sometimes called toxemia. The symptoms are sudden weight gain (more than 2 pounds per week), a swollen face and hands, a rise in blood pressure, and protein in your urine. Serious symptoms may also include severe headache, blurred vision, or severe abdominal pain. If you experience any of these symptoms contact your healthcare provider immediately.

Your circulatory system transports fluid within the body via its network of blood vessels. Your *lymphatic system* also absorbs and transports this fluid. The fluid carries oxygen and nutrients needed by the cells into the body's tissues. After the tissues use the nutrients, fluid moves back into your blood vessels.

Normally, your body maintains a balance of fluid, but with edema, either too much fluid moves from the blood vessels into the tissues, or not enough fluid moves from the tissues back into the blood vessels.

Edema is extremely common in the later months of pregnancy.

You may find that swelling is worse in the late afternoon and evening. The retained fluid could be nature's way of making sure a mother is protected if there's nothing to eat or drink during labor. Since some labors can last for many hours, or even more than a day, the reserved body fluid can serve to help keep you hydrated. You may find that the excess fluid collects in your fingers so you can't get your rings off, or in your ankles. The edema usually decreases overnight because elevating your legs helps the fluid get back into your circulation. Your healthcare practitioner will constantly monitor the level of your swelling by pressing into a bony area (usually your leg or the bony part of your ankle) to see what kind of indentation the pressure leaves. If the indentation stays for a few seconds, then you probably have edema.

WAYS TO REDUCE SWELLING

• **Eat more protein.** Increase the protein in your diet by including four servings of lean protein and four servings of soy milk or dairy products per day. The increase in protein will increase the protein pressure (osmotic pressure) of your blood and draw the fluid from your tissue back into your bloodstream.

- **Magnesium.** Sometimes fast-absorbing capsules of magnesium taken with meals can help to reduce edema. Ask your healthcare provider.
- **Natural fluid reducers.** Natural diuretics that help the body to excrete excess fluid include watermelon, cabbage, parsley, cilantro, dill, and cucumbers.
- **Feet relaxers.** Try to avoid standing for long periods of time. Keep your feet elevated at work so the pressure is taken off the back of your legs.

- **Lying down.** Lying on your side can help your body reabsorb extra fluid by taking pressure off your main veins.
- **Warm bath.** Taking a bath in warm water can help to compress your tissues and reduce swelling.
- **Swimming.** This is a great way for pregnant women to get exercise, and the pressure from the water helps squeeze the extra fluid back into your circulatory system.
- **Loose clothing.** Avoid tight-fitting clothes and shoes.

Tanning

Unless the tanning bed raises your body temperature, it's unlikely to pose any potential harm to the baby. But tanning (in a bed or in the sun) can be especially damaging to your skin during pregnancy and make you more prone to stretch marks, freckles, and other discolorations.

Ultrasound

Ultrasound uses inaudible sound waves to create video images of your baby's anatomy.

A sonogram is a freeze-frame of an image produced by ultrasound. Most ultrasound machines render sonograms with baby's bones as white and tissues as gray. Newer machines capable of real-time volume rendering (4-D machines) can produce images in a variety of tints.

Most women have at least one ultrasound in pregnancy, and it's becoming increasingly common for healthcare providers to advise two: a nuchal translucency screen at week 11 followed by a more detailed anatomy scan at weeks 18 to 20.

You also might have an ultrasound in early pregnancy if are not sure when the first day of your last period was, or you experience pain or bleeding.

In late pregnancy, ultrasound may be used to check amniotic fluid levels, the baby's position, and the condition and location of the placenta.

ARE ULTRASOUNDS SAFE?

The U.S. Food and Drug Administration says this: "Ultrasonic fetal scanning, from a medical standpoint, generally is considered safe if properly used when information is needed about a pregnancy. Still, ultrasound is a form of energy, and even at low levels, laboratory studies have shown it can produce physical effects in tissue, such as jarring vibrations and a rise in temperature.

"Although there is no evidence that these physical effects can harm a fetus, the fact that these effects exist means that prenatal ultrasounds can't be considered completely innocuous."

So while ultrasound is a valuable diagnostic tool, the U.S. Food and Drug Administration advises against the "over the counter" use of ultrasounds, like keepsake videos.

Vaginal Birth After a Cesarean (VBAC)

"Once a cesarean, always a cesarean" was the motto of many hospitals for many years. In 2009 a survey found that about half of hospitals would not allow vaginal births after a cesarean or didn't have doctors on staff that would perform them. But in 2010 the ACOG revised their guidelines to state that "*trial of labor* after previous cesarean delivery is safe and appropriate for most women with previous cesarean delivery, including some women with 2 previous cesarean deliveries."

A VBAC is not advised, though, if your baby is estimated to be larger than normal, if your baby isn't positioned head downward, or if there are inadequate facilities at your hospital for performing an emergency c-section should you need one. You and your healthcare provider will need to carefully review your medical records to study what caused your prior c-section. If it was the result of having a breech baby, having your placenta misplaced or coming loose (abruption), your baby having a cord accident, or because a previous baby went into fetal distress, you still have a 74 to 94 percent chance of a successful vaginal delivery. Your chances of successful vaginal delivery are lowered to between 35 and 77 percent if you had *cephalopelvic disproportion (CPD)*—a mismatch in size between your pelvis and your baby—or if you had an induction that failed.

Because of the small but real increased chance of rupture if you attempt a VBAC, you'll have to be more closely monitored during labor. Induction is not recommended, and you should not attempt to have your baby at home or in a birth center unless a blood supply has been set aside for you and there is a nearby hospital that has been notified in advance that can offer immediate help.

But as scary as that may sound, statistically a VBAC is safer for you than a repeat c-section, reducing your risk of infection and other complications related to a c-section. It's important that you have a healthcare provider who supports VBACs and will discuss the potential risks and

benefits with you and who attends deliveries at a hospital that is also supportive.

Vaginal Changes

Extra blood flow to your vagina and pigmentation may give it a

swollen, darker appearance. This is totally normal.

Varicose Veins and Spider Veins

Varicose veins appear as a swollen, purple, knotted network just under your skin. Usually they appear on your calves or thighs.

Varicose veins seem to be genetic, so if your parents or grandparents have them, there's a good chance you will too. *Spider veins* are small, dilated blood vessels that usually disappear after delivery. Most of the time neither are anything to worry about, but they may rupture if they're injured, so be kind to them and definitely don't try to massage them away. Let your healthcare provider know if the veins bleed or feel warm, sore, or tender; if your skin changes color; or if a rash develops nearby.

During late pregnancy some women develop varicose veins near the *vulva* or vagina. The major reason is that the body retains a lot of weight and fluid during pregnancy, and the baby weight compresses some parts of the pelvis, enlarging the veins. These usually go away after pregnancy.

Help for varicose veins:

• If you have leg veins, keep off your feet. Avoid standing for long periods of time, and sit with your feet elevated as often as possible. Keep your office chair in its lowest position, and use a footstool to take pressure off the back of your legs. If you have vaginal veins do the opposite: avoid sitting.

• Uncross your legs. Avoid sitting with your legs crossed. It only increases pressure on your veins.

• Exercise and stretch. Gentle stretching of your body can help blood to return to your heart so it doesn't pool in veins.

• Wear support hose. If the swollen veins are in your legs, you may want to try maternity support hose. Put them on in the morning before you get out of bed, while your legs are less swollen, to help to keep your veins from popping out.

• Avoid massage. Don't massage your veins or legs, which will push more blood into them and make them worse.

Vibrators

It's okay to use vibrators or sex toys during pregnancy—just keep them clean, use as directed, and never, ever insert anything in your vagina that's been used for anal penetration, because *E. coli* bacteria can cause severe urinary tract infections. There's no need to deprive yourself of orgasms, though; they keep your uterus and PC muscle toned and give the baby a happy hormonal rush (though of course the baby hasn't a clue what the source is).

Weight Training

Weight training can help you build muscle and stamina, and both will come in handy in late pregnancy and after, when you'll need to pick up your baby hundreds of times per day and lug strollers, diaper bags, and car seats. If you lift weights, here are some things to be mindful of:
• Lift with your spine in a neutral position—avoid arching, flattening, or twisting. The further along you are, the tougher this will get.
• When it comes to weight training, pregnant or not, form is everything. It is far better to lift lighter weights in perfect form than lift heavier weights and be out of alignment. Stay in control of the weights and don't use momentum.
• Take care not to cause joint injury; don't lock your elbows or knees while lifting, and don't stretch beyond your natural range of motion.
• Consider a session with a certified trainer who has experience with pregnant clients. The right trainer can help you adjust your form and alignment and devise a safe routine that will build core strength.
  Particularly good for pregnancy:
• Front, back, and side flies (raises and lowers) with free weights or resistance bands. Sitting on a yoga block or exercise ball can help you keep your spine neutral.
• Lunges and heel rises, with or without free weights.

X-rays and Radiation

The electromagnetic radiation of X-rays can cause gene mutations, so you want to avoid any unnecessary X-rays if you can help it, including dental X-rays.

X-ray radiation is measured (among other ways) in units of millirem (mREM), and 50 millirems per month is considered safe for a fetus. The average dental X-ray is about 1 mREM and a chest X-ray is about 8 mREM. Air travel also exposes you to cosmic radiation from subatomic particles in outer space: a cross-country flight exposes you to about 0.2 mREM an hour, and the full-body scans at the airport expose you to about 0.005 mREM. Tobacco is also irradiated, and each cigarette exposes a smoker to between 0.5 and 3 mREM, yet another reason to avoid smoke.

Yeast Infections, Vaginitis, and UTIs

YEAST INFECTIONS

The chances of your getting a vaginal yeast infection during pregnancy are high, due to hormonal changes that can affect the balance of bacteria. Fortunately, yeast infections are not associated with any kind of pregnancy complications or birth defects.

It's normal to have increased vaginal discharge during pregnancy. But if your discharge becomes thick, white, and creamy, and/or resembles cottage cheese, or you feel intense itchiness and irritation in your vaginal area, you may have a yeast infection. If you do get a yeast infection or experience any kind of vaginal itching or burning, or experience unusual discharge or painful urination, tell your care provider right away, and don't try to self-diagnose or medicate. Sometimes what seems like a yeast infection is actually vaginitis, and infections can sometimes progress into urinary tract infections, which can only be treated with prescription antibiotics.

While over-the-counter remedies such as Gyne-Lotrimin, Mycelex G, Femstat, and Monistat are generally thought to be safe in the last two trimesters of pregnancy, manufacturers recommend that they not be used during the first trimester.

In the first trimester, most healthcare providers opt for the antifungal antibiotics Nystatin and Mycostatin, which are not always as effective as the over-the-counter remedies. In any case, don't medicate yourself without first talking with your clinician.

To prevent yeast infections, eat plenty of probiotic foods such as yogurt made from live lactobacillus cultures. This good bacteria promotes a healthy vaginal (and intestinal) environment.

Wear loose, breathable cotton and synthetic fabrics. Steer clear of foods loaded with sugars, which encourage bacterial growth, and avoid long, hot baths, which create the perfect environment for the yeast to flourish. Try showers instead.

VAGINITIS

Vaginitis is the term for any infection that causes unusual discharge or redness, soreness, or itching around the vagina. While most vaginal infections are yeast infections, they can also have a number of other causes, including a streptococcal infection (see "Group B Strep," page 127) or a reaction to a product such as a soap or bubble bath. So if you have itching or unusual discharge, see your care provider, rather than trying to treat the problem yourself with an over-the-counter remedy.

Bacterial vaginosis is an infection caused by an overgrowth of bad bacteria in the vagina. If the infection isn't treated, you may develop an itchy discharge that can have a fishy smell. Because many women experience no symptoms, during your first pregnancy visit most care providers will use a cotton swab to take a sample of your discharge and check the sample to make sure that your vaginal bacterial balance is healthy.

URINARY TRACT INFECTIONS (UTIs)

Your urinary tract runs from your urethra to your bladder and then up to your kidney. Urinary tract infections (UTIs) are caused by bacteria that get caught in your urinary system and multiply. Some women appear to be more vulnerable to infection than others.

Pregnant women are at a higher risk for UTIs due to the softening of the urethra as a result of hormonal changes. When UTIs do occur, they tend to be more serious, possibly due to a variety of changes in the urinary tract. UTIs in pregnancy are more likely to develop into kidney infections, and kidney infections can increase your risk of preterm delivery. If you've had more than one UTI in the past, you're much more likely to get one in the future. The classic symptom

of a urinary tract infection is feeling like your bladder's constantly full, yet you're unable to pass much fluid when you get to the bathroom. Unfortunately, this is also a classic pregnancy symptom.

You may also have pain; a burning sensation when you urinate; bloody, cloudy, or foul-smelling urine; lower back or abdominal pain; or a low fever. Not everyone with a UTI has symptoms, however, which is why your care provider will periodically check your urine for signs of bacteria. It's important to treat UTIs right away because minor infections can lead to major kidney infections, which are painful and require hospitalization.

Ways to help prevent UTIs:

• Wipe from front to back to keep bacteria out of your urethral area.

• Wear cotton underwear. This will help absorb vaginal secretions.

• Avoid thong underwear—the thong part can create abrasions where bacteria can breed and helps bacteria migrate to the urethra.

• Avoid irritating products. Steer away from perfumed toilet paper, bubble bath, perfumed soaps, douches, or feminine hygiene deodorants.

• Urinate frequently. Don't hold it—go when you get the urge and as soon as possible after intercourse to rinse out your urinary opening.

• Nix caffeine. Caffeine is an irritant to the urinary tract.

Yoga

Yoga is a great way to lower your stress level during pregnancy and practice body and breathing awareness. Yoga classes specifically for pregnancy are a good find, but if you can't find one, take precautions:

- Let your instructor know you're pregnant, so he or she can help you modify poses, if necessary.
- In the second half of pregnancy, avoid any poses that have you lying flat on your back, or poses that strain or compress your abdominal muscles (such as deep twists, backbends, or upward bow).
- For balance poses, stand close to the wall or a chair in case you need to stabilize.
- Stretch only to the point of mild tension and avoid any poses that stretch your muscles beyond your usual range of motion. Pregnancy hormones soften your ligaments, making you more prone to injury.
- Avoid Bikram (also known as hot yoga), where the room is heated to 103°F or above. (See yoga poses on page 56.)

3

Managing Your Nutrition

Vitamins and Minerals 101

Every culture has its own ideas and superstitions about pregnancy nutrition. In West Africa, women are instructed to eat specially prepared types of clay. In traditional Chinese medicine, each month of pregnancy has specific dietary recommendations, like the fourth month for rice and fish broth and the sixth for the meat of muscular fowl and fierce beasts.

In America, we tend to assign magical properties to prenatal vitamins, believing that they can compensate for a diet of processed food. Not so. Your body absorbs nutrients from foods more efficiently than from pills, and also needs macronutrients (like protein, fiber, and carbohydrates) and lesser-known nutrients rarely found in vitamin supplements to maintain your health and pass on to the baby.

So no matter how perfect your vitamin-pill regimen, a **balanced diet** of whole grains, vegetables, quality fats, and protein is still essential. If your prenatal vitamin is making you nauseated to the point of not being able to digest a balanced diet, first try a different vitamin—sometimes two childrens' chewables with iron, taken twice per day, are plenty. But if all vitamins make you ill to the point of not being able to eat anything, talk to your healthcare provider about skipping the vitamin completely, then plan your meals carefully to make sure that all of your nutritional bases are covered.

RECOMMENDED DAILY INTAKE OF VITAMINS, MINERALS, AND MACRONUTRIENTS FOR PREGNANT WOMEN

Pregnancy recommended daily allowances (RDAs) are set by the Food and Nutrition Board (FNB) of the Institute of Medicine. For some nutrients there isn't enough information for the Board to make a recommendation for an RDA or upper limit, so the number you see below may represent what other researchers consider an adequate intake during pregnancy. Whenever possible, we provide the upper limit of intake, because when it comes to vitamins and minerals,

Pregnancy Menu

This is for a second-trimester pregnant woman who's 5'4" and 130 pounds and doesn't exercise. For a customized chart based on height, weight, stage of pregnancy, and level of activity, visit the USDA's Web site: www.choosemyplate.gov.
    Grains: 7 ounces, with at least 3 ½ ounces from whole grains
        Vegetables: 3 cups
        Fruits: 2 cups
        Milk: 3 cups
        Meat, beans and nuts: 6 ounces

"too much of a good thing" can put unnecessary stress on your system or even be toxic. Be particularly careful if you take multiple supplements.

If your prenatal vitamin is prescription, ask your pharmacist to write down or copy the label for you, so you know if your supplement has too little (or too much) of certain nutrients. Most prenatal vitamins don't contain calcium, for instance, because it can block the absorption of other nutrients. In some cases, like magnesium and vitamin A, there's no determined upper limit for the nutrient from food sources, but there is an upper limit for the synthetic versions found in supplements.

It's also important to note that nutrition, for all of the specific grams and micrograms, is not an exact science. While the recommended daily allowances are estimates based on averages, in real life everyone's nutritional needs are different, because everyone's body, genetic heritage, environment, and activities are different. Your nutritional needs will also change as you age. So listen to your body. If you crave a food, eat it (though if what you crave is a cookie, try to have one, not five). If a food turns your stomach, avoid it. Pregnancy is not the time to impose arbitrary dietary restrictions or rules on yourself, like a low-fat, low-carb, or raw foods diet. Your body needs a little of everything.

(When you're looking at supplement labels, note that micrograms is sometimes written as µg.)

If you can eat a diet that's a well-balanced variety of unprocessed or minimally processed foods every single day, as in the chart below, you won't need to take a prenatal supplement at all. But not everyone had access to nutritious food on a daily basis, which is why it's worth considering taking vitamins for nutritional insurance.

Macronutrients

Carbohydrates: 160–406 grams (g)

Fiber: 28 g, 29 while breastfeeding

Protein: About 60–100 per day, 25 more if you're expecting multiples

Water: 3 liters

Calcium: 1,000–1,300 mg (mg), no more than 2,500 mg

Choline: 450 mg, 550 mg while breastfeeding, no more than 3,500 mg (3.5 g) per day.[1]

Chromium: 29–30 micrograms (mcg) during pregnancy, 44–45 while breastfeeding, no more than 1.6 mg per day

Copper: 1,000 mcg, 1,300 while breastfeeding

Fluoride: 3.0 mg, no more than 10 mg per day

Iodine: 220 mcg, no more than 1,100 mcg per day

Iron: 27–30 mg, no more than 45 mg per day

Manganese: 2.6 mg, no more than 11 mg per day

Magnesium: 360–400 mg, no more than 350 mg per day from supplements

Omega-3 fatty acids (ALA, EPA, DHA): 300–1,000 mg, no more than 3,000 grams per day

Pantothenic acid: 6 mg, no determined upper limit

Selenium: 65 mcg, no more than 400 mg per day

Vitamin A: 770 mcg during pregnancy, 1,300 mcg while breastfeeding, no more than 8,000 mcg (2,500 IU) per day

Vitamin B1 (thiamin): 1.4 mg, no determined upper limit

Riboflavin (B2): 1.6 mg, no determined upper limit

Niacin (B3): 18 mg, no more than 35 mg per day

Vitamin B6: 2.2 mg, no more than 100 mg per day

Vitamin B7 (biotin): 30 mcg, 35 mcg while breastfeeding, no determined upper limit

Vitamin B9 (folate, folic acid): 600 mcg, for women who have had a fetus or infant with a neural tube defect, the recommended dose is 1,000–5,000 mcg per day

Vitamin B12: 2.2 mcg, no determined upper limit

Vitamin C: 60–300 mg, no more than 2,000 mg per day

Vitamin D: 5 mcg (200 IU), no more than 2,000 IU per day

Vitamin E: 15 mg (22.5 IU), no more than 1,000 mg (1 g) per day

Vitamin K: 65–90 mcg, depending on age, no determined upper limit

Zinc: 8–13 mg, no more than 40 mg per day

Calories and Weight Gain

When you're not pregnant you need about 1,800 to 2,000 calories per day, or more if you are especially active or tall. When you're pregnant you need about 100 more calories per day in the first trimester, and about 300 more calories in the second and third trimesters. Healthcare providers generally recommend a weight gain of about 2 to 4 pounds in the first trimester, and about a pound a week in the second and third, for a total gain of 25 to 35 pounds if you're of average weight. If you're underweight your healthcare provider may urge you to gain 30 to 40 pounds, if you're overweight or obese, 15 to 25 or less.

If you find you're gaining more than the recommended amount, a food journal can be a helpful way to figure out if too many empty calories are sneaking in. But still, don't let your daily calories dip below 2,000, as calorie-restricted diets have been found harmful to fetal brain growth. In general, from the baby's point of view, it's better to gain too much weight during pregnancy than not enough.

Water

You need about 3 liters of water a day while you're pregnant, which is the equivalent of about twelve 8-ounce glasses. Not all of this hydration has to be straight-up water, though: milk, juice, soup, seltzer, tea, and the water in fruits and vegetables count, too. Being under-hydrated during pregnancy can lead to nausea, headaches, and, more extremely, premature labor.

Tired of drinking water? Try:
- Flavored seltzer
- Half juice, half seltzer
- Decaf or low-caf iced tea or coffee
- Soup or broth
- Tomato or vegetable juice
- A Popsicle

Carbohydrates: 160-406 g

You don't actually need to eat any carbohydrates, believe it or not, but without them a body has to work harder to turn protein and fat into energy. Plus carbs

usually come with other nutrients. Unless you have severe nausea, eating too many carbs is more of a concern than getting too few. If you're diagnosed with gestational diabetes mellitus (GDM), then your healthcare provider will have you counting your carbs closely.

Aim to get the most nutritional bang for your carbohydrate buck: go for whole grains that will also have lots of other nutrients and fiber, and limit your intake of big sugar-and-white-flour bombs like mega-muffins, heaping bowls of pasta, cakes, and pies.

Table sugar or high-fructose corn syrup: 12 g per tablespoon
Cup of pasta: 24 g
12-oz. can of sweetened soda: 39 g
Cheeseburger: 28 g
Cup of ice cream: 64 g
Bagel: 70 g
Slice of carrot cake: 100 g

Protein: About 60-100 g per day, 25 more if you're expecting twins or multiples

Protein is an important building block of cells, and getting enough can help prevent fatigue, muscle soreness and body aches. Your body's requirements go way up during pregnancy, to 0.5 g per pound of pre-pregnancy body weight. So if you were 135 pounds pre-pregnancy you need about 67.5 g per day; if you were 165 pounds, 82.5 g. Because the body can store protein, though, it's not necessary to get that exact number of grams every single day, as long you average about that much over the course of a week.

Unless you're a vegan, or just retch at the thought of meat, eggs, or dairy, you probably won't have a problem getting enough. Animal products have a lot of protein, and so do beans, seeds, and soy and nut milks. If you're very queasy and can barely stand to eat, try adding protein powder containing whey, soy protein, or casein to a smoothie or beverage. (For more on vegan and vegetarian pregnancy, see page 168.)

Beef, chicken, lamb, pork, fish, or shellfish, about 17–30 g per 4-oz serving
Chickpeas, 14 g per cup
Cottage cheese, 2 percent fat, 15 g per cup
Cow's milk, about 8 g per cup
Lentils, 17 g per cup
Soy milk, about 7 g per cup
Hemp milk, about 5 g per cup
Almond milk, about 1 g per cup

Fiber: 28 g, 29 while breast-feeding

Fiber isn't considered an essential macronutrient, but it's important to good health nonetheless. It helps you digest and feel full, prevents constipation and hemorrhoids, lowers cholesterol, and slows down sugar absorption, reducing your risk of diabetes—all very good things while you're pregnant. All plant foods contain some amount of fiber, and some have more than others.

One downside: high-fiber foods can also give you gas. If this is a problem for you, try gas-prevention enzyme supplements like Beano, which are safe to take during pregnancy.

Fiber sources:
All-Bran cereal, 8.8 g per ½ cup
Blackberries, 7.6 g per cup
Oatmeal, 4 g per cup
Shredded wheat, 5.5 g per cup

One pear, about 5 g
Raisins, about 5 g per cup
Baked beans, about 10 g per cup
Lentils, about 1 g per cup
Almonds, about 3.3 g per oz

Docosahexaenoic acid (DHA): 200-500 g, no more than 3,000 g per day

DHA is a type of omega-3 fatty acid and the predominant fat found in brain cells.

ALA, also known as alpha-linolenic acid, is a type of fatty acid that's found in some vegetable oils and seeds. Flaxseed (also known as linseed) oil is rich in it, and so are kiwi fruit seeds, olive, canola and walnut oils, soybeans, and tofu. The body converts ALA into EPA (eicosapentaenoic acid) and then into DHA, so it's okay to take a supplement that only has DHA.

When it comes to DHA making fetuses into smarter babies, though, there's conflicting evidence. Some studies have shown higher IQs in babies whose moms took omega-3 supplements during pregnancy, but a large 2010 study found no cognitive benefit for babies.

DHA is found in fatty fish and certain types of coldwater seaweed, but because of concerns about pollution, it's probably best to get your DHA in a supplement made from fish oil or seaweed (called algal oil on ingredients lists).

Omega-6 is another family of fatty acids, found in palm, corn, soy, and sunflower oils. Omega-3, omega-6, and omega-9 acids compete with one another, and the Western diet is very high in omega-6 and -9. Too much omega-6 and -9 is associated with all kinds of health problems, including heart attacks and breast cancer,[2] so unless you're on some kind of fat-free or low-fat diet, if you take omega supplements you want to make sure they only have omega-3 and not the other fatty acids.

High amounts of omega-3 fatty acids have also been associated with an increased risk of stroke, bleeding, and reduced glycemic control in diabetics. So it's probably a good idea to avoid higher than the recommended doses of omega-3 supplements, particularly in the 2 weeks before your due date. Also be sure to ask your healthcare provider about the latest news on the safety of omega-3 supplements if you're diabetic. Note that research has found that DHA supplements may increase the length of gestation by an average of 4 days.

VITAMINS

Vitamin A: 770 mcg during pregnancy, 1,300 mcg while breastfeeding, no more than 8,000 mcg (2,500 IU) per day

This essential vitamin helps your vision and increases your resistance to viruses. It can be found in animal products, such as liver and butter, and in plant products that contain carotene, which your body converts into vitamin A. The body absorbs vitamin A about twice as efficiently from animal-product sources than vegetable sources. Carotene-rich vegetables are dark green, deep yellow, and orange: broccoli,

greens, green peppers, sweet potatoes, carrots, pumpkins, winter squash, apricots, carrots, papaya, cantaloupe, spinach, pumpkin, sweet potatoes, and mangoes. Vitamin A deficiencies are rare. If you take multivitamin supplements, avoid those that contain more than the recommended dose; large doses of straight synthetic vitamin A are associated with birth defects. However, supplements that contain vitamin A in the form of beta-carotene are safe.

B Vitamins

Several B vitamins make up the B-complex family, including folic acid, B6, B12, niacin, thiamine, and riboflavin. They're found mainly in animal products such as meat, eggs, and dairy, although (with the exception of B12) they can also be found in certain vegetables. The B vitamins are water soluble, which means that they are not stored in the body for long-term use, so it's important to get enough every day. If you take a daily prenatal vitamin, it should contain a full B complex.
Thiamine (B1): 1.5 mg per day. Thiamine, also known as vitamin B1, is used by your body to release energy from the carbohydrates in foods. Too little of it can make you feel listless. Pork is your best food source, with 0.7 mg per 3 oz, but B1 is also found in watermelon (0.23 mg per slice), avocados (0.2 mg per avocado), and peas (0.41 mg per cup).
Riboflavin (B2): 1.4 mg per day during pregnancy, 1.6 mg per day while breastfeeding. B2 plays a key role in metabolism, and is found in dairy products, green

leafy vegetables and legumes, kiwifruit, and avocados. It's also what makes your pee florescent yellow when you take vitamin supplements. If you drink 2 pints of milk per day, you'll be getting plenty of B2. Note that light destroys B2, so when you buy milk, opt for opaque containers instead of clear glass or plastic.

Niacin (B3): 18 mg, no more than 35 mg per day. Niacin, aka B3, helps your cells convert food into energy and regulates the balance of fats in your bloodstream. Salmon (14 mg per 3 oz), chicken (19 mg), peanuts, and enriched cereal are good sources.

Vitamin B6 (pyridoxine): 2.2 mg per day. Vitamin B6 is especially important for protein metabolism, and helps your body build proteins, including hormones, blood components, and enzymes. Your body also uses it to help regulate your blood sugar levels. Not getting enough can make you dizzy and cranky.

Some research has shown that B6 may be helpful in reducing pregnancy-related carpal tunnel syndrome and other aches and pains because the vitamin helps nerve cells to communicate properly. For some women, B6 supplements can also reduce the symptoms of morning sickness.

Whole grain cereal, bananas (0.7 mg), and chicken (0.8 mg per 3-oz serving) are good sources.

Biotin (B7): 30 mcg, 35 mcg while breastfeeding (no recognized upper limit). Biotin, also known as vitamin B7, is necessary for cell growth and the metabolism

of fats and amino acids. It also helps keep your blood sugar level steady (which may help ease mood swings and pregnancy-related nausea). Pregnant women are at a high risk of deficiency, so you want to make sure your supplement contains enough. Eggs, salmon, leafy greens, whole grains, and legumes are also good sources of B7.

Folate (B9): 600 mcg, no more than 1,000 mcg (1 g) per day from folic acid supplements. There is no health risk or upper limit for natural sources of folate found in food.

Folate is essential for fetal growth—it aids in the formation of genetic material and may reduce the risk of preterm birth. Folic acid is the synthetic form of folate. Natural folate is fragile, and is easily destroyed by heat, light, and the decomposition of vegetables. The body can only store a small amount, so it's important to get some every day, through a supplement or by eating raw leafy greens or citrus fruits. In 1996 the FDA began requiring folic acid be added to enriched breads and cereals because of evidence that it reduces birth defects if a woman has a sufficient amount in her system pre-conception. If you have previously had a baby with a neural tube defect, your healthcare provider may prescribe an additional folic acid supplement.

Sources of folic acid:
Lentils, boiled: 179 mcg per ½ cup (4 oz)
Oatmeal, instant: 150 mcg per packet

Asparagus, steamed: 131 mcg
per 6 spears
Spinach, steamed: 131 mcg per
½ cup
Chickpeas, canned: 80 mcg per
½ cup
Lima beans: 78 mcg per ½ cup
Orange juice from concentrate:
54 mcg per ½ cup
Broccoli, steamed: 52 mcg per ½
cup

Vitamin B12: 2.2 mcg per day.
Vitamin B12 is found exclusively
in animal products: milk, meat,
shellfish, and eggs. Unless
you're a vegan, you should
have no problem getting the
recommended 3 mcg of B12 per
day to maintain a healthy nervous
system. If you are a vegan, talk
to your care provider about
supplement options. Symptoms
of B12 deficiency, such as poor
neurological development, can
show up in the breastfed infants
of strict vegans.

Vitamin C (ascorbic acid): 85 to
300 mg. Vitamin C is necessary
for the proper function of your
immune system. The FDA
currently recommended daily
allowance of vitamin C for
pregnant women is 70 mg, but
recently the National Institutes
of Health has recommended
raising the recommended dose
to 200 mg. Because vitamin C
is water-soluble, it's just about
impossible to overdose because
your body will just pass what you
don't need through your urine.
But generally, your body can't
use more than 500 mg per day.
If you smoke cigarettes, though,
be sure to get at least 300 mg per
day, because your body depletes
its supply of vitamin C to fight

the toxins in cigarette smoke,
making it harder for you to fight
illnesses. Citrus fruits and juices
are good sources.

Vitamin D: 200 IU (5 mcg), no more
than 2,000 IU per day. Vitamin D is
necessary for calcium absorption,
and it helps prevent illnesses
(possibly including cancer and
heart disease). Most Americans
are deficient. Your skin makes
vitamin D when exposed to
sunlight, but most people don't
get enough sun to make sufficient
amounts, especially in the winter
months. Most milk and some
orange juice have vitamin D
added (though butter, cheese, and
other dairy products usually do
not). Salmon and cod liver oil are
also good food sources. If your
baby is exclusively breastfed, you
may also need to give her vitamin
D supplement drops.

Choline: 450 mg. Choline is a
water-soluble essential nutrient
that helps maintain cell walls.
Too little choline has been
associated with neural tube
defects, preeclampsia, low birth
weight and prematurity. Eggs,
meat, and milk are good sources,
as are cruciferous vegetables
like cabbage, cauliflower, and
broccoli. It's a good idea to
make sure your prenatal vitamin
contains some choline, too.
Protein sources:
Large hard-boiled egg, 113 mg
One tablespoon soy lecithin, 250
mg
Quart of 1 percent milk, 173 mg
Pound of cauliflower, 177 mg

Selenium: 65 mcg, no more than
400 mcg per day. Selenium is an
essential trace element necessary
for thyroid function. Nuts,

cereals, meat, fish, and eggs are all good sources. High amounts of selenium can be toxic.

MINERALS

Calcium: 1,000-1,300 mg, no more than 2,500 mg

Have you heard the rumor that babies take calcium from their mothers' teeth? While that's not technically true, any calcium you take in will go to the baby first, with you getting whatever's left. So it's important to get at least 1,000 mg of calcium every day for the sake of your own bone density (and 1,300 mg a day if you are breastfeeding or under 18). Prenatal supplements usually don't contain much calcium because it can hinder the absorption of other vitamins and minerals. You can get your calcium through food, additional supplements, or a combination. If you take calcium supplements, avoid taking them an hour before or after your prenatal vitamin and don't bother taking more than 500 mg at a time, because your body isn't able to absorb more than that all at once.

Calcium sources:
Skim, lowfat, whole, or chocolate milk: 300 mg per 8 oz
Calcium-fortified orange juice, soy, rice, or almond milk: 200–400 mg per 8 oz
Broccoli, cooked: 180 mg per cup
Swiss cheese: 272 mg per oz
Cheddar cheese: 204 mg per oz
American cheese: 174 mg per oz
Cottage cheese: 77 mg per ½ cup
Yogurt: 345–415 mg per cup
Canned oily fish with bones: 200–300 mg per 3-oz serving such as salmon and sardines
Tofu prepared with calcium: 50–250 mg per 3-oz serving chloride or sulfate
Leafy greens such as kale, collards, or turnip greens: 100–170 mg per ½ cup
Mineral water: Gerolsteiner 80 mg per cup; San Pellegrino 50 mg per cup

Chromium: 29-30 mcg during pregnancy, 44-45 mcg while breastfeeding, no more than 1.6 mg per day

Chromium is a mineral used to metabolize food. Deficiencies are pretty rare, though, so don't worry if your prenatal doesn't contain any. Good food sources include whole grain breads and cereals, lean meats, cheeses, and some spices, such as black pepper and thyme.

Copper: 1,000 mcg, 1,300 while breastfeeding, no more than 7.8 mg per day

Copper is another essential mineral needed for food metabolism, and pregnant women are susceptible to deficiency because demand increases. Deficiency can lead to anemia and fatigue. Copper overdose is rare, but cooking acidic foods in copper cookware can lead to excess amounts over time. Good food sources include oysters, beef or lamb liver, Brazil nuts, blackstrap molasses, cocoa, and black pepper.

Fluoride: 3.0 mg, no more than 10 mg per day

Fluoride is another essential mineral. It helps strengthen teeth and bones. Because fluoride is added to the water supply in many places, though, deficiencies are pretty much unheard of.

Iodine: 220 mcg, 290 while breastfeeding, no more than 1.1 mg per day

Iodine helps keep your thyroid functioning, and plays an essential role in lactation. Because most salt is fortified with it (iodized), deficiencies are pretty rare. Any food from the sea (like fish, shellfish, or seaweed) will also contain some.

Iron: 27-30 mg, no more than 45 mg

Iron is used to make red blood cells, and as your blood volume goes up during pregnancy, so do your body's requirements. Most women, pregnant or not, don't get enough iron. During pregnancy, you'll need 30 mg of iron per day. (Non-pregnant women need 15 mg, and a nursing mom needs 19 mg.) The National Academy of Science recommends that expectant moms in their second and third trimesters take a daily iron supplement containing 30 mg of iron. Unfortunately for vegetarians, it turns out that iron from plant-based foods is not as well absorbed as the iron from meat. The carbonates, oxalates, and phosphates in foods such as tea, cranberries, rhubarb, spinach, and soda block your absorption of iron to some degree. Consider drinking soy, almond, or cow's milk with 3 tablespoons of blackstrap molasses (found in health food stores) each morning and evening. Vitamin C enhances iron absorption from plant sources, so try drinking orange juice with iron-rich foods, or combinations like spinach with diced red peppers.

Iron sources:

Cereal, ready to eat, fortified: 1–16 mg per cup
Clams, canned: 11.2 mg per ¼ cup
Braunschweiger (liver sausage): 5.3 mg per 2 oz
Beef liver, fried: 5.3 mg per 3 oz
Molasses, blackstrap: 5 mg per tablespoon
Baked beans: 5 mg per cup
Oysters, cooked: 3.8 mg per oz
Sirloin steak: 2.9 mg per 3 oz
Baked potato, with skin: 2.8 mg per medium potato
Soup, lentil and ham: 2.6 mg per cup
Burrito, bean: 2.5 mg each
Soup, beef noodle: 2.4 mg per cup
Rice, white, enriched: 2.3 mg per cup
Pop-Tart, fortified: 2.2 mg per pastry
Enriched pasta: 2 mg per cooked cup
Ground beef, lean: 1.8 mg per 3 oz
Tofu, firm: 1.8 mg per ½ cup
Apricots, dried halves: 1.7 mg per 10
Cashews, roasted: 1.7 mg per oz
Spinach, frozen: 1.5 mg per ½ cup
Bread, whole wheat: 1.2 mg per slice (varies with brand)
Broccoli, fresh cooked: 0.7 mg per ½ cup
Egg: 0.7 mg per egg

Manganese: 2 mg, no more than 11 mg per day

Manganese is another essential mineral, and not the same as magnesium. It's needed for bone growth and keeping glucose levels steady. Nuts, beans, whole grains, and tea are good sources. Requirements go up during pregnancy, but deficiencies are rare. Overdose may be a concern if you take multiple mineral supplements, though.

Magnesium: 360–400 mg, no more than 350 mg a day from suppliments

Magnesium is needed for more than three hundred biochemical reactions in the body and is needed for bone and tissue cell function. It helps maintain normal muscle and nerve function, keeps heart rhythm steady and bones strong, and some studies suggest it can lower your risk of preeclampsia and low birth weight. Getting enough of it can spare you the pregnancy irritations of leg cramps, mental disorientation, and even depression. Magnesium is found in some amount in all unprocessed plant foods. Not all prenatal vitamins contain magnesium, so check labels.

Magnesium sources:
Avocado, Florida: 206 mg per
    medium avocado
Almonds: 86 mg per oz
Mixed roasted nuts: 66 mg per oz
Spinach: 65 mg per cooked ½ cup
Peanut butter: 50 mg per 2
    tablespoons
Banana: 30–45 mg per medium
    banana
Chocolate bar: 31 mg per oz
Kiwifruit: 53 mg a cup

Zinc: 11–14 mg, no more than 40 mg per day

Zinc is important for maintaining your immune system and helping the fetus grow, and low levels have been associated with low birth weight, prematurity, and other serious complications. Zinc is found in shellfish and red meat, and also in nuts and legumes, though it's less easily absorbed from plant sources. One study found that zinc supplementation during pregnancy was associated with a 14 percent reduction in premature deliveries. Zinc needs vary by age: if you're 18 or younger you need 13 mg per day while expecting and 14 mg while breastfeeding; if you're 19 or older you need 11 mg per day during pregnancy and 12 mg while breastfeeding.

Zinc sources:
Six cooked oysters: 76 mg
Beef, 3 ounces: 6 mg
Turkey, dark meat, 3 ounces: 3.8 mg
Baked beans: 1.8 per mg per ½ cup

Vitamin E (tocopherol): 15 mg (22.5 IU) during pregnancy, 19 mg per day while breast-feeding, no more than 400 IU per day

Vitamin E protects the body from tissue damage. Deficiencies are rare and supplements appear to increase the risk of excessive bleeding, so it's better to avoid vitamin supplements that contain extra E.

Vitamin K: 65–90 mcg (higher amount for women under age 19)

Vitamin K is necessary for blood clotting and maintaining bone density in adults. Deficiencies are rare, except in the case of people with liver disease. Newborns have low levels of it, which is why they're given an injection soon after birth (for more on this, see page 429).

Is Organic Food Worth It?

Organic food is grown or raised by farmers who don't use synthetic pesticides or fertilizers made of synthetic ingredients or sludge from sewage treatment plants. Organic meat, poultry, eggs, and dairy products come from animals that are given no antibiotics or growth hormones. Herbicides, pesticides, and antibiotics consumed by cows can be passed along through their milk. Before a product can be labeled "organic," a government-approved certifier inspects the farm where the food is grown to make sure the farmer is following all the rules necessary to meet USDA organic standards. These higher standards mean that organic foods are more expensive for consumers. Should you spend the extra money on organic foods? For fresh fruits, grains, vegetables, and dairy products, it's a good idea to pay a little more to lower the risk of your and your baby's exposure to unnecessary chemicals and pesticides. Chemicals such as dioxins are carcinogens considered to be potentially associated with cancer and with birth defects in animal studies. The foods most likely to be contaminated with pesticides are strawberries, rice, oats, milk, bell peppers, bananas, green beans, potatoes, and spinach. Many of these crops come from overseas, where farmers may not be well monitored in their use of dangerous pesticides. Wash all fresh vegetables well, even organic ones.

Vegetarianism and Veganism

If you're a vegetarian (that is, you don't eat meat but do eat eggs and dairy products) you don't need to take any special nutritional measures during pregnancy. Eggs, dairy products, fortified cereals, and nuts can supply the extra protein, iron, zinc, B vitamins, and fats that you need.

If you're a vegan, though, it's vitally important to pay close attention to your diet on a daily basis. You will need to take supplements to supply vitamin B12 plus the extra iron, calcium, and zinc pregnancy requires. Don't try to go without supplements—you can risk brain damage to your baby as well as potentially fatal excessive blood loss during delivery. Note that it will take an awful lot of beans and nuts to get the protein you need—3 cups of tofu or 3½ cups of cooked lentils per day. It can also be a challenge to get enough calories. Make sure that your healthcare provider knows you're vegan, and work with her to develop a nutritional plan to follow during pregnancy and breastfeeding.

Food Safety

Worrying about food safety during pregnancy can be a little crazy-making: be sure to eat fish—but not certain kinds and not too much. Fresh fruits and vegetables are vital for good health, but by the way, they're the foods most likely to be contaminated with foodborne illness and pesticides. It can get to the point where you're scared to eat anything. And there's good reason to worry: one CDC study found that 1 in 6 Americans is stricken with a foodborne illness every year.

What can you do?

First, note that most food is contaminated during processing. The more a food is handled, the greater the risk that it will have come into contact with bacteria or viruses. You can reduce the risk by processing food yourself: instead of buying deli cold cuts, cook and slice your beef, ham, or turkey breast at home. If you want a hamburger, grind chuck roast yourself, instead of buying preformed patties or beef that's already ground. The CDC estimates that every year about 80 percent of food poisoning cases are from food prepared in "commercial or institutional establishments" and only 20 percent are from food prepared at home.[3]

Wash all of your fruits and vegetables well, even if they're organic or are pre-cut or pre-washed.

Handle raw meats as the potential infectious agents that they are. Don't use wooden cutting boards for meat: the wood can absorb juices from raw meat and pass them onto other foods. If you bring home meat packaged on a Styrofoam tray and plastic-wrapped, lower the odds of meat juice drips by putting the packaged meat inside another plastic bag before putting it in the fridge.

Keep your surfaces clean. Fill a spray bottle with one-tenth bleach and nine-tenths water, and use it to clean your food prep surfaces and cutting boards used for meat. Leave the solution on the surface for about 3 seconds before wiping off any excess moisture.

Wash your hands often with hot, soapy water when you're cooking, and dry them with a clean hand towel or paper towel, and/or invest in disposable latex gloves to wear for food prep.

Banish vermin. Mice and insects can track germs all over your food prep surfaces with their little feet, and their feces are too gross to mention (one word: hantavirus). If you see one mouse or cockroach, assume there's about a hundred more in the wall you don't see, so as soon as you spot vermin, call an exterminator and be sure to give your kitchen a thorough bleach-and-water scrubdown while wearing gloves and a face mask before you cook there again.

Cook foods thoroughly, especially animal products like meat and eggs. In restaurants, ask that burgers or steaks be cooked to at least medium temperature.

Keep your hot foods hot (65°C or 149°F) **and your cold foods cold** (4°C or 40°F). Bacteria grows most readily at the temperatures in between. Make sure your fridge is set at a temperature of 4°C or 40°F or less, and check your fridge's temperature with a thermometer every so often. If you take meals to school or work and don't have access to a refrigerator to store it in, put a cold pack in your lunch bag.

When you do eat out, never eat at a restaurant with a dirty bathroom. Also avoid buffet-style restaurants, where food is often kept at bacteria-encouraging temperatures.

Don't reheat leftovers more than once, and don't refreeze defrosted food.

Probably needless to say, don't eat any suspect or unappealing food. If in doubt, throw it out!

If you suspect food poisoning— you have more-intense-than-usual nausea, stomach cramps, diarrhea and/or vomiting, or you can't eat or keep any food down for longer than 12 hours—call your healthcare provider right away.

④

Birth

When your baby finally decides to arrive, it's only normal to have mixed feelings. On one hand, you can hardly wait to get over your cumbersome pregnancy and finally get to meet that active little one who's become so much a part of your life. On the other hand, it's normal to be anxious, even terrified, in the face of the prospect of giving birth, especially if this is your first baby. Like all new experiences, even though you can study all the angles, it's hard to imagine exactly what being in labor and delivering a baby will be like until you actually go through it.

Knowing what's going to happen ahead of time can make the strangeness of the unknown a little more familiar and less anxiety-producing. In this chapter, we will give you all the important information you need to know to prepare yourself for a hospital or a home birth. It will help you take a realistic look at what typical birthing experiences are for moms these days, and it will provide you with an arsenal of research findings to help you navigate what's in the best interest of both you and your baby.

The Stages of Labor

In medical circles, labor is usually described having four distinct stages. From your point of view as a patient, the stages will probably pass through in a blur, since you'll simply be engrossed in the strong sensations and signals your body

is sending you. But being aware of the *stages of labor* and its complexities can help you feel more in control and less anxious.

The first stage of labor is the process of the uterus drawing up to make the cervix open up so the baby can be born. This stage has three parts: latent phase, when you first begin to notice contractions and realize that they mean business; active phase, which is hard work, and finally, the toughest part of labor, transition phase, when the cervix becomes fully thin (effaced) and wide (dilated) to let the baby out.

The second stage is the pushing, or bearing down, stage when the uterus and pelvic muscles push the baby through the birth canal to the outside.

The third stage is expelling the *afterbirth*—the placenta, membranes, and so on—and the uterus starts to shrink back to its regular size.

The fourth stage is after-birth recovery, when the uterus contracts back from watermelon to grapefruit size.

How Is Labor Managed in the Hospital?

If you give birth in a community hospital, where most babies in the United States are born, your labor will be overseen by your private healthcare provider, and if she is not physically present, it will likely be managed by a labor and delivery nurse using your caregiver's standing orders and instructions for procedures, monitoring, and interventions.

Most labor and delivery areas in hospitals are also guided by a set of protocols based on current practice guidelines established by national professional organizations in medical specialties, including obstetricians, family practice physicians, midwives, pediatricians, and labor and delivery nurses.

Monitoring Your Progress

Once you're checked in to the hospital, your vital signs, including your temperature, pulse, respiration, and blood pressure will be taken. Your contractions and your baby's heart rate will also be listened to with a *fetoscope* or Doppler, and you may have a belt strapped around your abdomen to take readings of your contractions and your baby's heart rate using a small sensor box connected to an *electronic fetal monitor* (EFM).

You may be given a routine blood test to check if you're anemic, to confirm your blood type, and possibly to determine if you have blood clotting problems.

As part of your labor evaluation, you will probably be given a quick pelvic exam to determine if your cervix has started to thin (efface) and begun to stretch open (dilate). If your amniotic sac has ruptured, the nurse or practitioner will don sterile gloves and collect a sample of the fluid with a cotton swab. It will be examined on a slide under a microscope to confirm the rupture and look for signs of meconium or infection.

If you are dilated 4 or more centimeters (cm, about 1½ inches), you will likely be labeled as being in active labor. On the other hand, if you are having regular contractions, but are not dilated to that magic mark, you may be given the option of strolling around the hospital for an hour or so (or may even be told to go home) and return to labor and delivery to be reexamined to see if you have reached 4 cm.

If you're in active labor, the nurse on duty may want to place

Measuring Dilation

Your baby's progress through your birth canal will be measured by how wide your baby's body, usually her head, is stretching the mouth of your uterus, the cervix. The stretching happens as the uterus pushes and squeezes your baby downward through your pelvic bones. The process is called dilation. The thinning and softening of the cervical wall is called effacement.

In the latter weeks of your pregnancy, your cervix may stay tightly closed, or it may begin to gradually stretch open by a few centimeters (cm). (One inch equals 2.54 cm.) By the time your baby is ready to be born, your cervix will have changed from barely being open to about 8 centimeters dilation to full dilation of about 10 cm in the final part of the first stage.

Your insides and the thinning and widening of your cervix will be inspected repeatedly with a gloved hand during your labor to see how far down your baby is, how effaced and dilated your cervix is. Here's how to interpret what you'll be told:

1 cm = width of a Cheerio
3 cm = slice of banana
4 cm = Oreo cookie
5 cm = lid of a small juice can
7 cm = lid of a soda can
10 cm = width of a small bagel

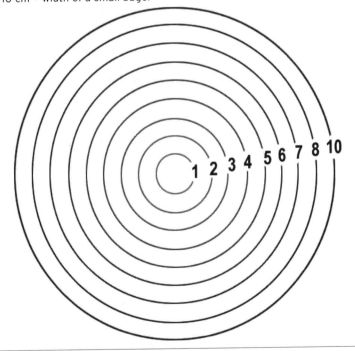

a tiny tube with an anticoagulant in it (to prevent blood clotting) on the back of your hand, called a hep-lock. This gives caregivers constant access to your veins in case they want to give you an IV of intravenous fluids. You can decline the hep-lock or postpone it, since many women find it uncomfortable and irritating.

Even if it's in your birth plan that you don't want a hep-lock or continuous fetal monitoring, it's up to you to inform the nurses on duty at every shift change. Hospital policies may vary when it comes to monitoring—after an initial monitoring period you may be able to get up and walk around with your contractions and baby's heart rate checked every hour or so. If you're being induced and/or getting an epidural, then the hospital may mandate more frequent monitoring.

STAGE 1

What's Happening

Picture your uterus as a large, upside-down pear. The neck of the uterus (stem of the pear) faces downward toward your vagina. The neck and tip end of the uterus are called the cervix, the Latin word for neck. During this stage, the cervix softens and becomes thinner and wider.

Effacement is expressed as a percentage, with 50 percent effaced meaning the cervix is halfway through its thinning process, and 100 percent, or fully effaced, meaning the cervix has become paper-thin and has almost disappeared. The effacing process can happen over hours, or even days, of mild, irregular contractions.

During this stage of labor, contractions draw the sidewalls of the uterus upward, causing the diameter of the cervix to widen. A woman is considered to be in active labor when her dilation reaches approximately 4 centimeters (3 fingers), and fully dilated when it reaches 10 centimeters (5 fingers).

Once full dilation happens, you enter the second stage of labor. As with effacement, it can take hours, or days, for the cervix of a first-time mother to make it to 4 centimeters (approximately 1½ inches). Cells in the uterus actually learn how to work together, and with each labor the process gets more efficient. It also takes the uterus two to three times longer to dilate the cervix 1 centimeter during early labor than it does later on. The dilation process usually moves slowly at first then increases as you near 10 centimeters.

During first births, effacing and dilating are usually two separate processes, with effacement (effacing) happening first before dilation begins. For mothers who have previously given birth, effacement and dilation often happen simultaneously. Some healthcare providers and anesthesiologists prefer to wait to administer an epidural until the latent stage has passed, while others allow mothers to have epidurals whenever they request it.

How Long the First Stage Lasts

How long the entire first stage lasts varies widely, but typically takes about 6 to 18 hours from the time labor starts for first-time mothers, and between 2 and 10 hours for mothers who have given birth before.

How the First Stage Feels

Labor contractions don't just come and stay; they have a pattern of tightening, releasing, resting, and then tightening again. At first, they may resemble waves of strong menstrual cramps, except that they come and go.

Labor pain often starts in the back and moves around to the front, and sometimes radiates into the upper thighs. There are regular pauses between each contraction. Contraction cycles usually become stronger and more intense as labor goes on, with discomfort peaking for a few seconds halfway through each contraction, then easing off, giving you time to recoup and rest in between.

Unmedicated contractions usually don't last longer than 1½ minutes, while the breaks in between contractions go from 5 minutes at the start of labor to less than a minute toward the end.

How this stage will feel to you will depend upon how you've elected to deal with labor pain. If you've decided to forego painkilling drugs, try walking around, breathing evenly through contractions, and assuming various positions for comfort. (For more on that, go to page 181.)

If you've decided to have an epidural and it took properly, you'll be lying down and probably won't be feeling pain, though you may be aware of pressure, and in rare cases may experience nausea, itching, or other side effects from the drugs.

If you've chosen to have narcotics, you'll probably feel groggy and a bit out of it.

What to Do During the First Stage

Here's a primer on how to handle your first stage of labor:

- **Relax through early contractions.** There's no need to go crazy with labor positions or breathing exercises you learned in childbirth class unless they really help. Try to not wear yourself out too early in the process.
- **Breathe.** Inhale through your nose and out your pursed lips with deep breaths during contractions, but don't pant or hyperventilate. Try to breathe deeply to the bottom of your lungs. Making low-pitched noises may help.
- **Move around.** Moving around can help to stimulate nature's own painkillers, *endorphin*s. If you're not connected to monitoring lines, change positions frequently, especially if your contractions appear to be getting weaker or further apart.
- **Try a birth ball.** Sit on it (supported) or kneel and hug it.
- **Sit on the toilet.** Staying on the toilet for a while can help to open the pelvis and rotate the baby. Use a footstool to prop your feet.
- **Try temperature and pressure changes.** Warm or cold compresses to your back or lower abdomen may help in the middle of a contraction. Getting a shoulder massage or having pressure applied to your back or hips may be temporarily soothing.

- **Make the most of your hospital bed.** If you're stuck close to bed because of monitor wires, an IV, or an epidural connection, try to sit as upright as is comfortable and request extra pillows for support. You can also lie on your left side if that feels comfortable to you, but avoid lying flat on your back (being supine). Doing so can affect your blood pressure and could deprive your baby of needed blood circulation and oxygen.
- **Urinate frequently.** Drink sips of water between contractions to make up for your sweating and panting. Make sure to urinate frequently to keep your bladder empty so there's more room for your baby to move down. If you've had an epidural, you may have a catheter

inserted, which will do the peeing for you.
- **Don't give up.** Although transition may be intense, it means you're getting closer and closer to having your baby. Let a doctor, midwife, or nurse know if you have pinching pain anywhere in your hips or pelvis.
- **Ask for help.** If pain becomes overwhelming and you can't cope anymore, ask for relief.

STAGE 2: FROM TRANSITION TO PUSHING

The Phases of Stage 2
How the Second Stage Feels
It may take a few contractions for you to figure out what your body

The Phases of Stage 2

STAGE 2 PHASES	HOW LONG THE STAGE LASTS	WHAT'S HAPPENING
Passive stage	Approximately 15 to 20 minutes	Your cervix has dilated between $8^1/2$ and 10 centimeters. Your baby is in the process of descending downward and is getting aligned for birth.
Expulsive (active or bearing down) **stage**	20 to 30 minutes (an uncomplicated active stage can last an hour, or longer, and still be normal)	Your baby has moved deeply into your pelvis and is putting pressure on your lower body and vaginal area.

is doing. The *urge to push* will become very compelling on its own, and when it does, it will be difficult to do anything but push when the contractions hit.

Most of the discomfort you'll feel at this point will be from the pressure of your baby's head stretching your lower body and vaginal tissues.

You may feel the sensation of pressure even with an epidural.

"A ring of fire" is what midwives use to describe the burning, then tingling, then numbing from the pressure of the baby's head as it presses forward and recedes backward near the end of the second stage.

During this stage, the bones at the base of your pelvis, including your tailbone, will need to be free to flex outward instead of being pressed inward toward the front of your body, as they are when you lie down or sit. A variety of positions can help your pelvis to efficiently expand. Sitting up works well for some mothers, as does a temporary squat or semi-squat.

If you're experiencing *back labor*, continuous pain in your lower back, pushing while you're down on all fours may be the most comfortable for a while.

If you're exhausted from long hours of contractions, lying on your left side for this stage will allow you rest between contractions without hampering your stretching.

CONTRACTIONS	WHAT TO DO
Contractions slow down.	Rest, and collect yourself. Don't attempt pushing unless you have a strong urge to do so.
Contractions are accompanied by a sudden, strong urge to push, and you may find yourself making loud groaning sounds.	Go with your instincts. There's no need to hold your breath and push to a count of ten. Light pushes three to five times per contraction are more natural.

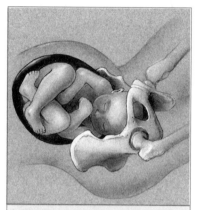

Getting through your pelvis is your baby's hardest job.

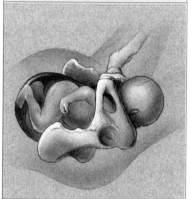

His whole body will rotate to make it through.

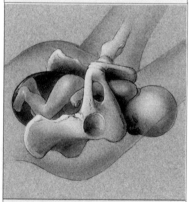

Finally his head will free itself and his shoulders will emerge one at a time.

What to Do During the Second Stage

- **Request time to rest and regroup.** Even though you're fully dilated, if you haven't felt the urge to push yet, ask for time to rest and let the baby descend until you feel the urge to push.
- **Breathe deeply and evenly between contractions.** Take deep breaths between your contractions to help maintain good oxygen levels for your baby. Finally his head will free itself and his shoulders will emerge one at a time. Getting through your pelvis is your baby's hardest job.
- **Don't worry about soiling the bed.** Yes, it may happen, because the baby's head will be exerting pressure on your rectal area. But there's no need to be embarrassed—birth attendants have seen it many, many times and will discreetly wipe anything away.
- **Try to stay upright.** It will help the baby descend and you'll be able to push more effectively if you are in an upright position rather than lying flat or semi-reclined.

  Have the back of the bed raised, and use the sidearm of the bed or towels tied to the sides to pull yourself up.
- **Get off your tail(bone).** Having your tailbone (coccyx) compressed by the weight of your body may be uncomfortable.
- **Push effectively.** While you're pushing, relax your perineum, and try to direct your bearing down toward your lower pelvis, rather than concentrating your pushing forces from your chest area.

Will You Need an Episiotomy?

An *episiotomy* is a surgical procedure that involves cutting into the connective tissues and muscles in the area between the vagina and the anus to widen the birth canal in order to ease the baby out.

For a long time, episiotomies were a routine procedure for childbirth. Healthcare providers thought that giving a woman a surgical *incision* would ease her delivery and avoid the deep, jagged tears that might happen. It was also thought to prevent urinary incontinence, to keep the muscles of a woman's pelvic floor from becoming too lax, or to prevent a prolapsed (dropped) uterus, but research has failed to prove that having an episiotomy can prevent any of these things from happening.

In fact, recent research now shows that having an episiotomy actually increases a woman's chances of severe tearing, excessive bleeding, infection, and swelling. It can cause severe discomfort after birth and make sex painful.

Episiotomies today are most often performed when forceps or vacuum extraction are used. Having an epidural increases a woman's risk for needing to have these instruments used to help pull her baby out. There are times when babies are in dire trouble and may need to be delivered quickly. In that case, an episiotomy may be important.

Ask your healthcare provider to discuss the pros and cons of having an episiotomy. Let her know your preferences, and ask what strategies might help you to avoid the procedure. Your caregiver may perform massage of your perineum, use care in supporting your baby's head, or apply warm compresses to help your vaginal area relax and stretch in order to reduce the risk of tearing. You can also master breathing techniques that will help you hold back should your baby be arriving too quickly, which can reduce your risk for tearing.

Research vs. "Purple Pushing"

In hospital rooms across the nation (and on reality birth shows), nurses can be seen commanding mothers in the second stage to push: "Ready, take a deep breath, now hold it and push, push, push!" Then, the count begins: "1...2...3...4...5–" until the number ten is reached and the purple-faced mother is allowed to gasp for air before the push command and the counting begin all over again. This can help if an epidural blocks the urge to push, in which case it can help to let the epidural wear off a little.

In 2000, the Association of Women's Health, Obstetric, and Neonatal Nurses (AWHONN) issued an evidence-based guideline recommending that breath-holding or forced pushing be avoided during this stage. It suggests that mothers be free to rest and not push in the early part of this stage, even if they are fully dilated; that they be allowed to rest through some contractions if they wish; and that they be allowed to push in any way they feel comfortable, such as pushing for only 4 to 6 seconds with only a slight exhale.

STAGE 3: BABY IS BORN!

What's Happening During the Third Stage

This stage of labor begins immediately after the birth of your baby and ends with the delivery of your placenta. (If you have a C-section, you'll skip this stage of labor.)

All during your pregnancy, the placenta has been anchored to the wall of your uterus by hundreds of capillaries and supportive connectors.

These anchoring threads are bathed in a pool of blood. After the sudden decompression caused by your baby's evacuation, several contractions will quickly close off the placenta's attaching fibers to help stop bleeding.

You may be asked to push when your care provider sees the first signs of the placenta detaching.

Expelling the afterbirth usually takes less than 15 minutes but can take as long as 30 minutes.

Once the placenta arrives, it will be examined to make sure nothing is still remaining in your uterus that could cause infection. After you pass the placenta your uterus will begin shrinking and hardening. You'll be able to feel the top of it near your navel. Nursing your baby will encourage your body to release *oxytocin*, which will help your uterus remain firm, or you may be given an IV of Pitocin or an injection to help it contract. In the meantime, ask that your baby be put on your chest. Unless there's a medical emergency, you can ask that newborn procedures like weighing and measuring be delayed so you can have a few moments to bond as a new family.

How Long the Third Stage Lasts

Five to 30 minutes.

How the Third Stage Feels

With the excitement of seeing and holding your baby for the first time, you may be mostly oblivious to this stage of delivery, unless your care provider presses the top of your uterus as your placenta comes out, or massages your uterus immediately after the placenta is born, in an effort to help close off open blood vessels. That can be painful.

COPING WITH PAIN DURING LABOR

There are lots of solid reasons for simply having your labor and giving birth without painkilling medications. Here are some of them:

- **Just when you think you can't stand it any longer, it's nearly over.** Many a woman has decided to get an epidural at the very moment when the first stage of labor is coming to a close, only to be too numb to push effectively. Just before giving birth, it's not uncommon for a woman to utter something like, "I think I'm going to die," or "Please give me a c-section," at which point everyone in the room smiles knowingly, because that means the baby will be born very soon.
- **When it's over, it's over.** Once your baby is born, you'll have

some post-birth contractions to expel the afterbirth and shrink the uterus, but other than that and *afterpains* (which can range from vague to intense), you'll be done. Unless you've lost a lot of blood, you'll be able to get up, get in the bed on your own, eat a big meal, whatever you choose to do.

• **Safer and easier recovery for baby and you.** Although medications may appear to be benign for babies, virtually every drug that enters a mother's body is also transferred through her bloodstream to her baby. Babies have very poor resources for processing and eliminating chemicals. Research is lacking on the potential long-term effects of epidurals or narcotics on a baby's delicate brain and nervous system, particularly if the effects don't show up until later, although there is currently no evidence of harm to babies.

Using medications sparingly during labor, or not at all, can protect your baby and help to maintain efficient contractions. That, in turn, will help to protect your baby from being oxygen-deprived, particularly if medications lower your blood pressure or speed up or slow down your contraction. Plus, you'll have more freedom of movement and avoid unpleasant drug-related side effects, such as drug-induced nausea and vomiting, itching, or having a hangover afterward.

• **No worries about side effects.** Even though most epidurals succeed in removing the pain of labor, an epidural can cause you to have problems urinating, numb

your lower body to the extent that your balance and ability to walk safely are affected, mute your natural urge to push during the second stage of labor, and change your sensations and awareness of giving birth. Sometimes epidurals work unevenly or not well for some women, and the drug mix can cause nausea and itching or, more rarely, serious side effects, such as drastically lowering your blood pressure, affecting your sense of being able to breathe, or leaving you with a severe, prolonged headache. (Newer techniques are helping to combat that.) Some opiate-derived narcotics can cause constipation, making your first bowel movement after having your baby a painful ordeal.

BIRTH WITHOUT DRUGS

Today's obstetrical mind-set is that labor is painful, and no mother should have to suffer through it if she chooses not to. While this may be true, it's also true that with comfort measures and support many women report feeling empowered by their ability to cope with labor.

There are a host of nondrug alternatives available to help you in dealing with the pain of labor. Most nondrug approaches rely on giving the body alternative sensations during contractions can help to interfere with the delivery of pain signals to the brain. But nondrug strategies only serve to distract you from pain signals; they don't have the power to completely eliminate the pain.

During transition, most mothers are cranky and have a compelling need to be left alone and untouched by others. In that case, any effort to do things to you, mechanical or human, may only serve to raise your level of irritation. But once you know that's where you are and that you'll soon be pushing your baby out, even transition can become bearable.

Some strategies are practical and easy to apply, such as the use of warm compresses or ice packs, standing in a warm shower, or sitting in a tub of warm water. (See Water Birth and Hydrotherapy, page 186.) Other techniques require practice or the help of an expert.

Even if you plan to take an epidural or use other drug options for pain, it makes sense to have some effective nondrug pain management strategies up your sleeve. They will come in handy when you're at home, in early labor, and managing afterpains.

Continuous Support

The gold standard for coping with the discomforts of birth is to have someone accompany you through your experience who will be there for you, encourage you, acknowledge your progress, and make you feel protected and nurtured. That person could be your life partner, your sister, or someone else of your choosing, such as a calm and reassuring friend or, best of all, a doula or labor assistant who knows the ins and outs at your particular hospital or birth center.

Bear in mind that many physicians don't appear until you get close to time for delivery. For most labors, support, such as it is, will come from multiple labor and delivery nurses on rotating shifts. So planning to have someone there for you the whole time is the biggest step you can take toward a lower-stress birth.

Massage

A woman who is experiencing lower back pain during labor may find deep massage of her lower back between and just above the buttocks using the heels of the hand or pressing of the pelvis on both sides during a contraction can bring relaxation and temporary relief.

Firm massage of the hands or feet can also be very soothing and help a mother stay relaxed. Rolling pins and small paint rollers are sometimes handy for helping with back pain. Having someone stand behind you and press your hipbones firmly from both sides can also help ease discomfort.

Reflexology relies upon reflex points on the feet that correspond to organs and structures of the body. By gentle manipulation and pressing certain parts of the foot, the sensation of pain during labor can be reduced.

Movement and Positioning

Movement and frequent position changes are age-old (and instinctive) comfort measures for labor. Mothers-to-be have historically used standing, swaying, and leaning forward or backward with support from others as a means for getting their babies out.

During late pregnancy, changes in hormones help to relax the ligaments and connective tissues of the pelvis so that the joints and bones that support the pubic area can stretch to accommodate your baby.

Moving around a lot—rocking your pelvis, swaying, walking, squatting, or raising one leg and supporting it on a chair, and bending forward while being supported in the front or the back—can all help the bones and cartilage of your pelvis to realign positions and stretch. In addition, being upright helps work with the force of gravity, rather than against it, which happens when you're lying down and your pelvis is reclined. Upright positioning and movement also make contractions more efficient. When a mother lies on her back, the baby must negotiate an angled exit, but when a mother stands, sits upright, or bends forward, a straight pathway is formed. Mothers often report that being in an upright position and being free to move around also makes their contractions stronger, but less painful.

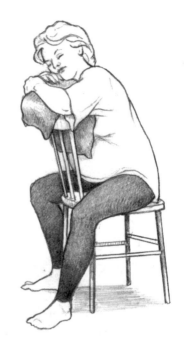

There are numerous positioning strategies you can use, even if you're in a cramped space. You can position yourself leaning over an adjustable hospital table with a pillow for support, sit on the toilet backward while using a pillow to support you under your arms and head, use a birth ball to posture yourself, lean back on your partner while being supported under the arms, rock in a rocking chair, or use modern-day birthing aids such as a suspended strap or labor bars.

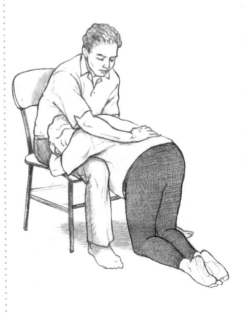

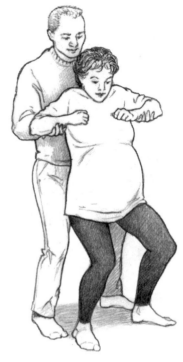

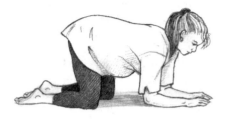

Relaxation Breathing

The way you breathe can affect your baby's oxygen intake, and it can also help you make it through contractions by altering your awareness of pain. Think of breathing as bringing in oxygen to send to your baby. Breathing too rapidly and shallowly, either on purpose or because you're fearful and anxious, will change your body chemistry and contract the blood vessels that feed your brain, which in turn will affect the flow of oxygen to your body and to your baby.

Breathing too fast can also increase a feeling of anxiety during labor, which then leads to increased tension in the body, heightening the sense of pain. In turn, a chain reaction gets started: fast breathing, more anxiety, and more pain sensations.

Slow, deep breathing using the muscles of your abdomen delivers air into your lungs and oxygen into your body and to your baby. Here's how it works: As you breathe in, move your diaphragm, the muscle deep at the bottom of your lungs, downward while pushing out your belly. This increases the volume of air flowing into your lungs by

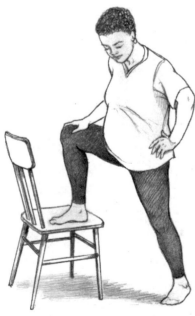

creating a partial vacuum to suck air in. Then, when you breathe out, your diaphragm muscle should rise back up into your chest while your abdomen sinks down to push out air.

It's easiest if you take air in through your nose and then breathe it out through pursed lips, although you can do both inhaling and exhaling through your nose or both through your mouth if your nose is congested. Take 5 to 6 seconds for each inhalation, and slow down from fifteen to seventeen breaths per minute to five to seven breaths, exhaling gently for the same amount of time after each breath.

Your chest should be relaxed, rather than tense. Most of the movement during breathing should be in your abdomen as it expands first, followed by your chest as it contracts to let out air. Air exchange should be flowing and relaxed with no pausing or holding your breath at any point.

Mastering the art of deep breathing will come in handy in the midst of labor. Try practice sessions three or four times per day where you change from shallow chest motions into the deeper breathing pattern that engages both your chest and your abdomen. Try to make your breathing slow, steady, and regular.

Again, if done correctly, your abdomen will rise when you breathe in, and contract and fall as you breathe out. Gradually, your everyday breathing habits will start to change. For help and support in getting your breathing straightened out, take a prenatal yoga class, attend a meditation group, listen to tapes on breathing, or join groups practicing chi-kung (qigong) or tai chi, both of which emphasize breathing skills.

Hypnotherapy

Being able to enter a hypnotic state can help your body relax, so your muscles and your uterus can work at peak efficiency. You can be taught self-hypnosis techniques in advance of going into labor that you can then employ during contractions. Hypnosis techniques are actually very simple and rely on focused concentration. You will learn with practice how to put yourself into a very relaxed state of mind in which your attention is deeply focused, yet you can remain highly aware. With proper training, you can learn to come in and out of your hypnotic state at will.

Hypnosis bypasses the active, critical part of the mind and gives suggestions for eliminating fear and pain. Through instruction or tapes, you can learn how to use a hypnotic cue, sometimes called an anchor, to help you enter the hypnotic state. Cues can also be used to help you feel anesthetized and numb to help in relaxation and comfort.

Since fear and tension increase the sensation of pain during labor, you will be shown ways to release fears so that you can enter into birth positively with visualizations of birthing comfort and breastfeeding success.

Mothers give hypnosis in birth a high rating for satisfaction, and current research suggests that hypnosis may be effective in reducing pain during labor. Studies show that mothers who use hypnosis are less likely to require drug-related pain relief, less likely to have their labors augmented, and more likely to have vaginal, rather than cesarean, deliveries. (See hypnosis sources in the Resources.)

Water Birth and Hydrotherapy

Women who have used warm water tubs and/or showers during labor sometimes report it to be more effective for pain relief than medication.

Studies show that as many as 90 percent of mothers who gave birth in water rate their birth experiences extremely positive.

Water birth is especially popular in France and the United Kingdom, where thousands of mothers have given birth underwater in spacious, portable pools available in most hospitals.

The ideal time for entering the tub or pool is when a mother is dilated between 5 and 6 centimeters. Entering the pool earlier than that can cause labor to slow down.

The water exerts an even pressure on the body, which is thought to discourage tearing during birth, and it gives the mother's body buoyancy, which makes it easier to find comfortable positions than on land. It is also useful for mothers with conditions such as physical disabilities or asthma.

Water birth requires careful monitoring of the baby's heart rate and the mother's condition and should only be used by mothers with normal labors that are progressing as expected. The baby must be *full term*, and not preterm or post-term, and in a normal,

head-down (cephalic) position. Water birth should not be used if there are signs of fetal distress, such as irregular or slow heart rate, or when your baby is passing meconium (stools). Mothers who have been given painkilling drugs should not attempt to labor or birth in water, nor should it be used if there are any complications for either mother or baby during the process of birth, such as a baby with insufficient oxygen during the second stage of labor, or for babies known to have cleft palates or other anomalies.

Mothers experiencing breech births or whose waters have been broken for more than 24 hours also shouldn't attempt water birth.

Although parents are concerned that their babies could drown during a water birth, babies have a dive reflex that enables them to hold their breath until their nose and face are exposed to air; plus, they're still being supplied oxygen from their umbilical cord.

Within seconds after a baby is born under water, he will be immediately lifted up and out of the water so that he can take his first breath.

Sterile Water Injections

Injecting sterile water directly under the surface of the skin has been used to eliminate lower back pain for mothers experiencing back labor, and research has found no known side effects and excellent results. The injections are done at specific points below the base of the spine (the sacrum) and are followed by the formation of a small, temporary swelling (weal) where the injection was done. Pain relief follows within 2 to 3 minutes and lasts up to 2 hours or longer.

If hospital policies permit it, nurses can administer the injections. First, the back is wiped with antiseptic, and then a small amount of sterile water is injected in four places. Ideally, the procedure is done with two people administering the injections on both sides simultaneously.

The injections cause an intense burning and sensation of pain that lasts 30 to 90 seconds. Relief from the procedure follows within 2 to 3 minutes.

It's not clear exactly why the injections are so effective, but it is thought to do with the way nerves can act as gates, closing off the transmission of pain to the brain when there is more than one competing signal. Although effective for lower back pain, the injections don't appear to have any effect on front labor—the discomfort of contractions.

If you'd like to have the technique available as a part of your pain relief arsenal, discuss it with your care provider.

Prayer

Many mothers report that prayer was one of the most powerful tools they had to get through labor. If faith and prayer can move mountains, it could very well move babies too. Certainly, if prayer is an important part of your religious faith, then it also belongs in your hospital room.

Conscious Relaxation

Being able to relax during labor is vital. If you are stressed and keep your muscles tense, you will exhaust yourself, and the hormones secreted in response to stress can affect the efficiency of contractions. When stress and tension last for a long time, it can reduce the oxygen supply to your baby in the same way that stress can affect your digestion, or it can speed up your heart rate, alter your circulation, or give you a headache.

Learning how to consciously relax can help you monitor your own tension levels. Good relaxation techniques will help keep you centered and focused so you feel more in control of your labor.

One relaxation system has been widely used in Europe for decades. It is called the autogenic method, or Schulz method, named after Dr. Johannes Schulz, who was the first to describe this technique. Schulz discovered that focusing on specific body sensations, such as imagining feelings of heaviness and warmth, can help the body to relax.

To apply the Schulz system, the student must master a series of relaxation techniques that are applied to various parts of the body. The client is guided to focus on feeling a sense of heaviness in the arms and legs, starting with the dominant side, followed by sensing a feeling of warmth in the arms and legs, then warmth and heaviness in the heart area, in the breathing, in the abdomen, and ending with coolness in the forehead.

Slow breathing accompanies each step in this progression, and a silent phrase is repeated five to seven times with each formula, such as "my arm feels heavy," "my heart feels warm," before you open your eyes and stretch. It is recommended that each focus area be mastered individually before moving on to the next by using twice daily repetitions. The concept is to be an alert but passive observer of body sensations. Some people have visual imaginations that easily can picture what is being asked and respond to it, but others may not be able to.

Most childbirth education courses offer parents helpful relaxation strategies. For example, the **Bradley Method** teaches a series of relaxation techniques coupled with deep breathing exercises to encourage physical, emotional, and mental relaxation during the stress of labor. There are a number of other forms of meditation and relaxation, including Transcendental Meditation (TM), Buddhist practices, and yoga breathing techniques, that can be applied not only to labor and giving birth, but also to the everyday stresses of life.

Making Sounds

A birthing mother's throat and voice can be useful tools for encouraging the progress of labor. Opening your throat, making whatever sounds come, and visualizing or saying the word "open" can connect your mind and body to encourage progress.

MEDICATION FOR LABOR PAIN RELIEF

There are a variety of pain relief options that use medications to help mothers with the pain of labor and birth. **Analgesia** is the term used for drugs that mask pain or change a mother's mental state so that pain becomes less anxiety-producing.

Analgesia is usually administered in labor through an injection or fed into your veins through an IV line. Besides making you drowsy, analgesia can affect the baby and cause him to be sluggish or have trouble breathing after birth.

Anesthesia refers to a category of drugs that numb pain by altering the transmission of pain signals from the mother's nerves to her brain.

Regional anesthesia injects medications into a mother's spinal column, cervix, or vaginal ring to produce a loss of sensation in that specific area.

General anesthesia administered through a face mask renders a mother completely unconscious and is usually reserved only for emergency cesareans where speed is of the essence.

Local anesthesia (a local) is directly injected into a specific part of a mother's body to provide specific numbing to that body area. An epidural, which allows for a continuous flow of numbing medication into the epidural area of the spinal cord, is by far the most popular painkilling method for labor. It can provide almost total relief from labor pain while allowing a mother to remain awake and aware.

Spinal anesthesia (getting a spinal) is similar to an epidural but uses a lower dose of medication injected in the space under the membrane that covers the spinal cord. It is usually used for cesarean sections when rapid painkilling effects are needed. More recently, spinals and epidurals are being combined, which is called a CSE (combined spinal epidural).

Regardless of the pain relief options you choose for labor, it's important to weigh the side effects on both you and your baby. Some medications can cause nausea and vomiting; others make a baby sluggish and may interfere with breathing immediately after birth.

Some have been shown to place the mother at greater risk for having her labor augmented or having to have forceps or vacuum extraction used to deliver your baby.

There are a variety of ways to learn about pain-relief options. Your healthcare provider should be your number one source, but many childbirth preparation courses discuss these options.

All About Epidurals

In the 1900s, pain relief in childbirth was a progressive feminist cause, and middle- and upper-class women sought out obstetricians who offered the latest scientific breakthrough, twilight sleep, which was a combination of morphine and scopolamine that let women give birth either without pain or without the memory of the pain (no one is quite sure which). But twilight sleep turned out to have some pretty heady side effects, not just completely removing a mother from the birth experience, but dangerously suppressing the baby's breathing. Fortunately, spinal anesthesia technology, developed in the 1920s, became progressively safer and more refined and eventually became routinely used to relieve labor pain.

Epidurals are by far the most effective painkilling method for labor and birth, and as many as 90 percent of laboring mothers in community hospitals are opting for epidurals or spinal blocks.

Some medical situations may require an epidural. For example, an epidural, spinal, or CSE will be used in place of general anesthesia for cesarean sections, except during dire emergencies when speed is of the essence. The type of medication and dosages may be different for these situations than during labor.

A healthcare provider may also recommend a mother have an epidural if she appears to be in extreme pain, or if her labor has lasted for many hours, she seems to need time to rest, or she has been given a labor-inducing drug to make contractions intensify.

How it feels to have an epidural. Healthcare providers have different policies about the best time during labor to administer an epidural. Some prefer to postpone it until a mother's dilation is 4 centimeters or more, so there is no possibility it will interfere with the delicate balance of labor becoming established.

Prior to getting an epidural, an IV line will be inserted into the back of your hand, or in your arm, and taped down to keep it in place.

A blood sample will be taken from your arm into a tube to test the clotting speed and to obtain your blood count. An IV bag will be attached to a hanger beside your bed and connected to the neck of the catheter taped to your hand to administer fluids to prevent a fall in blood pressure.

An anesthesiologist or anesthetist will perform the actual epidural, and getting one usually takes between 10 and 20 minutes, sometimes longer if he has a problem finding a workable location for inserting the needle between the vertebrae of your lower back. If you are petite, be sure to remind the anesthesiologist of your height, since being less than 5'4" may affect the strength of your dosage.

The anesthesiologist will wear gloves, a mask, and sterile gown to help prevent infection. You will be asked to sit upright and then to lean forward with your legs dangling from the bed or supported by a stool, or you may be instructed to fold your legs in front of you on the bed. Some mothers are instructed to lie on their sides in a curled-up fetal position. All of these positions are to round your back and help to enlarge the space between the small bones of your lower back.

Your back will be wiped with an antibacterial liquid, after which you will receive a numbing injection near the insertion site a little lower than halfway down your back. You may momentarily feel a stinging or burning sensation. After the area becomes numb, a long, thin needle will be inserted between spaces in the vertebrae of your lower back until the epidural space that surrounds the spinal cord is located.

An extremely thin tube (catheter) will be threaded through the needle, and the needle removed. The tube will be secured on your back with tape to keep it from moving. A syringe will be fastened onto the other end of the tube to administer a drug, or a combination of drugs, such as bupivacaine, a numbing anesthetic, and possibly a narcotic (such as fetanyl) used to strengthen and lengthen the effects of the drugs. After it's inserted, you probably won't be aware that the tube is there.

Once the epidural is in full effect, you may feel euphoria from having the pain taken away, and want to simply take a nap (and if you can, you should). As your epidural takes over, your legs will begin to feel heavy, warm, or tingly. Then your lower belly and hips will also start to become numb, but you will continue to feel pressure signals for your lower body and have total movement and sensation from the waist up.

Medical reasons for not having an epidural. If you have any of these problems, make an appointment with the anesthesiologist or nurse-anesthetist who will be handling your epidural prior to going into labor to discuss potential complications. Here are some medical reasons for avoiding an epidural:

- **You're taking blood thinners.** If you have been taking anticoagulants because of heart or stroke problems, it could affect the healing of your epidural injection site.
- **You have a skin condition or infection.** An infection on your lower back near the injection site could cause problems.
- **Blood-clotting problems.** If you have blood-clotting problems, your epidural may have problems healing.
- **Spinal deformities.**

Abnormalities in your spine could affect the ability of your anesthesiologist to administer the epidural in your spinal column and could affect the spread of the medication.

• **Nervous system disorders.** Since an epidural affects the way your nerves transmit pain signals, a CNS (central nervous system) disorder may make having an epidural unadvisable.

Potential epidural side effects. An epidural may cause one or more of the following:

• **Itching and nausea.** Approximately 1 out of 5 mothers experiences itching caused by synthetic opioids related to the morphine/heroin family used to strengthen the epidural and make it last longer. Symptoms for most mothers are mild and temporary, but very rarely, symptoms can be extreme. Medications are available to treat them.

• **Fever.** Epidurals can cause epidural fever, a rise in a mother's temperature not related to infection. First-time mothers are five times more likely to have a fever higher than 100.4 than mothers who have previously given birth, and it is estimated that 24 percent of first-time mothers will experience fever. A baby's body generally remains 2°F warmer than the mothers', so when the mother's body heats up, the baby's will too, which in turn speeds up the baby's heartbeat.

Fever could also signal an infection, which is of serious concern and could be treatable. Both mother and baby may be treated with antibiotics as a precaution against infection, and the baby may be shipped off to the nursery for a workup and observation.

The baby may be given blood tests and possibly a spinal tap. One study of newborns whose mothers had epidural fevers were almost twice as likely to undergo *sepsis* evaluations than mothers who didn't and had to stay in the hospital a day longer than babies whose mothers did not have a fever.

• **Sudden drop in blood pressure.** Epidurals can cause *hypotension*, a sudden drop in a mother's blood pressure, which can affect the baby's oxygen supply. Treatment includes administering extra fluids and drugs known as vasopressors, such as ephedrine or phenylephrine, through an IV, which constrict small blood vessels to restore blood pressure to normal.

• **Longer labor.** Unless epidural medications are reduced during the second stage of labor when it's time to bear down, mothers having epidurals may not feel the urge to push. Mothers having epidurals will generally take longer to push the baby out than those who haven't. They are also more likely to be given oxytocin (Pitocin) or other drugs that make contractions stronger and closer together.

• **Increased rate of instrumental and cesarean deliveries.** There is an increase in the number of deliveries with forceps or vacuum extractions during the bearing down stage. Some believe that epidurals are associated with an increase in cesarean section for dysfunctional labor (*dystocia*), but it is not clear from current research whether epidurals actually lead to more cesarean sections, or mothers with longer, poorly progressing labors are more likely to use epidurals and require cesareans.

- **An out-of-position baby.** Studies of epidurals have reported a 20 to 26 percent incidence of babies being out of position or failing to rotate normally during birth. *Malpresentation* can prolong labor and lead to instrumental delivery using forceps, vacuum extraction, or cesarean section.

- **Headache.** Spinal headache, or post-dural puncture headache (PDPH), affects approximately 1 out of 100 mothers who have epidurals. Symptoms can last from 2 to 10 days or longer. It is caused by the leaking of spinal fluid from the membrane that surrounds the spinal column and is treated with a procedure called a *blood patch*.

- **Extremely rare complications.** Some mothers experience prolonged tingling and weakness in their legs, and very rarely, temporary or permanent paralysis in the legs that affects walking. Some patients having epidurals have *convulsion*s (seizures). While epidural-related deaths are extremely rare, potentially life-threatening complications are estimated to occur in about 1 out of 4,000 cases. When major neurological and brain damage has occurred in patients, it has been associated with oxygen deprivation caused by profound drops in maternal blood pressure.

There are also rare reports of enduring spinal nerve damage.

Your baby's position and other vital signs will be monitored throughout your labor to ensure that he is doing well. One way that a baby's progress during labor is tracked is through noting the baby's position in his mother's body.

Symptoms of an Epidural Headache

- Stiff neck.
- Pain that radiates to your neck.
- Pain in your forehead and back part of your head that increases when you're sitting up or standing, but decreases when you're lying flat.
- Pain that lessens when pressure is applied to your abdomen.
- Nausea and vomiting accompanying the headache.
- Vision problems, such as sensitivity to light, seeing double, or difficulty focusing.
- Auditory symptoms, such as a loss of hearing, ringing in the ears, or extreme sensitivity to noise.

Your Complete Cesarean Section Guide

Cesarean sections are now the most common major surgical procedure performed in the United States. According to the estimates available at the time of this publication, 36.7 percent—more than 1 in 3 women—in the U.S. undergo c-sections every year.

Higher c-section rates may have much to do with a changing population. Women giving birth today are, on average, older and more likely to be overweight, two factors likely to lead to a complicated delivery for a variety of reasons. An increase in the use of fertility drugs has also led to more multiple births, which often necessitates a c-section. And induction of labor has also been on the rise; according to the Centers for Disease Control and Prevention (CDC), between 1990 and 2006 the use of labor induction has increased from 10 to 22 percent of all deliveries, and induction is associated with double the risk of c-section delivery.

And, finally, c-section rates are high because about half of c-sections are repeat c-sections. Though the ACOG revised their practice guidelines to encourage providers to allow women to give birth vaginally after a previous c-section, many hospitals and healthcare providers still won't allow VBAC.

"Nonreassuring fetal status" is the main reason you may be urged to have a c-section, and is the given reason for about a third of cesarean deliveries. This means that the baby's vital signs are indicating a possible problem—the baby's heart rate is abnormal or a test of the fetal blood shows that the baby is not getting enough oxygen. Your healthcare provider may ask you to change positions, give you oxygen, or if you're using Pitocin, lower the dose. If none of this helps and the baby is still showing signs of distress, then you may need to have a c-section. In most cases the baby is fine, but providers of course want to err on the safe side, since a lack of oxygen to the baby can be serious.

Failure to progress is when a woman doesn't give birth after being in labor for a certain amount of time—either dilation doesn't happen, or the baby is unable to descend. About 18 percent of c-sections are attributed to a lack of progress in labor.

If there are no signs that your baby's in trouble and you're willing to wait for a vaginal birth, yet you're being told something along the lines of "if you're not dilated by X centimeters in the next X minutes, you're going to need a c-section," ask for more time and try walking around or changing position, drinking water, or sitting on the toilet or a birth ball to stay upright. A 2007 survey of moms found that one-fourth of those who'd had c-sections felt like they'd been pressured into it by hospital staff. To keep that from happening to you, if you're told that you might need a c-section, make sure that you know and understand the reason. If the baby's showing signs of distress, of course you don't want to take chances. On the other hand, though, a *fetal heart rate* that seems too fast, slow, or irregular by itself is not necessarily the sign of a problem.

If you need to, ask for a second opinion from the on-duty head of obstetrics or a specialist in maternal-fetal medicine.

If your primary healthcare provider is a midwife, she won't be doing the surgery; it will instead be performed by the obstetrical backup on call at the hospital, and your midwife should still be able to suit up in scrubs and come in the delivery room to talk you through what's happening, if you wish.

THE CESAREAN SECTION EXPERIENCE

In preparation for surgery, your pubic hair will be clipped from the area where the incision will be done, and you'll be wiped down with antiseptic. You will have a catheter, a small tube, placed into your urethra to make sure your bladder stays empty. If you haven't had an epidural or spinal yet, the insertion can be uncomfortable, and you can ask that it not be done until your epidural or spinal goes into effect.

If you have sufficient pain relief, you should not feel the incision. If you do feel the doctor cutting, or any pain, inform your anesthesiologist immediately.

The table you are on will be tilted to the left or a pillow placed under your right lower back to keep the pressure of the weight of your uterus from pressing down on important arteries.

Your arms will be loosely fastened down on each side of you to prevent them from contaminating the sterile operating area. A sheet about eighteen inches high will be draped like a tent in front of you at about chest level so you won't be able to see the surgery. But your partner may be allowed to take pictures or a video of your baby when she emerges from your belly.

You'll also have a blood pressure cuff on your arm to keep track of your blood pressure, EKG leads to monitor your heart rate, a hep-lock in the back of your hand to administer IV fluids or medications, and a clip on the tip of your finger, called a pulse oximeter, to keep tabs on the oxygen levels in your blood.

All of this can feel quite disempowering, which is why it's so important to have someone in the room who is telling you what's happening.

The whole procedure is remarkably quick: it will take 5 to 10 minutes to remove your baby.

Here's what happens on the other side of the drape: your abdomen will be opened with an incision through your skin and abdominal tissues along the lower abdominal crease a little above your pubic bone. The opening will be pulled apart, with muscles and tissues separated either with tools or with the surgeon's fingertips.

Once an adequate opening has been made, your obstetrician will reach inside your uterus and place a hand under your baby's head. Your baby's head will be exposed first, and then the doctor will gently ease out the rest of the baby's body, which will feel like a sense of pressure followed by a strong tug as your baby's body emerges through your incision.

Some hospitals offer to hold a mirror so a mother can see the baby being pulled out. It's normal to have temporary feelings of vulnerability or fear. Having your partner or labor assistant telling you what's going on will help.

Your baby will be taken to a warming cart and his mouth and nose will be suctioned. The baby will finally begin to cry, and your baby will be given an Apgar rating. Your baby's weight, length, and time of birth will be recorded. You may then be aware of the pushing and pulling of tissues and organs as they are being handled after delivery. The placenta will be delivered while the surgeon feels inside to make sure that the entire placenta has been removed, so no pieces of tissue are left inside to cause infection, and you will be given oxytocin intravenously to help your uterus contract back to pre-pregnancy size.

The next step will be to repair the incision made into the uterus, then sewing together the layers of abdominal tissue cut during the surgery. Your incision will be closed with stitches, usually in two layers, and the whole process usually takes less than a half-hour.

After surgery the interior stitches will dissolve on their own. Staples may be used along the outside of the cut; they will be almost painlessly removed later.

Sometimes surgical tape or a dissolvable suture is used instead to seal the incision.

Once the surgery is complete, you will be rolled into a recovery room, and in some cases, you may be transferred onto another bed by nurses or orderlies who will pick up your sheets and slide you across from one surface to another.

You'll be covered with a warm blanket and are likely to stay in the recovery room for an hour or more, while your blood pressure and other vital signs being monitored. You may continue to be hooked up to an IV solution hanging from a pole on wheels, and still have a catheter in your back from the epidural. You'll have a bandage taped over the stitches to protect them, and a tight elastic band around your waist to keep the incision site from being jostled. You may also have a pad and possibly cold packs in your underwear for any fluids and to reduce any swelling.

Some hospitals also use inflatable leg cuffs that blow up and deflate, which encourages blood circulation.

In the postpartum recovery room, hospital staff will be coming in often to check your blood pressure and temperature and make sure you're not experiencing any complications from your surgery.

An anesthesiologist will come in to remove the catheter in your back, and the IV will be removed at some point as well, though staff may want to keep your hep-lock in for a while in case they need access to your veins.

If you were given general

anesthesia for an emergency c-section, you'll probably feel groggy and just want to nap.

If you choose to breastfeed, you'll need help with positioning. Ask the nurse or a lactation consultant to help you arrange pillows and get a good latch.

YOUR RECOVERY FROM CESAREAN SECTION

The first sign that your epidural is wearing off will probably be a pins-and-needles feeling in your legs and pain at your incision site. How quickly you start to get your sensations back will depend on the type of analgesia you had, how strong a dose was used, when you received your last dose, and your own body's response to medication.

Don't be shy about asking for more pain medication if you need it: painkillers work best when you take them before pain gets unbearable. Make sure your nurse knows that you plan to breastfeed, since some medications aren't recommended for nursing mothers.

The next day you may also begin to feel stomach cramps from trapped gas, which is common after any sort of abdominal surgery. Pulling in your abdomen and grunting as you exhale helps expel the gas. Just as with mothers who have given birth vaginally, you may become aware of your uterus cramping as it squeezes shut and shrinks as it recovers from birth.

You may be encouraged to suck on ice chips or be offered clear liquid or juice to drink. Later, you may be offered regular foods.

The purpose is to stimulate your intestines and colon so your bowels will start acting again. Avoid carbonated beverages, though, because they may lead to more gas pain.

Soon after delivery, you may be asked to do simple foot exercises to help prevent blood clots from forming in your legs, and deep breathing exercises to help clear your lungs.

At some point the nurse will come in to remove your catheter. Although you probably didn't feel the catheter being put in, you may have momentary, mild discomfort and a burning sensation while it is being removed. You may have difficulty urinating for a while after removal. Bruising and swelling can block your *ureter*, the 4-centimeter-long tube that goes from your bladder to the urinary opening. Drink plenty of water and try warm water from a squirt bottle on the upper part of your vagina as you try to urinate. If that still doesn't work and your bladder is unpleasantly full, buzz and tell the nurse.

You'll also be encouraged to get up and walk within hours after your surgery, unless your legs are too wobbly to support you. It can be really painful as you start to sit up and your abdominal muscles contract into the incision site, and nurses should be there to help you when you get up and walk to the bathroom for the first time.

If you've had a c-section you can expect to remain in the hospital for 72 hours after the time of delivery, as opposed to the 48 hours mandated for a vaginal birth. If you have complications, your stay may be extended even more. You'll also be more likely to be re-admitted to the hospital in the weeks following birth.

After you get home, you're going to need help for the first weeks after your surgery. If your partner is unable to stay with you to help you around the clock, consider enlisting the support of other family members or hiring a nurse or postpartum doula. You should never be left alone in the house with the baby until you've recovered enough to get out of bed on your own and pick up and carry your baby.

The surface of your cesarean incision will heal around 6 weeks after your surgery. You may initially have numbness at the scar site, and some mothers develop scar tissue, called keloids. A cesarean is major abdominal surgery. It will take at least 6 weeks for you to recover, and some mothers experience pain at the incision site much longer. Some amount of permanent numbness around the scar site is also normal.

POTENTIAL CESAREAN SECTION COMPLICATIONS

A cesarean is major surgery, and with it come risks. Rarely, the surgery can be life-threatening, leading to hemorrhage (severe bleeding), blood clots, and infections of the uterus or the incision area. (Most women are routinely given antibiotics as a preventive measure.) In some cases c-section mothers develop twisted and blocked intestines in the years that follow the surgery as the result

of scarring and the formation of scar tissue (adhesions).

Pain is also an issue with cesareans. It is more intense and longer-lasting in the days and weeks following surgery than giving birth vaginally. Even picking up your baby in the early days can be tough. You will be likely to be using pain medication to help you cope with that; make sure that you bring medication home from the hospital. In some instances mothers who have had cesareans suffer from ongoing pain in the lower abdomen, probably due to scarring from the surgery.

In rare instances, women with cesareans are more at risk for undergoing an emergency hysterectomy (removal of the uterus) in the early weeks after birth. They are also more likely to have blood clots, or suffer cuts and nicks of the bladder.

C-SECTION RISKS FOR FUTURE PREGNANCIES

Surgical birth leaves scars behind and affects the strength of the uterus, which can impact future births. Women who have had c-sections are also slightly more likely to have difficulty conceiving in future pregnancies and to have ectopic pregnancies.

Placenta misplacement is also more common with women who have had cesarean sections, due to scars and weakening of the uterine wall. Previous c-sections also increase the risk of stillbirth in future pregnancies.

In addition to physical

risks, c-sections take their toll emotionally on mothers, who reported in a survey conducted by the Childbirth Connection (*www. childbirthconnection.org*) that they tended to be less satisfied with their birth experiences, and felt that they had less control over their births. They were also more vulnerable to depression after birth (***postpartum depression***, or PPD). If you find yourself having flashbacks to your c-section or are feeling angry, depressed, or hopeless in the weeks after you come home from the hospital, it's important to let your healthcare provider know and to seek support—there are c-section recovery support groups online, and many hospitals and birth centers host postpartum support groups for new moms that can be a valuable lifeline during recovery.

Having a Home Birth

If you are expected to have an uncomplicated labor, having your baby at home may also be an acceptable alternative to a hospital or birth-center birth, though in the U.S. less than 1 percent of mothers give birth outside of a hospital setting, with about 27 percent of these moms in free-standing birth centers and 65 percent in a residence).[1] Home birth is not as safe an option if you have a preexisting physical condition that could negatively affect your labor, such as a history of stillbirths, bleeding problems, a prior cesarean section, or other preexisting physical problems associated with complications.

Should complications arise that could not have been anticipated in advance, you may need to be transported to the hospital for specialized care. Know that there are rare but potentially serious risks associated with the delay in access to hospital care that could happen should you experience a major complication like placental abruption, fetal distress, or other serious problem during homebirth. It's estimated about 12 percent of moms who attempt home or birth-center births are transferred to a hospital during or soon after labor and birth. If you're going to go for a home birth, enlisting the services of a trained, certified midwife is essential. One overview of the outcomes of six studies of 24,000 planned home births found home birth to be an acceptable alternative to hospital care for selected low-risk pregnant women.

Mothers who had a home birth had fewer medical interventions.

Having a home birth is also your least expensive option and will provide you with uninterrupted privacy in the comfort of familiar surroundings.

If you elect to have a home birth, you can find excellent sources online to help you in preparing for your big event, including the equipment you should have on hand and what your midwife will probably supply. (See Resources at the back of this book.)

Giving Birth to Twins or Multiples

Twins occur in about 3.2 pregnancies out of 100, triplets about 1 in 10,000, and quadruplets in 1 out of every 512,000. The use of *in vitro fertilization (IVF)* and fertility drugs is increasing the chances of mothers having multiples. Women ages 30 to 40 are also more likely to give birth to twins, as are African-American mothers. *Monozygotic* (identical) *twins* come from the same egg splitting in two, while *dizygotic* (fraternal) *twins* come from two eggs fertilized by two different sperm, but other than having genetic testing, or discovering your babies are different sexes during a sonogram, there's no way to know which type of twins your babies are until they're born.

Twins may share one placenta but have two different amniotic sacs, or each of your babies may have its own placenta. Twins and multiples bring a number of risks. They may be low birth weight; they may suffer from twin-twin transfusion, in which one twin steals blood from the other; they may have a greater risk of preeclampsia (toxemia), placental problems, or cord accidents; and they may be out of position for birth. The greatest risk is that your twins will set off the labor process early and be born prematurely before their body systems have had adequate time to mature. If both babies are positioned head downward, which happens with 45 percent of twin pregnancies, and your babies are full term and a good size, you will probably be able to deliver them normally. Twins often weigh less than normal because they've had to vie for space inside. They typically arrive between weeks 36 and 37 of pregnancy, and between 10 and 15 percent of twins are born by 28 weeks.

You have a 45 to 50 percent chance of needing a cesarean if you have any risk factors, such as placenta previa or *intrauterine growth retardation* (IUGR), if your babies are out of position for birth, or if you start labor early, rather than making it to full term. If you're carrying three or more babies, then it's almost certain you will be delivered by cesarean section.

Even if both of your babies are in the right position, your labor and delivery may be more difficult than normal. For example, your second baby may have trouble getting down the birth canal. An epidural may be suggested for you, which will let you have a quicker transition into a c-section if something goes wrong. It will also allow your healthcare provider to manage a breech birth or to massage your uterus should there be excess bleeding.

Vaginal delivery for your first twin has been shown to be safe for both mother and baby, and for your second baby, if he is large enough to make it through safely. But if your babies are both breech (bottom down) or are in other odd positions, then your healthcare provider may feel that it's wisest to allow you to carry your babies as long as possible, and then schedule a cesarean section.

Your birth experience will be the same as mothers giving birth to singletons, except things may take a little longer. Whether you give birth vaginally or your babies are delivered by c-section, they will be temporarily named "Baby A" and "Baby B," depending upon which baby comes out first.

Carrying multiple babies will cause your pregnancy to be considered high risk because multiples raise the potential for complications during labor, including premature delivery. As with other conditions, careful monitoring will help to ensure that your pregnancy and labor progress normally and that you and your babies aren't endangered in the process.

Your Baby After Birth

Once your baby arrives, there will probably be a deafening silence in the room. Everyone will be waiting for your baby to breathe: the most important, first step of surviving in this world. After what may seem like an eternity, at last you will likely hear sputtering, gasping, and then the lusty wails of new life. Most babies will breathe within a minute after birth, and everyone heaves a collective sigh of relief. The baby's breathing! The baby's okay! It's a girl! (or) It's a boy! You'll find yourself elated by that news, even though a sonogram may have told you that months ago.

Your newborn will be gently suctioned with a rubber bulb with a pointed end to remove blood and fluid from mouth and nose.

Your baby's chest will be watched to see that breathing is normal and regular, and his heart rate monitored to see if it speeds up to about 100 bpm or more. His color will be assessed from blue to pink, and he will be checked for how well his muscles flex by looking at how tight his fists are.

He will be dried off quickly to reduce heat loss and chilling from evaporation. Many care providers now place the baby in *skin-to-skin contact* with you and then try the baby on your chest. At last you get to meet this little person who has been squirming around inside for so long.

FIRST BREATHS

While your baby was still in the womb, he floated inside a warm balloon of amniotic fluid with his lungs filled with a mildly salty liquid. Babies swallow the liquid and take practice breaths from time to time, but that's a far cry from inhaling the icy cold air of planet Earth for the first time. Those first breaths are critical and sometimes can make the difference between life and death. During your baby's trip down the birth canal, up to one-third of the fluid filling his lungs will be expelled from the pressure exerted on his small chest. Lung tissues will absorb the remainder of the fluid.

As your newborn gasps in

air with every scream, his skin coloring will rapidly change from a rich, purplish blue into a bright, cherry red as his circulatory system changes from getting oxygen through his placenta and umbilical cord to getting it through his lungs. Sometimes whether a baby needs extra help or not can't be determined until after he is born.

At other times, certain signs are used to tell if a baby might need help right after birth. These include the baby being born before 34 weeks of pregnancy; too slow or irregular baby heartbeats during labor; fresh stooling from the baby (meconium) that arrives before the baby does; a baby's having retarded growth during pregnancy; twins and multiples; abnormal *presentation*s, such as feet first; a birth that requires a forceps delivery or vacuum extraction because he gets stuck; a baby born by cesarean section; when a baby and mother have blood incompatibility; and when a mother's been put to sleep with general anesthesia.

If a baby needs help, he will be laid on a special padded cart with the bed tilted so his head is slightly lower than his feet to help fluids to drain out. The equipment on the cart includes a heater, an oxygen supply, suctioning devices, a stopwatch, a resuscitation bag to pump air into the baby's lungs, a baby-size face mask, a laryngoscope for peering down the baby's throat, special tubes for suctioning and draining, and drugs for stimulating the baby's system if needed.

CLAMPING AND CUTTING THE CORD

Within a few minutes of birth, your baby's umbilical cord will be squeezed together by a plastic clamp, and then painlessly cut off, leaving a stump. Usually the stump and the umbilical area will have medication put on it to help protect it from infection, which may make the stump purple.

It will take 2 to 3 weeks for the cord to dry and wither before it falls off on its own, leaving the belly button behind. As it dries, it may have an unpleasant odor, but don't try to manipulate it into coming off early—that can cause bleeding and make your baby more vulnerable to infection. In the meantime, newborn diapers with a U-shaped belly cutout will help keep the diaper from irritating the cord. If you're using cloth diapers, you can simply make a fold to be sure the stump is exposed to air.

Some healthcare practitioners suggest gently cleaning the stump with a cotton ball dipped in plain water, or they may suggest rubbing alcohol, which could cause your baby discomfort because it burns. Be sure to contact your baby's healthcare provider if there is any bleeding, pus, or swelling that suggests an infection. The way your baby's cord is cut has nothing to do with whether your baby will have an "inny" or an "outy" belly button. That's determined by the muscular structure of your baby's abdomen.

WHAT HAPPENS RIGHT AFTER BIRTH

Your baby will be weighed and measured, evaluated (see Apgar score), given an ID bracelet or anklet (or both), given a shot of vitamin K, have antibiotic ointment applied to his eyes to ward off infection, and have his footprints recorded. A sample of blood from his umbilical cord will be sent for tests. Ask the hospital staff for a copy of the footprints as a memento.

If you're in a hospital, you may be given an IV of Pitocin to stop postpartum bleeding and help your uterus contract. If you had an episiotomy and/or tearing, you'll be given a shot of a local anesthetic and stitched up, usually with dissolving stitches hat won't need to be removed but will need to be kept clean.

Your Baby's Apgar Score

Soon after your baby is born, your healthcare provider may tell you that your baby was given a 7, a 9, or a 10 Apgar score. The score will be written down in your baby's record. It is used to help birth attendants assess how well a newborn is doing right after birth in order to make a decision about rescue operations, such as helping the baby to breathe.

The word Apgar is derived from the name of Dr. Virginia Apgar, an anesthesiologist in obstetrics who developed the scoring system more than 50 years ago. By interesting coincidence, each letter of Apgar's last name—A–P–G–A–R—stands for things birth attendants observe in the baby immediately after birth—Activity, Pulse, Grimace, Appearance, and Respiration. Your baby's score will be calculated twice—1 minute and 5 minutes after he's born. More recently, the score refers to a baby's color, respiration, heart rate, reflex irritability, and tone.

Experienced practitioners make the calculations in their heads. The score at the 5-minute point is the most telling. If the baby's score is 7 to 10, everything is progressing normally. A score of 4 to 7 says the baby may require some extra measures to help him breathe. Babies with scores of 3 or less are in serious trouble and need emergency care, such as CPR or deeper suctioning to clear their lungs of fluid. In some cases, babies with very low scores may be showing the first signs of lasting problems, such as damage from oxygen deprivation or birth defects, but many babies with very low scores at first turn out to be perfectly normal over time.

Your Recovery from Birth

Soon after giving birth, you may remain in the delivery room for a little while, then you'll be transferred from the labor and delivery area to your own postpartum recovery room. If your baby is rooming in, he will be given a bassinet in your room. If the baby is in the nursery, he will be brought to you at least every 3 hours for feeding. If he is in your room, nurses, residents, and occasionally doctors will come in to check the baby's vital signs a few times a day.

What to do during the first hours after birth:

- Rest. Hospitals are noisy, interruptive places. Your sleep may be broken by a nurse wanting to take vital signs, check your pads or stitches, or give you medicine.
- Drink water. Keep yourself hydrated, especially if you lost a lot of blood.
- Page a nurse if you need help. That's what they're there for! At first you may need help getting to the bathroom or lifting your baby in and out of bed for nursing and diapering.
- Use painkillers. Ask for medication if you are in pain. Your healthcare provider will prescribe a medication schedule for you, and you may need to remind nurses of the schedule.
- Get good breastfeeding advice. At most hospitals you'll get a visit from a lactation consultant, who will help you position your baby and make sure he is latching on well. (For more about breastfeeding, see the next chapter.)
- Watch for symptoms. Report any of the following symptoms immediately: a fever, a headache, a gush of blood or passing large clots, feeling faint, sharp pain and swelling or heaviness in one leg, unusual pain in your chest, not being able to urinate.

If you had a vaginal delivery you'll have a pound of cold packs, padding, and gauze in your underwear, and stitches if you had an episiotomy. Keep your stitches clean by spraying or pouring warm water over your perineal area following urination. Then gently pat (don't wipe) dry from front to back with toilet paper, a damp warm washcloth, or wipes premoistened with witch hazel.

Other tips for managing healing *perineal sutures*:
- Use a small footstool to reduce strain on your stitches.
- If sitting hurts, try an inflatable doughnut-shaped "peri-pillow," available in pharmacies. Also, some mothers find sitting in a hard chair more comfortable than in a mushy one.
- Tuck and hold in. Tense your buttock muscles and Kegel before you sit down or stand up so that you pull your sore parts in and up.
- Practice Kegels to encourage your muscle and tissues to heal.
- Ask for a stool softener to prepare for your first post-birth bowel movement.

If you had a c-section your lower stomach will be wrapped in bandages and elastic. You'll need help getting in and out of bed for the first few days, because the surgery cuts through the connective tissues of the abdomen and stretches out the lower abdominal muscles. You'll also have staples and strips of medical adhesive (called Steri Strips) holding the suture together. As your pain relief medications wear off, the stitches may hurt or itch.

Many moms report a delay in milk production after a c-section. If your baby shows signs of dehydration or loses more than 7 to 10 percent of his or her body weight in the first 24 hours and pumping produces only a few drops of colostrum, your nipples are sore, and you're exhausted, it's okay to let the hospital staff give the baby a bottle-feeding or two until your milk comes in—one or two bottles of formula will not prevent you from being able to breastfeed.

Speaking of formula and breastfeeding, hospitals often send mixed messages about them. On one hand, nurses report that some hospitals now have a policy of refusing to give a baby formula the first time a mom asks and sending in the lactation consultant instead. On the other hand, the hospital will likely send you home with a plush diaper bag of formula samples and coupons, courtesy of a formula company that they have a marketing agreement with. It's also not unheard to get conflicting advice from different people in the hospital.

Our advice is to listen to the lactation consultant over other member of the hospital staff when it comes to breastfeeding and do your best to breastfeed, but also stand up for your own needs. If you want a nurse to give the baby a bottle so you can rest up to heal and check out of the hospital, that's okay. You can still try again to breastfeed in a few hours or the next day. And while breastfeeding is healthier for you and your baby, if you choose to bottle-feed your baby will still be fine.

Anyway, getting back to recovery, vaginal or c-section, in the hours and days after birth, new moms may also experience:

• **After pains.** Your uterus begins shrinking right after the placenta is delivered in order to shut off open blood vessels. Within 30 minutes after birth, it reduces to the size of a large grapefruit. It will return to a more normal size within 6 weeks after birth. In the meantime, especially in the first 3 to 4 days after birth, you'll experience after-contractions that feel like menstrual cramps and can range from mild to intense.

• **Sweats.** After birth your hormones shift and cue your cells to release all of that extra fluid they were retaining to sustain the baby. So during the first week postpartum you may find yourself waking up with the sheets soaking wet, even if your room is a comfortable temperature. A waterproof pad can help keep your mattress clean.

• **Breast discomfort.** During the second to sixth day after birth, as your breasts begin milk production, they can feel full and sore, which is called engorgement. This can be particularly uncomfortable if you elect not to breastfeed or if your baby's not positioned correctly at your breast. The stretching and friction of your baby's mouth and tongue action can also cause nipple pain. Putting cool cabbage leaves in your bra can help. (Really! Cabbage has anti-inflammatory properties.) Let your healthcare provider know if breast pain persists past the first week postpartum.

• **Breast changes.** Giant nipples, stretch marks . . . will your breasts ever be the way they were? As long as you're breastfeeding, your breasts will be full and the same cup size as they were a few days after the baby was born. After you wean, your breasts will gradually lose weight and become flatter, and they may hang lower than they did pre-pregnancy. This "deflation effect" can even make them appear smaller than before. (This happens to mothers who bottle-feed too.) Fortunately, the changes may be so subtle that no one notices them but you. Any stretch marks on your breasts will gradually fade to a lighter color, although they may never disappear completely. After you wean, your nipples will return to their normal size and color over time. Your Montgomery glands, the white spots on your nipples, will stay enlarged for a while. Eventually they'll shrink, but they may remain more visible than before you became pregnant.

• **Achy pelvis.** You may have pelvic pain if your baby was very large or arrived in an odd position, your pelvis was very narrow or unusually shaped, or your tailbone (coccyx) was injured during delivery. There is no way to splint a broken or injured tailbone; it will simply have to heal in time.

Most hospitals have a policy of getting new birth moms up as quickly as possible to help speed recovery and to protect them from forming blood clots in the legs. Don't be surprised if you're weaker than you imagined.

You may be terrified of having your first bowel movement after birth. If you had a c-section, you won't be released from the hospital until you've passed gas. You'll probably be supplied with a small, plastic squeeze bottle to fill with warm water for rinsing off your sore perineum every time you go to the bathroom.

It's okay to ask your nurse to take your baby to the nursery when you need a rest. Also, call the nurse to take the baby to the nursery if you need to take a shower or leave the room for any reason. If your hospital has lactation consultants on staff, take advantage of their skills. You'd think that, like most bodily functions, breastfeeding would be self-explanatory, but if you've never done it before, it can be tricky and frustrating. Trust the advice of the lactation consultant above all others—even postpartum nurses have been known to give conflicting or erroneous advice.

Ask if the hospital has a number that you can call later if you have breastfeeding questions or problems. (Also see our discussion about breastfeeding on pages 238–246.) If your baby is being observed or treated in the NICU, you and your family members should be allowed to don sterilized scrubs and visit.

Your care provider, or a partner in the same practice, will check on you. She will feel your uterus to make sure it's contracting properly, check your stitches or incision site, and, startlingly, may "honk" your breast to make sure you're making milk. Your care provider should also instruct you on how to care for any stitches or incisions.

She should also check to see if you have hemorrhoids, and give you cream to use for them, if necessary. Make sure that your partner has installed a car seat in time for the ride home. Most hospitals won't let you drive off without one.

Five Postpartum Don'ts

Once you and your baby get home, make an appointment with your healthcare provider for your first checkup, which most schedule about 6 weeks after birth. You may need to be seen sooner if you develop problems. Until your post-birth appointment, here are the basic five don'ts suggested by most healthcare providers:

1. Don't drive if your stitches are still painful or you're under the influence of opiate or narcotic painkillers.
2. Don't lift anything heavier than your baby.
3. Don't have intercourse before you've healed.
4. Don't use douches or tampons.
5. Don't do strenuous household chores.

STAGE 4: SENSATIONS AFTER BIRTH

What's Happening

Your uterus is starting to firm up and shrink. Open blood vessels and capillaries in the uterus are closing off. Your hormones are beginning to shift. Your milk-making glands start to activate, which stimulates your breasts to produce high-protein colostrum. Your milk will come in within a couple of days. Your body starts processing all of the fluids and tissues of pregnancy so it can return to its non-pregnant state.

How Long the Fourth Stage Lasts

The official dimensions of this stage are 24 to 36 hours during the immediate postpartum.

Actual recovery takes about 6 weeks for your body to become completely functional and up to 6 months to feel like your normal self again.

How the Fourth Stage Feels

After your elation and adrenaline rush wears off, you may begin to feel deeply tired and achy. Your **perineum** will be sore and swollen, and you will probably experience aches and pains. If you've had an epidural, you may start to have a pins-and-needles feeling in your legs and hips as the painkillers wear off. (If you've had a c-section, see page 196.) You will have heavy bleeding from your vagina and require maxi-pads for a while. Your breasts may become swollen and hard after about a day, called **engorgement**. Walking may make you feel weak and dizzy, but you will be encouraged to get up and walk within hours of birth to discourage blood clots. Your body will stay in its pregnant size for quite a while, and your belly will probably stay mushy for months.

Tiredness and temporary **baby blues** are typical.

It's only human to shy away from pain. Most of us would do anything to not have to endure it. And, yes: childbirth hurts. For most mothers, it's more than the discomfort that birth instructors once labeled the sensations of labor in order to minimize mothers' fears. Pain has a utility in birth. It's a powerful signal for a mother to find a safe place and to encircle herself with caregivers.

Your Body Postpartum

Immediately after birth, your healthcare provider will declare the official birth time, and while the baby is being weighed and measured, given eye drops, and having his or her reflexes tested, your doctor or midwife will be putting you back together again by stopping any excess bleeding and stitching up any c-section or episiotomy incisions. The noise, bustle, and intensity of hospital delivery rooms can be so disorienting that if you've had an epidural, you might even forget for a moment that there's a baby involved until you suddenly hear a small, catlike cry.

Once all's well, then comes to golden moment when your healthcare provider places your baby on your chest and you can finally look into one another's eyes.

Your baby will know who you are right away from your unique smell and the sound of your voice. Enjoy this moment as long as you want to, and don't let anyone rush you through it. After your baby beholds your face for the first time, he or she will start turning his or her head from side to side, *rooting* for a nipple. In case that's not enough of a hint, your nipples may also start tingling, itching, or even burning. Your healthcare provider or a nurse should help you position yourself and baby for the first feeding, which will not only nourish the baby and start building his immune system, but will also cue your uterus to start contracting

from the size of a watermelon to the size of a pear.

After the first feeding, if you're in a hospital, you will likely be moved from the large, relatively plush birthing suite to a smaller, more Spartan postpartum recovery room, while your baby is taken to the nursery for shots, heel-printing, and a bath. If there are any shots or tests you don't want performed on the baby, or if you want to delay his bath, make sure you or your partner communicates that to the pediatric nurses before they take him to the nursery.

Some hospitals will make sure you empty your bladder before you leave the delivery room, and will catheterize you if you're too swollen to pee on your own. If you had an epidural you may experience tingling or other side effects as it wears off over the next 2 to 4 hours.

From the turn of the century until the mid-90s, most hospitals kept babies in one big nursery room, only bringing the baby to mom by her request. But these days more hospitals practice rooming in, which is keeping the baby with you in your postpartum room unless you ask to have the baby taken to the nursery. Or, if your baby needs extra help or monitoring, he or she may be sent to the NICU (neonatal intensive care unit).

Right after delivery, in spite of having been awake for days and exerting yourself to the limit, you may find yourself hyped-up and unable to sleep. Try to eat and drink something if you can, and let nurses or your partner take care of the baby while you get some rest. If your hospital practices rooming in, you'll need to call the nurse to have the baby taken to the nursery if you want to try to have an uninterrupted stretch of sleep or a shower, or if you need to pick the baby up but can't due to a c-section or painful stitches.

Once the initial adrenaline rush and the excitement of finally giving birth is over, the hormones will die down, and you may begin to feel some of these other sensations:

- **Exhausted.** You may feel as if you just ran a marathon or went for a round in the boxing ring.
- **Sore and swollen.** Your vaginal and perineal area has undergone a lot of stretching and trauma, and if you got stitches from an episiotomy, they may hurt. The pain is worse when you sneeze or cough, and at first when you sit down or walk. ("Please, don't make me laugh!")
- **Crampy.** You'll have contractions or after-pains as your uterus shrinks back to its pre-pregnancy size.
- **Woozy and trembly.** Especially if you've lost a lot of blood, you may feel woozy and shaky.
- **Headache-y.** Tell your nurse right away if you have a headache. If it's severe, it could be a side effect of your epidural, or it could be a sign

of preeclampsia, especially if it's accompanied by swelling in your face, fingers, and ankles.

- **Uncomfortable going to the bathroom.** Urinating the first time may be difficult if you had a catheter inserted during a cesarean or epidural. Most women are also constipated for a few days after birth. Drinking a lot of water may help. Note that opiate-derived painkillers, such as codeine, may make constipation worse. If you're too shaky to get out of bed, you'll be given a bedpan.
- **Sweaty.** Much of the fluid you retained in the weeks before birth will be sweated out in the days after birth. You may wake up with the sheets soaking wet. You may be too unstable to shower for a little while too. Many new moms report that the first postpartum shower is the best of their lives.
- **Achy.** Your muscles may be strained from the exertion of labor and pushing. Your tailbone area (coccyx) may hurt.
- **Bruised.** It's not uncommon to have bruises on your body that you don't remember getting. If you had an IV, epidural, and/or injections, you could have bruises from them too.

5

You and Your Baby

Here's a brief summary of newborn basics: what they look like, what they do, and what to do with them.

Newborn Looks

The baby models you see on television and on greeting cards are usually pudgy 6-month-olds. Typically, a newborn looks reddish, splotchy, and puffy. Babies born by cesarean section will have rounder heads; babies delivered vaginally will have elongated heads from the squeezing of the birth canal. In the first few days baby's head will return to a more rounded shape.

Your baby's skull will have two sunken places, which are the *fontanels*, or soft spots. The spots are where the bones of the skull have not yet fused. You will see a diamond-shaped indentation on the top of the head and a smaller triangle-shaped one toward the back of the skull. The soft spot may have a pulse, but the membrane and skin over the fontanels are pretty tough, so you need not worry about it getting punctured. The triangle-shaped one will fuse together first, at between 2 to 12 weeks of age, while the larger one on the top of the head will close by around 2 years of age.

Babies born in the later weeks of pregnancy will have chubbier cheeks and more hair. Babies born prematurely are often wrinkly because they haven't had time to develop a fatty layer beneath their skin and may have few or no eyebrows or lashes.

WEIGHT

The average newborn weighs 7½ pounds; between 5½ pounds and 10 pounds is considered a healthy range. If your baby is smaller or larger than 90 percent of babies his same gestational age, it could be that you and your baby's father are very small or large people, or it may signal a physical problem.

A loss of 5 to 7 percent of birth weight is normal in the first 72 hours after birth. Weight loss of more than 9 percent in the first week is a sign that breastfeeding needs to be evaluated—your *letdown* may have been delayed because of medications or a physical problem, or the baby is not latching properly.

Babies should regain any lost weight and be back to birth weight by 10 to 14 days after delivery. Your baby's pediatrician will check baby's weight, length, and head circumference at the first appointment.

Baby Weight-Gain Guidelines

0-4 months: 5.5-8.5 ounces per week
4-6 months: 3.25-4.5 ounces per week
6-12 months: 2.0-4.0 ounces per week

Growth spurts announce themselves with a baby's increased appetite and the strong demand to nurse more frequently. They usually occur when a newborn is 7 to 10 days old and later at 3 to 6 weeks of age.

Babies who are born smaller than normal are called small for gestational age (SGA). That means the baby is smaller than 95 percent of all babies born that same number of weeks of pregnancy.

A baby may be small because he has small parents. But in some cases this small size can signal that the baby did not get adequate nutrition during pregnancy, or because labor was induced or a c-section scheduled too early. If poor nutrition is the cause, the baby may have had intrauterine growth retardation (IUGR).

IUGR can be caused by chromosomal abnormalities, poor functioning of the placenta, or the mother's illness or smoking during pregnancy. A tiny baby may have trouble breathing and low oxygen or blood sugar levels, or trouble keeping warm, and he may require support in a neonatal intensive care unit (NICU).

Exceptionally small babies are sometimes more vulnerable to breathing problems and other complications, while a larger-than-normal baby may signal a problem with blood sugar levels and need extra feedings to help control the problem.

A baby is labeled as large for gestational age (LGA) when he is larger than 95 percent of babies the same gestational age. Some babies may be too large to safely be birthed by their mothers, and a cesarean section may be required. Many babies are big because their parents are large, too. Besides inheritance, the most common cause of LGA is a mother with diabetes, which causes her to pass high blood sugar levels onto her baby. This causes the baby's body to produce extra insulin, which results in excessive baby weight and size. After delivery, the baby's blood sugar may rapidly drop, which may make the baby fussy, jittery, and ravenous for feeding. A heel prick may be recommended to test the baby's sugar level, and the baby may be given sugar water or formula, or fed through an intravenous line.

SKIN

Some newborns develop peeling skin after birth, especially on their palms and soles, and some are born covered with a downy layer of hair called lanugo on their shoulders, down their backs, and sometimes on their faces, too. It will soon disappear.

A newborn's skin is very thin, almost translucent, and changes color with shifts in temperature. It may appear cherry red, mottled, or sometimes bluish or even bruised from his trip down the birth canal. All babies, even if they have dark skin, appear pinkish and fair-skinned at first until the skin's natural pigment develops. Your baby will redden all over if he has been crying, if you're changing his diaper and clothes, or if he's urinating or straining at a bowel movement. You may glimpse blue veins underneath his skin that are transporting blood back to his tiny heart and lungs for oxygen.

At birth, your baby's skin will probably be coated with streaks of a creamy white substance called vernix, especially in folds and creases. The vernix served as a protective ointment while your baby floated in his mildly salty amniotic bath during your pregnancy, and it has antiseptic properties. If left alone, the vernix will naturally be absorbed into your baby's skin or be rubbed off. Hospitals bathe babies soon after birth because the vernix and amniotic fluid are considered body fluids that could potentially contain infectious agents. If you ask to delay the baby's bath, nurses and doctors will have to wear gloves while handing him until he's bathed, which is a mild inconvenience for hospital staff but a double-win as far as the baby's concerned.

A newborn's skin is very sensitive to dryness and may peel and be vulnerable to rashes, particularly if his skin comes in contact with irritants, such as the chemicals and perfumes in detergents used to launder his clothes and sheets or those found in premoistened diaper wipes and baby skin products.

Some babies are born with birthmarks, skin discolorations or semi-permanent bumps that generally go away on their own.

Stork bites, sometimes called salmon patches or angel kisses, are reddish or pink patches that often can be found above a baby's hairline, at the back of his neck, on the eyelids, or between the baby's eyes. They are caused by collections of tiny capillary blood vessels close to the skin that darken when your baby cries. They generally fade within the first 2 years.

Mongolian spots are large, blue-gray, bruise-like marks, often on the lower back or buttocks, most often found on babies with dark skin. They generally fade over time, although in some cases they never disappear entirely.

Café-au-lait spots are permanent birthmarks that are light and coffee-colored and usually occur on a baby's torso, arms, or legs, while *strawberry marks* are soft, raised marks that will turn red usually at about a month of age. Sometimes strawberry marks grow larger over time, but they almost always disappear before a child reaches age 10.

EYES

You may notice that your newborn's eyes are very sensitive to glare. Shielding his eyes from the lights in the delivery room may encourage him to open his eyes wider to gaze at you. During the first weeks after birth, newborns don't generally shed tears when they cry. After 3 to 4 weeks, your baby's eyes may start to appear glassy and there may be a tear or two when he cries. In time, he will shed copious tears, mostly when crying.

A newborn's eyes can appear puffy and swollen for a day or so, the result of natural fluid accumulation from having lived in the amniotic sac for so long coupled with the pressures of birth. You may also notice red streaks in your baby's eyes caused by broken blood vessels from birth pressures. All of these eye problems quickly disappear.

All babies are born with lighter-colored eyes than they will wind up with eventually, because the color-producing cells of the eye haven't started working yet. Your baby's eyes will reach their mature shade of blue, green, or brown between 1 and 3 years of age.

Babies are also born unable to focus on objects at a distance: they can see about 12 inches—the exact distance for focusing on your face when he's nursing. Your baby's ability to understand visual signals and to focus his eyes matures rapidly during the first few months of life.

By the time he is 6 or 7 months old, his vision will have sharpened from 20/500 (legal blindness) to 20/50. Then he will be able to recognize you when you walk into the room, tell the difference between day and night, and discern whether objects are close or far away.

Some newborns have eyes that don't appear to work well together. One eye may wander in a different direction than the other, or both eyes may appear crossed. True crossed eyes are rare in babies. If your baby's eyes are actually crossed, light will not reflect the same way from both eyes. More often, the appearance of crossed eyes is an illusion caused by having a wide bridge between the eyes and thick folds on the upper eyelids. Most eye alignment problems resolve themselves in the first 12 weeks of life. After the first 12 weeks, if one eye appears crossed or turns outward while the other doesn't, your baby may have weak eye muscles on one side. If after the first 4 months you suspect your baby's eyes are crossed or not working together, confer with your baby's healthcare provider.

If a visual problem is suspected, your baby may be referred to a vision specialist (ophthalmologist). In rare instances, a baby may be given small glasses to balance the visual input from both eyes so that the brain learns how to process signals evenly, or, more rarely, surgery may be suggested to correct more serious eye coordination problems.

HEAD AND NECK

Your baby's head will appear to be attached almost directly to his chest at first, and as he matures, his neck will begin to elongate. Some babies have uneven neck muscles that cause them to hold their heads cocked to one side. This is called *torticollis*, and it may result in an oddly shaped head from uneven pressure in the back. It can be caused by the baby's cramped quarters inside the uterus, or it may result from injury during birth.

The shortened neck muscle that pulls the head to one side may seem swollen in the weeks that follow birth, or it may have a small lump the size of an olive. After 2 or 3 months, this condition usually resolves on its own. Sometimes babies develop torticollis following birth from remaining in the same position while sleeping or riding in the car. You can help your baby's shortened neck muscle to lengthen and become more flexible by gently changing his head position during sleep or in his car seat.

NOSE AND BREATHING

A newborn's nose is flat, which helps him to breathe and nurse at the same time, even when a mother's breasts are pillowy and

large. Babies' breathing may be noisy even though it is perfectly normal. While young children normally breathe twenty to thirty times a minute, newborns breathe twice as fast—forty to sixty times a minute. Your baby's breathing will naturally get faster if he has a fever, which is his body's way of trying to cool down.

Signs of infant breathing problems are:
• Flaring the nostrils with each breath.
• Contracting and releasing of the muscles of the neck with each breath.
• Chest pulling (sinking) between his ribs or under his rib cage while struggling for breath.
• The belly moving up and down in an exaggerated way with each breath.

All these things are normal if your baby is crying, but not normal if he isn't. If you sense your baby is having serious breathing problems, or his lips become blue around the edges, go to the nearest emergency room. Do not try to feed him anything until you get help.

FACIAL EXPRESSIONS AND HEAD CONTROL

Newborns don't have control of their facial muscles as older babies do. They can grimace and yawn, and there may be spells of hiccupping. (Remember those bounces from inside when you were pregnant?)

Between birth and 4 weeks of age, most babies are able to briefly gaze at their parents' faces before blinking or dozing off to sleep. You're most likely to elicit this response from your baby if you position him face to face with yourself with about 12 inches of distance between the two of you. Sometime during that first month, your baby will also master briefly holding his head up when he's in a facedown position lying on his stomach. You also may notice that your newborn suddenly pauses at the sound of your voice or music, or he may awkwardly turn his head in the direction of your voice as you speak to him, as if he is trying to locate you.

Baby smiles or cooing when you smile, talk, or play with him don't usually appear until between 3 weeks and 2 months. Between 5 weeks and 3 months of age, your baby will be able to hold his head up for a long time when lying on his stomach, and he may turn himself over, at first by accident and then on purpose, between 2 months and 5 months of age. Your baby will gain head control when supported in an upright position sometime between 6 weeks and 4 months of age, but he won't be able to sit up on his own without toppling over for several more months after that.

Your baby may laugh and squeal by 6 weeks to 4½ months of age. Keeping a journal of your baby's emerging body skills and antics could be something you'll treasure in years to come.

HANDS AND FINGERS

You may be able to get your newborn to grasp your finger or a rattle or other object in his tiny fist, but he probably will be oblivious to what you're doing. A baby's toes can grasp too, especially if you elicit the **Babinski reflex** by gently caressing his arches. A newborn's grasping skills are probably left over from more primitive times, enabling a baby to cling tightly to the hair of the caregiver who is toting him. A hungry newborn has the power to propel his body toward your breast, and babies also change positions in their cribs by digging their small heels. Your baby will be able to bring his hands in front of him between 6 weeks and 3½ months of age, and to grasp a rattle placed in front of him by about 2½ and 4½ months. Some babies are born with scratchy fingernails. Until you can cut them, baby gowns with fold-over mittens may help to protect baby's face from getting scratched. Use baby-size fingernail clippers, and clip his nails when he's asleep. To make fingernail cutting easier, sit in a chair with a good light. Position your baby with his back to your chest so that his fingers will be in the same position as your own. Some parents, afraid of cutting tiny fingers, elect to file the nails with an emery board.

NIPPLES

Newborns of both genders may have puffy-looking breasts and can even secrete fluid from their nipples during the first weeks of life. This so-called **witches' milk** is a reaction to the massive dose of hormones babies get near the time of birth. These hormonal effects will disappear in the first few weeks after birth.

UMBILICAL CORD

All during pregnancy, your baby was nourished inside your uterus by the umbilical cord that fastened him to the placenta. When the baby is born, the cord is cut an inch or so out from the baby's body, and it may be bandaged. There is evidence that delaying cutting the cord for 2 or 3 minutes until it stops pulsating can help boost baby's iron levels.

The fleshy stump that remains will begin to dry up and darken in the days after birth. In about 2 to 3 weeks, it will fall off on its own. You shouldn't tamper with it or try to do anything to make it come off before it's ready. That could cause unnecessary bleeding and could lead to infection.

The best way to prevent infection is to keep the cord clean and dry. Use a cotton swab dipped in warm water to gently wipe away any moist debris and scabbing material that forms next to the belly. Give the cord lots of fresh air by keeping the diaper peeled away from it to help it dry up and heal.

Some babies are born with "outies"—belly buttons that are destined to stick out rather than turning inward. There's nothing you can do about that, so there's no need to fuss or worry. It's futile to use bandages, wraps, or other gimmicks to make it stay inward. They don't work and may irritate your baby's belly.

HIPS

Newborns don't have hipbones with sockets like those of children and adults. The socket for their hipbone is nearly flat, and the head of the hipbone must stay in the right position for the joint to form around it.

About one out of every hundred babies is born with flat hip sockets that may not form correctly as the child matures. Your pediatrician will check your baby's hips by holding your baby's knees and pressing down on the hipbones and then rotating the bones in their sockets. It's not painful, but if a "clunk" sound is heard, it means that the baby's bone (femur) is not in the appropriate place because the socket is too flat. This condition is called developmental dysplasia of the hip, or DDH. If your baby is diagnosed as having DDH, an X-ray or ultrasound exam may be recommended in order to determine a course of treatment. It may be as simple as double-diapering your baby, or a special harness to hold your baby's hip in place. In more severe cases, a cast or surgery may be recommended.

GENITALS

Your newborn baby's genitals may be swollen and red from the rush of hormones that your baby experiences as birth nears. Female newborns may also have a whitish vaginal discharge or a small amount of bloody spotting from withdrawal from the hormones she was exposed to in utero.

If you leave your son's *foreskin* intact, his penis will require no special care. Remember this handy rhyme: "If intact, don't retract, only clean what is seen."

If your son is circumcised, don't wash his penis with water until the incision site has healed completely, which should take 7 to 10 days. In the meantime, change his bandage every time you change his diaper, and your pediatrician may recommend putting a dab of Vaseline on the site to keep it from sticking to the diaper. Under normal circumstances your infant daughter's genitals don't require extraordinary care either.

Girls form a white substance in the folds of the *labia*, called *smegma*, and it's beneficial and necessary. If fecal matter gets into the vaginal folds, wipe from front to back with a warm, damp washcloth or baby wipe, or if the umbilical cord site has healed, dip her bottom in a warm bath. One important thing to remember about changing your daughter is to always wipe from front to back. Fecal bacteria (*E. coli*) in the urinary tract can lead to painful urinary tract infections in girls of any age.

Circumcision

Circumcision is the surgical removal of the part of the shaft skin of the penis that folds over the *glans* when the organ is in a flaccid state. If you choose to have your son circumcised in the hospital, the surgery is typically performed the day after birth, before you leave the hospital. The surgery can also be performed in a private doctor's office, or if you are Jewish, by a *mohel* who is medically trained to perform circumcisions as a part of a Jewish ceremony known as a bris. (Note that Medicaid in your state may not pay for this procedure).

Reasons for circumcision:
- **Religion.** If you're Jewish, then a brit milah is considered a commandment from God, though there is no requirement for how much skin must be removed to fulfill it.
- **Appearance.** Some parents prefer the look of a circumcised penis. The most common reason parents give for circumcision is that they want the son of a circumcised father to "look like Daddy."
- **Lower risk of HIV transmission in adults.** Circumcision appears to halve the risk of female-to-male transmission of HIV during unprotected sex. It's important to note, though, that the odds of a man becoming infected with HIV after one episode of penile-vaginal intercourse without a condom are 1 in 5 million (1 in 50 million with a condom), and even with a partner who is HIV positive are about 1 in 500. So the chances that the circumcision will someday prevent an infection are pretty tiny.
- **Lower risk of UTIs.** This is often cited as a benefit of circumcision, but the risks of surgery do not outweigh the potential benefit, says the American Academy of Pediatrics. (Most UTIs can be treated by a round of antibiotics.)

Reasons against circumcision:
- **Medical advice.** Every major medical organization, including the American Academy of Pediatrics and the American Medical Association, does not recommend routine circumcision. While circumcision may slightly

reduce the risk of certain diseases like penile cancer, the benefit does not offset the risks of the surgery. For every case of penile cancer prevented, an estimated forty-one babies die from surgical complications. Research has also found conflicting evidence for the claim that circumcision reduces the rate of HIV. Says the AMA, "Virtually all current policy statements from specialty societies and medical organizations do not recommend routine neonatal circumcision . . . The low incidence of urinary tract infections and penile cancer mitigates the potential medical benefits compared with the risks of circumcision."[1]

• **Ethics.** It's not easy to justify performing cosmetic surgery on a child who is not able to consent.
• **Permanence.** The surgery is irreversible.
• **Pain.** While there are ways to reduce the pain a baby experiences during and after the procedure, no method, not even a *dorsal penile nerve block*, eliminates the pain completely. Even today, the majority of circumcisions are performed without anesthesia.
• **Declining popularity.** While in the 1980s about 80 to 90 percent of newborn boys were circumcised, that rate dropped to 48 percent in the early 1990s. Some studies suggest the rate in the United States may be as low as 32.5 percent.[2] Worldwide only about 30 percent of men are circumcised.[3]
• **Complications.** While the immediate post-operative complication rate of newborn circumcisions is low (about 1 in 476)[4] some complications can be serious, including infection, hemorrhage, or uneven removal that requires additional surgery, and, very rarely, death from excessive bleeding.
• **Financial.** Not all insurance plans or state Medicaid programs cover the cost of surgery.
• **Sexual.** Circumcision removes the most sensitive parts of the male organ and the penis' protective covering, reducing penile sensation by a lot (which is exactly why it became popular in Victorian-era America in the first place).[5] It also reduces lubrication and sensation for a man's partner.

Your son's circumcision experience. If you elect to have circumcision performed in the hospital before you go home, it's a good idea to request to personally meet the person who will perform it and to discuss what kind of anesthesia will be used. Some hospitals relegate the surgery to relatively inexperienced surgical residents, and some do not provide pain relief unless parents expressly request it. Ask the surgeon about their level of experience and ask that your partner or other family member be with your baby during the procedure.

For a hospital circumcision, a nurse will come by before the procedure to make sure that you've signed the proper consent forms and to pick up your baby. The procedure should only be performed on healthy babies in stable condition.

Your baby's penis may be numbed, most often using a topical cream that is applied to the penis half an hour to an hour before the procedure. This cream, however, only numbs the surface of the skin and does not numb the pain from the tightening of the clamp used to hold the skin in place or from the incision. A dorsal penile nerve block (DPNB) uses a needle to inject numbing agents around the base of the baby's penis.

A newer method, called a subcutaneous nerve block, injects the painkiller directly into the penile shaft and has been found to be very effective in blocking pain with fewer side effects than other methods. Ask the person who plans to perform circumcision what numbing agents will be used.

Your baby will have his diaper taken off, and he will be strapped onto a board, called a "circumstraint," that spreads and restrains his legs and covers his body so that only his penis area is exposed. Since a newborn's foreskin is not fully developed and is tight, the doctor will stretch the skin away from the penis head and pull it forward. A metal clamp will be used to capture the skin to hold it in place so that the foreskin can be slit and trimmed away. There may be bleeding following the surgery, and the device purposely remains in place long enough for it to stop.

Following the surgery, your baby may be fussy and not interested in eating for a few hours. The end of his penis will be red, and after awhile, a yellowish crust may form around the incision site. Depending upon the procedure used, your baby's penis may have a dressing and gauze on it that will need to be changed when you change the baby's diaper. You'll be given written instructions about what to do. Normally, a baby's circumcision site will heal within 7 to 10 days. In the meantime, don't bathe him, other than with a washcloth or sponge.

Circumcision Emergencies

Call the doctor or go to the emergency room after a circumcision if your baby has:
- Discoloration of the penis
- Bleeding
- Pus, spreading redness, or fever
- No wet diapers for more than 3 hours
- Inconsolable crying

What if my partner and I disagree about circumcision?
Based on what we've heard from many moms, if your partner is circumcised himself and has never mentioned his feelings about circumcision one way or another about it, odds are he will want his son to also have the surgery.

And it also happens from time to time (though less frequently, in our experience) that moms will be for the surgery and dads are against it.

If you, the mom-to-be, feel that you don't want this surgery to be performed on your son, there are two tactics you can choose from: Bring it up with your partner, see what he says, and argue your points if you disagree. Or, you can opt to let your healthcare provider know you do not consent to the surgery and address the issue if and when your partner brings it up.

If you go with plan 1, there are no lack of materials out there to help you make your case. Just Googling "circumcision video" is usually plenty for most guys. You can also order an information packet from one of many online anti-circumcision groups, such as cirp.org, and there are nonfiction books on the history of the practice at your local library.

But before you whip out an audio-visual presentation with handouts, take a minute to consider how this might make your partner feel. Imagine if half of women in the world had cosmetic vaginal surgery as babies, you were one of them and had always assumed your husband was fine or even preferred the look of your lady parts. If he suddenly came at you with, "this surgery is a terrible thing and I don't want our daughter to have it," even if you agreed with the logic, it might also make you feel self-conscious and defensive.

So consider letting your partner bring it up if it matters to him, and make your case then. He may not even mention it.

If he does bring it up, let him make a convincing argument for the surgery. The same applies if you are a dad who's against the surgery and mom is for it. Lawsuit-wary hospitals won't perform a circumcision unless you both consent, so there's really no need to resort to extreme tactics or months of debate when a "nah, I can't consent to that" will do.

Should a parent who's against circumcision surgery consent to

it so the pro-circumcision parent won't sulk? That's a relationship question lots of moms (and some dads) have grappled with since the practice began.

If you and your partner are at a serious impasse on whether or not to have the procedure performed on your son, another option is to decide to delay the decision for a specific amount of time—after you arrive at the hospital, for instance, or before your son turns 2.

Uncircumcised penis care. Uncircumcised baby penises don't require any special care or cleaning. Don't try to retract the foreskin or clean under it or let doctors or nurses do so; forcible retraction can cause injury. The foreskin will naturally become fully retractable when your son hits puberty, usually between the ages of 11 and 16. Once the *prepuce* is retractable, your son will need to wash under the foreskin with plain, un-soapy water.

> **TIP**
>
> After circumcision, most hospitals sell the discarded foreskins, which can be cultured into *stem cells* and used to make skin grafts and wrinkle creams, and for cosmetic testing.

Babies Who Need Help

All parents look forward to bringing their new babies home with them from the hospital, but if you have a baby or babies who are premature, or if your baby is full-term but has health issues, she may be transferred to a neonatal intensive care unit (NICU, pronounced "nick-ewe"), a specialized baby-care facility found in larger hospitals.

A NICU's staff is made up of specially trained nurses, doctors, doctors-in-training, and other healthcare professionals to take care of your baby. The list may include a clinical nurse specialist who is an RN with a master's degree in nursing; a *neonatologist*, a pediatrician with special skills and training in caring for premature and sick newborn; a neonatal nurse practitioner (NNP); and special nutritionists and therapists to help manage your baby's needs.

There may be a social worker assigned to you too, trained to counsel you and your partner through the experience, including managing healthcare arrangements and financial issues. Some hospitals also have support groups for parents of babies in the NICU.

Walking into the NICU after your baby has been whisked away is a scary and surreal experience, completely different than what you probably imagined it would be while you were pregnant. You will be instructed how to wash your hands and arms, and you may need to wear a special gown inside. Instead of cuddling with your baby in a hospital bed surrounded by flowers and balloons, you're surrounded by bright lights and babies with all sorts of health challenges, each hooked up to beeping and flashing machines. Your baby may be hooked to wires and tubes and a mask to assist with breathing, and you may not be able to hold her at first. Most hospitals also don't allow children in the NICU, too, which can be difficult if you have other children who are eager to meet their sibling.

The emotional experience of having things go awry for your baby can be incredibly wrenching. Everyone reacts differently to stress. It's not unusual to be strong and in control while a crisis is going on, then break down later when the immediate crisis has passed. Having to go home or back to your room and leave your baby behind is an indescribably empty feeling. It can help to know that the NICU staff really care and that your baby is in the safest possible place with people who are best trained to help her, and that the *prognosis* for babies who are premature or have health issues has never been better.

Depending on what your baby's health issue is, you may or may not be able to hold her. Skin-to-skin contact (aka *kangaroo care*) can have powerfully positive effects on newborns. Even if you can't hold your baby, a gentle, still touch, like a light hand on your baby's back or belly, can have comforting effects. Talking to your baby can also soothe her—she will hear and recognize your voice. And though it's difficult to do, you may also be able to help by pumping breastmilk. If your baby is premature, you may meet with a specialized nutritionist to help you feed your baby in a way best suited to her needs. Depending on your baby's health issues, before you check out of the NICU you may need to take a specialized preemie-care and/or infant CPR course, and your baby may need to pass a car seat test, where she's monitored for a time while strapped in her car seat to make sure she can get home safely. If your baby is very small, you may need to get a new car seat that is rated to accommodate her size.

Before you leave the hospital:
- Make your baby's first pediatrician appointment.
- Get a copy of your medical records. At some point you may have questions about what happened during delivery, and this information will also be especially valuable if you ever decide to get pregnant again (never say never!). Also write down your birth experience and any questions you want to ask your healthcare provider while the experience is fresh in your memory.
- Also get a copy of your baby's medical records, especially if your baby had health issues or was in the NICU for any reason.
- Put your discharge instructions, medical and legal records, and newborn's footprints in a safe place.
- Make sure your baby's car seat is installed properly.
- Take home any prescription medications you might need, and make sure you have the right number of refills prescribed.
- Bring home any opened packages of diapers, sanitary pads, breast pads, breast pump bottles and tubing, slipper socks, and other personal care items.
- Leave the *formula* samples if you plan to breastfeed, but check the formula company's goody bag for any other coupons or other supplies you might want.

YOU AND YOUR BABY, ALONE AT LAST!

The First Week at Home

Yes, birth is beautiful spiritually, but bodily . . . not so much. Even if your birth was uncomplicated, your major muscle groups have gone through hours of work, the skin on your stomach and bottom has been stretched to the maximum, and you may not have eaten or slept for 24 hours or much, much longer. In the days after birth you'll be bleeding and bruised, and if you're in a hospital, woken up around the clock, punctured, groped by various doctors, nurses, and/or lactation consultants, and, by the way, completely responsible for the life and major medical decisions of a tiny, helpless infant. These are the times that try women's souls. It's no wonder that moms come out of the hospital feeling weak, rattled, and shell-shocked. And if your baby needs intensive care you may be operating in crisis mode for a lot longer than you'd anticipated.

A home-birth experience will be a quieter and more intimate, but no less tiring, experience.

Here's what you need to know to get you through the first days and weeks after birth.

Your labor is over, you've given birth, and now it's time to return home to start recovering and

exploring life with your new baby. As you'll soon discover, getting over childbirth and coping with a newborn is extremely challenging, but doable.

Your Recovery

The five most important things to know about the early postpartum period:

Call your healthcare provider or the nurse on duty right away if you develop a fever or blurred vision, if you have problems urinating or having a bowel movement, if you pass blood clots larger than a quarter, or if your bleeding increases or soaks more than a pad an hour.

Also call your healthcare provider if your breasts develop red streaks or lumps or you develop sore spots; these could be the signs of infection or a plugged or infected milk duct. Nipple pain at the start of breastfeeding is normal, but call your healthcare provider about any nipple pain that persists beyond a week postpartum. And call if you develop:
- Pain in your calves, which can be a sign of a blood clot or inflamed vein
- Breathlessness
- Swelling in your face or fingers
- Unpleasant-smelling vaginal discharge
- An inflamed incision
- Abdominal pain that doesn't go away

You'll need help at home, someone to stay with you to help you out for at least a week or more after you leave the hospital. If your mom, partner, or relative can't be

home with you, ask your healthcare provider or pediatrician to help you find a postpartum nurse or doula to stay with you and get you through the recovery period.

It's a good idea to avoid vigorous exercise, lifting anything heavier than the baby, and vaginal intercourse for at least 6 weeks postpartum. And if you have a c-section, expect to be mostly bedridden for about a week (though you should get up and walk around one floor of the hospital or your house several times per day to help speed healing).

You *will* sleep in unbroken stretches again someday, after your baby's stomach grows enough to hold more milk and her sleep cycles become established. But in the meantime, for the first 6 weeks to 4 months, wanting to be held and waking up every 60 to 90 minutes or so is completely normal, to-be-expected behavior.

Other things to expect during the postpartum period:

Vaginal bleeding, discharge. *Lochia* is heavy period-like discharge that starts immediately after birth and stops sometime between 4 and 6 weeks. Basically, it's the wall of your uterus sloughing off stuff from the placental site so it can grow a new lining. You may experience more flow while you're nursing too, from the hormonal stimulation to your uterus, so it's a good idea to put on a fresh pad before you sit down for a feeding. When you're sitting or lying down the fluid can pool and thus may gush out when you stand up, but don't panic, this is not a sign that you're hemorrhaging. It's also normal to pass blood clots the size of dimes or quarters. Contact your healthcare provider immediately if you're worried.

From the third to the tenth day after delivery, lochia will begin to lessen and get lighter in color. Some doctors wipe down the lining of a woman's uterus following a c-section, and if your doctor did that, you'll have lighter flow that disappears more quickly.

Lightheadedness. Your blood volume, which increased 20 percent during pregnancy, will return to its normal levels within a week after birth. You may temporarily feel lightheaded when you sit up or stand quickly. Lightheadedness can also be a sign of anemia, so let your healthcare provider know if you feel lightheaded more than once or twice. A severe headache in the first week after birth may be a dangerous symptom of preeclampsia, especially when it's accompanied by blurred or double vision, so call your healthcare provider right away if you experience severe pain or vision disturbances.

Weight changes. After delivery, you'll only be about 6 to 10 pounds lighter than you were before you had the baby, but you'll lose another 10 pounds or more in the first weeks after pregnancy as your body drops all of that extra water weight.

Hemorrhoids. The pressures of pregnancy and birth can make hemorrhoids (swollen veins around your anus) larger and more uncomfortable, and sometimes they may bleed after a bowel movement. Hard stools are your enemy. Most healthcare providers will prescribe a stool softer as part of a new mom's medication schedule. Topical creams can also help, as can witch hazel wipes and compresses—you can make a cold compress by saturating a pantiliner with witch hazel and freezing it.

Sleeping on your side may help to relieve hemorrhoid pressure, as can avoiding standing or sitting for long periods of time. Eventually most hemorrhoids shrink and disappear (at least until you get pregnant again). In the meantime, eat plenty of fiber-rich foods, drink plenty of fluids, and don't strain on the toilet. If a bowel movement doesn't happen in 2 minutes, get up and try again later.

Hair loss. Hormones during pregnancy keep your scalp from shedding hair as it normally would, which leads to a more luxuriant head of hair while you're expecting. Once your baby is born, though, hormones make your hair's growing-and-shedding cycle go back to its usual patterns, and you may notice a little more hair coming off on your brush or in the shower.

Depressive feelings. As your estrogen levels drop sharply in the hours and days after birth, you may experience mood swings, weepiness, irritability, and a diminished sex drive. About 60 percent of moms report some depressive symptoms in the first 2 weeks after birth. For most moms these "baby blues" will pass in a week or so, but 10 to 20 percent of moms settle into clinical depression, which has the same symptoms as the baby blues, but lasts longer—usually from 3 to 6 months after the baby's born, and sometimes longer if left untreated. And truthfully, not all negative feelings after birth deserve to be blamed on hormones. Recovery can be a tough and painful time.

They say the most stressful jobs are those where you have no control over the process and total responsibility for the outcome, and that just about sums up the parenting experience, especially in the newborn phase. Family interaction can affect how you feel too. Women who have negative relationships with their partners or their own parents and those with financial problems are at a higher risk of the blues becoming deeper and lasting longer.

Newborn Routines

Sleep, eat, poop, pick up, put down . . .

Fortunately, if you ever worried "whatever am I going to do with a baby?" you'll find that a baby's needs are usually simple and obvious.

Feeding, sleeping, and dirtying diapers will be your baby's three main activities, which means that breastfeeding or mixing bottles, trying to sleep, and changing diapers will be yours, along with trying to stay fed, clean, and clothed yourself. Did we mention you'll need and want a lot of help during this time? Before you went into labor you may have cringed at the thought of your mother-in-law staying with you for a whole 2 weeks; now you'd beg her on your knees to stay for a month, if you could only get out of bed.

DIAPER CHANGING 101

In the first year alone, you'll be doing diaper changes about two

thousand times. Newborns hate to have their diapers changed. It upsets them. So watch out, there are apt to be howls of protest and chin-quivering cries.

If you've never changed a diaper in your life, here's what to do. (We'll assume that you're among the 95 percent of parents who use disposables.)

1. Prepare by getting out a clean diaper and a wipe or two. Usually the design on the diaper will indicate where the front is.
2. Lay the baby down on his back on a changing pad or towel, being sure to support the head and neck at all times.
3. Remove the old diaper. If it has Velcro tabs, you can roll it up and use the tabs to make it a tidy package.
4. Use a damp washcloth or a pre-moistened baby wipe to clean off the baby, being sure to wipe from front to

back, and keep all fecal material out of the urinary tract area.

5. Apply diaper rash ointment or kaolin clay powder if your baby's bottom looks red.

6. Lift up the baby by the ankles, and slide the new diaper under his rump.

7. Peel off the tabs that cover the tape, pull the diaper firmly around your baby so it will stay on, and press the tape into the soft, patterned area of the diaper. Voilà. You'll become so expert at it that you can do it in the dark with your eyes closed by the end of the first month (or sooner).

BOWEL MOVEMENTS

Baby bowel movements can change from one day to the next, and can be very different from one baby to another. Most babies will have their first bowel movement, called meconium, soon after they're born. It will be dark, sticky, and tar-like. In the weeks and months that follow, your baby may have a bowel movement eight times a day, or he may not have a bowel movement for days on end. As long as his stools are soft, rather than hard like pellets, everything is probably okay.

How bowel movements look and smell depends upon whether a baby's breastfed or bottle-fed. A breastfed baby's stools are almost liquid (but not the same as diarrhea). They aren't smelly, resemble small curds, and range from mustard yellow to light brown in color, sometimes with small speckled solid pieces that look like mustard seeds. Breastfed babies will pass stools almost every time they nurse. In the early weeks, that may mean as many as 8 to 10 stools in a single day.

A bottle-fed baby's stools are usually green, but they can be yellow to brown. They are usually firmer than a breastfed baby's, similar to thick pudding, and they may change appearance if your baby changes formula brands. The stools will have a stronger, more unpleasant odor than those of a breastfed baby. Your bottle-fed baby will pass fewer stools than a breastfed baby, too, and the stools will be larger. Stools may change color temporarily if your baby becomes ill, but contact your baby's healthcare provider if they turn bright red, are filled with mucus, or are white or bloody or have a coffee-grounds consistency.

Around 4 to 6 weeks of age, your baby's pooping pattern may slow down, and by the time he reaches a year of age, bowel movements and diaper changes will be much less frequent. By that time, breastfed babies will have about four bowel movements a day, while formula-fed babies will have two a day. Some babies may go 3 or 4 days before having a movement and be perfectly normal. If you're concerned that your baby hasn't had a bowel movement in a long time, or the stools are hard, then contact your baby's healthcare provider.

Once your baby begins eating solid food, at about 6 months, his stool colors (and odor) will change in response. Stools may be green, orange, yellow, or brown depending upon the foods your baby has eaten. Some foods that the baby can't digest will be passed intact, which can be odd and sometimes surprising to parents.

A breastfed baby's stools will likely get firmer as he moves to solid foods, while a formula-fed baby's stools may do just the opposite and become looser.

HANDLING AND REFLEXES

Newborns are born with strong reflexes, and it can take some practice to pick the baby up, put him down, and dress him without setting them off. No one knows for sure why babies are born with the reflexes they have, but, interestingly, all healthy newborns have certain reactions in common.

Rooting, also known as the search reflex, is probably the first reflex you'll see: as soon as your breast touches baby's cheek, he will automatically turn to that side, open his mouth, and extend his tongue in readiness to nurse. The reflex can backfire, though, if you try to guide your baby to your nipple by touching his cheek, but he instead turns towards the touch of your hand. For a good latch, you'll want to keep clothing or blankets from brushing his face as he feeds.

The startle reflex (also known as the Moro reflex) is another important one for parents to look out for. For the first 4 or 5 months, if your baby hears a loud noise or thinks he's falling, he'll jump, his arms and legs will jerk out and in, and he'll usually start to cry.

So when you put baby down, you want to go slowly and gently, only sliding your hands out from under his head and bottom after he's been placed down.

Other noteworthy newborn reflexes include:
- **The Babinski reflex.** When you touch the sole of your baby's foot, he spreads his toes.
- **The Palmer reflex.** When you touch the palm of his hand, he'll grasp your finger.
- **The stepping reflex.** If you hold him upright on a flat surface, he'll make stepping motions.
- **The crawling reflex.** When placed on the floor on his tummy, his arms and legs will make crawling motions, even though he won't be able to crawl for many more months.
- **The righting reflex.** If he is held in an upright position and is tilted, his head will move in the opposite direction to the body tilt.

NEWBORN COMMUNICATION

Your newborn is acutely aware of your voice and is prepared to respond to it. Even when he is only a few days old, he will turn his whole body around to orient to the sound of your voice calling his name from across the room. Your baby will move in synchrony with your voice's inflections. Only a few weeks after birth, he will move his lips and tongue in response to your talking. In moments of alertness, he may imitate you when you make a facial grimace, stick out your tongue, or shape your lips into an

O. He is capable of responding to your speaking to him by changing his breathing and making cooing noises.

SILLY BABY GAMES

The limited attention spans of young babies means that they will only be able to attend to you for moments at a time. As your baby matures, the amount of time he can spend paying attention to you will expand. But there are some tricks that even babies less than a week old can do that might be fun to try once your baby's fed and diapered but is still awake and staring:

- **Rattle watching.** Babies are attracted to movement if it's close enough (about 12 inches from the face) for them to focus. Slowly pass a bright rattle, ball, or other toy back and forth in front of his face and watch how his eyes try to track it. Your baby's eye movements may be jerky, and he may seem cross-eyed, but still you can see that he is trying to watch.
- **"Monkey see, monkey do."** Babies sometimes will imitate the facial gestures of adults. Again, move into an eye-to-eye position, about 12 inches from baby's face, and stick out your tongue, or open your mouth widely. Do this slowly and deliberately, and see if your baby returns a similar facial gesture.
- **Marching.** Babies only hours old will make marching steps if they are supported in an upright position. Hold your baby with your hands around the chest, under the arms. Hold the baby

over a tabletop so that the soles of his feet are pressed gently onto the surface. Then tilt your baby a little to one side and then the other so that one foot and then the other touch the table. Your baby will lift alternate legs.
- **Palm trick.** Pressing your thumbs gently into your baby's palms will likely cause him to open his mouth.

WHAT ABOUT DAD?

The postpartum period is no piece of cake for moms, and it can be tough on dads, too. Surveys have found that about 20 percent of dads suffer some sort of depression in the year after a baby's birth. Watching someone they love go through the discomforts of childbirth, while at the same time feeling helpless to do anything about it, can feel disempowering, and not all men (or women) are comfortable expressing feelings of weakness.

A lot of fathers also have hard-to-express feelings of being left out, or fears something should happen to the mother of their child. And, like moms, dads can beat themselves up when they don't feel how they think they ought to be feeling: a new dad should feel manly and powerful, not helpless and exhausted! And the self-blame can add an extra layer of stress to the situation. For some men, too, the new responsibility of fatherhood can translate into a sudden feverish devotion to work, which can seem to a mom like emotional distance at the worst possible time. Far from bringing a couple close together, trading off baby-care shifts can make it feel like you rarely see one another. Fathering also requires a whole different set of skills than husbanding, and things that used to seem like minor foibles, like, say, watching sports for hours or not pitching in with chores, can become capital cases to a new mom. Given all of these challenges, it's no wonder that the majority of divorces are initiated in the first 2 years after a baby's birth. You may not be able to "baby proof" your marriage completely, but here are some time-tested tips for getting your relationship through this challenging phase:

- Don't make it a contest: who has the harder job, who sleeps less or does more (we all know mom does).
- Let your partner to relate to the baby in his own way. Your baby and his dad have to form their own relationship separate from you, and mothering and fathering styles are usually very different. Even though your partner may appear relatively physical, awkward, or loud around the baby, don't micromanage his baby handling skills unless you really feel your baby is in danger. As long as a baby's head and neck are supported and nothing obstructs breathing, your baby can adapt to all kinds of styles. More important than dad doing everything exactly "right" is for him to build his confidence and for him and baby to bond. Otherwise you'll never get a minute's peace.
- Explore new ways to express affection other than sex. It's not unusual for new mothers, and sometimes fathers, to lose all sexual interest for as long as a year after birth. Some of it is hormonal and physical, some is feeling "all touched out" by their babies, and some is plain old tiredness. Until the sexy comes back, find new ways to be close, like snuggling, hugging, or taking time out to relate in other ways.
- Take a shift. One of the major ways a new dad can help a new mom is to pick up the burden of home responsibilities so mom can recover and tend to the baby. On the practical level, this translates into offering to fetch the baby when she cries, diapering and dressing, rocking the baby between feedings, strapping the baby into a soft carrier for walks, letting the baby have tummy time on dad's chest to give mom a break, and while baby is with mom, cleaning up whatever needs cleaning, preparing food, and so on.
- Consciously divvy up responsibilities. Most dads are willing to do what they can to help out, but it helps to be clear about who is responsible for what. Don't be afraid to be upfront about what needs to be done: "I need you to take over doing the dishes/laundry/vacuuming/paying bills," rather than hinting or silently fuming if he doesn't take the initiative. When your partner does chip in to help, be sure to say thank you (even if he doesn't always thank you for all the things you do, and even if you still don't think he's doing enough).

- Recognize that the situation is temporary. Stressful times can bring out the best and worst in all of us, but these times will pass. If you feel on the verge of saying something you might regret later, take a breath, have a snack, wait until the baby's asleep. (And remember, cleaning services are cheaper than couples' therapy or a divorce lawyer.)

WHEN CAN BABY LEAVE THE HOUSE?

Because illnesses in newborns can be very serious, most healthcare providers recommend avoiding crowd situations and germy places for at least the first 6 to 12 weeks after birth. That doesn't mean you have to hide in your house. Just avoid places where germs lurk, like the mall, airports, and bus terminals, and if you do go out, keep baby close to you, in your arms or a soft carrier. If you're planning a welcome-baby party or naming ceremony, wait at least 6 weeks before you welcome a house full of people, and make sure guests wash their hands thoroughly before handling the baby. Ask anyone with obvious cold symptoms to not handle your baby.

YOUR 6-WEEK CHECKUP

Most care providers schedule a postpartum visit for their patients within 6 weeks after birth to make sure they're healing properly. Don't hesitate to call your healthcare provider sooner if you have any questions or things don't seem to be going well for you. But believe it or not, by 6 weeks, you'll probably be well on your way back to your old self—physically, anyway.

Your postpartum bleeding will have begun to disappear, and any perineal incisions or any tearing should be healed. Bring your baby along in a carrier to your checkup if you want to—your care provider and the office staff will be happy to see her!

During this exam, your care provider will:

- Check your perineum to make sure any tearing or incisions have healed.
- Check your abdominal incision, if you've had a cesarean.
- Examine your breasts for any lumps, which may signify a clogged duct.
- Feel your stomach to make sure that your uterus has returned to its normal size.
- Give you the go-ahead to resume exercising (or not). Ask if you need to restrict or modify your activities for any reason. You may also want to ask your care provider to suggest local postpartum exercise classes.
- Give you the go-ahead to resume sexual activity (though you don't need to tell your partner that if you don't want to!).
- Discuss birth control options. Don't leave your healthcare provider's office without a plan to prevent pregnancy until you feel mentally and physically ready for another child. Note that many birth control pills aren't recommended for breastfeeding mothers. Other options include an IUD or condoms.

Your Postpartum Abs

A lot of new moms get a condition called **diastasis recti**, which is a separation of the long muscle that runs down the center of the abdomen. All women who've had c-sections will have some degree of separation, though it happens to mothers who deliver vaginally, too.

Here's how to tell if your abdominals have separated: Lie on your back with your knees bent and your feet flat on the floor. Gently lift your head and shoulder blades off the floor using your abs. Place the fingers of one hand on the abdomen underneath your belly button. If your recti muscles have spread apart, you'll be able to feel the soft space in the center with hard muscle running from the top down on both sides. If the gap in the center is more than an inch or so, then your muscle has split. You'll also know you have it if it's impossible to do a sit-up from a lying-down position without someone holding your feet down.

Some simple exercises, like mini-crunches and low leg lifts, can help you coax your split rectis muscles back together.

SLEEP

In Babyland, there is no normal. The only language spoken here is crying (sometimes your baby's, and sometimes yours). As you wade through feeding, diapering, burping, rocking, sleeping, and feeding, "ad exhaustium," clocks are useless and only make you aware of how much sleep you're not getting. Even when you do sleep, it's not the nice, unbroken stretches the babyless are accustomed to. The up-and-down can make it seem like a fog has slipped over reality—2 days seem like 2 weeks.

At first, most newborns will sleep about 16 to 18 hours out of every 24 and they need to feed often, at least once every 4 hours (if not every 90 minutes). Adding to the surreal quality of Babyland, it can sometimes be hard to tell a sleeping newborn from an awake one. It might look like your baby's fallen asleep while nursing, but as soon as you try to put her down, her eyes will snap open. Or a sleeping baby may make noises, move, or even have her eyes half-open.

The good news is, as your baby's stomach grows, feedings will become further between, and by 6 months to a year most (though not all) babies will settle into a routine of sleeping through the night and taking predictable naps during the day.

In the meantime, sleep is the most precious commodity in the home of new parents, and having a partner willing to divide up the tough shifts will be more valuable than a diamond-studded tiara. Your recovery will be a million times easier if you can stay in bed for a full 8 or 9 hours of sleep, with someone bringing you the baby for feedings or giving her a bottle of pumped milk (for more on milk pumps and pumping, see page 243). And note that the closer you keep your baby, the less awake you will have to get to feed.

But best place for a baby to sleep is not an easy call. If you and your partner are light sleepers who don't smoke and have a baby-proofed bed, bed sharing is a great way to keep your milk supply up, get more sleep, and bond as a family, and it may help prevent SIDS. But many pediatricians are dead against bed sharing, because hundreds of babies are killed accidentally every year in unsafe parent-bed situations. (As one pediatrician put it, "once you've seen one baby that's been smothered in a parents' bed, you don't ever want to see another.") Sharing a bed with the baby will also become less and less restful for parents as baby becomes bigger and squirmier at night.

A compromise, and what's recommended by the American Academy of Pediatrics, is to have the baby sleep in a bassinet in the parents' room, so parents can be on hand. But this doesn't work for everyone—the baby wants to be in physical contact with mom and is no happier 2 feet away than 20. And with the baby in your room, it's tough to resist the temptation to just lie down in bed with baby after the second or third feeding of the night. Some babies also make a lot of noise in their sleep, which can keep light-sleeping parents awake.

Having the baby sleep in her own room and crib is most parents' end goal, starting out having the baby sleep in her crib from the first day makes sense. But this means a parent (usually mom) will be getting up to walk to another room every couple of hours, trying to feed the baby while sitting up, then trying to convince the baby to go back to asleep again in the crib, or falling asleep in the chair, which is statistically even more dangerous for the baby than the parents' bed. Cribs also pose dangers of their own, with the American Academy of Pediatrics reporting that crib-related injuries send an average of 9,500 babies to the emergency room every year in the United States.

It's not surprising that polls of parents show that lots start off putting the baby in the crib but end up having the baby sleep in a combination of places, from cribs to bed to bouncy seats or car seats, and getting very little rest themselves. We say, whatever gets you through the night—the important thing is the baby is safe.

Straight Talk on Safe Sleep

Research of SIDS cases has found that often in the past what medical examiners had classified as SIDS may have actually been accidental deaths. So it's important to know how to keep baby safe from sleep hazards.

- Don't bring the baby into your bed if you or your partner smokes. The research associating cigarette smoke exposure and SIDS is strong. Amazingly, even if you or your partner only smokes outdoors and never around the baby, there are still enough harmful chemicals remaining in a smoker's exhaled breath to increase a baby's risk.
- Do use a fan in the room where your baby sleeps. Studies have found that having a fan in baby's bedroom reduces the risk of SIDS by a whopping 72 percent.

- Don't let baby sleep in a bouncy seat or swing unless you're awake to keep an eye out. Swing- and bouncy-seat straps and padding can create suffocation and entrapment hazards.
- If your baby sleeps well in her car seat that's okay, do be sure to put the car seat on a stable surface like the floor on in the crib (not a table, countertop, or chair).
- Don't bring your baby into bed if you or your partner has been drinking or taking sedating medications, or if you're a heavy sleeper. If your partner is the heavy sleeper, put the baby on your side of the bed and use a bed rail to prevent roll-off.
- Unless you're positive you will never, ever let your baby into the adult bed, do be sure to give your bed a thorough check for entrapment hazards. Gaps between the mattress and headboard or between the bed and nightstand or wall can create places for your baby's head to get wedged if she rolls off. The safest parent bed is a mattress or futon on the floor and no bed frame.
- Don't leave a baby alone in an adult bed. Even newborns can scoot themselves off if they wake up and discover mom isn't there.
- Don't use a baby sleep positioner in a crib, bassinet, or adult bed. They can create pockets of exhaled air, a suffocation hazard.
- Ban the fluff. Plushy crib bumpers, pillows, quilts, and stuffed animals can also create dangerous carbon dioxide pockets and suffocation hazards, so keep them out of baby's sleep area. Dress the baby in a sleep sack, pajamas, or a swaddled blanket to keep baby warm in the crib.
- Don't swaddle the baby or use a sleep sack in an adult bed—your baby needs to be able to kick off any bedding that might fall on her face accidentally.
- Do be very cautious to keep pillows and blankets away from your baby's face if your baby comes into the adult bed.
- Always respond to baby's cries, and don't try to keep baby on a feeding schedule or make her cry herself to sleep for at least the first 6 months (if ever). If you're trying to establish breastfeeding, you can't feed too often but you can feed too little. For the first week, your baby should nurse at least every 4 hours (if not more often), day and night. After the first week, though, don't wake her up to feed if she sleeps more than 4 hours overnight.

The good news for tired parents is that the baby-sleep situation is temporary.

Sometime between about 6 weeks and 6 months, the hormones that cue your baby's sleep-and-wake cycles will start to assume more regular day and night patterns, and you'll start to see a natural sleep schedule emerge. But before that happens, you'll be treated to what's known as the 6-Week Crying Peak.

What tends to happen is this— your baby amazes you by pulling some long sleep stretches all of a sudden—5 or 6 hours or more. But with more sleeping comes more crying—often starting in the late afternoon and going on . . . and on. While 3-week-olds cry an average of

1.7 hours per day, 6-week-olds cry 2.2 hours per day. The good news is that these crying jags almost never mean that a baby has *colic*, or gas, or is allergic to your milk or that there's anything seriously wrong.

Instead, the crying is actually a good sign that your baby's sleep hormones are starting to flow in a regular cycle in response to the weakening afternoon sunlight.

SIDS—The Silent Killer

Sudden infant death syndrome (SIDS) is the sudden, unexplained death of a baby who is less than 1 year of age. SIDS usually occurs when babies are sleeping. For babies less than a year old, it is a leading cause of death after the first month.

The exact cause of SIDS is still unclear, but there are numerous theories about what happens. One is that babies at risk for SIDS have underdeveloped carbon dioxide sensors in their brain that fail to arouse the baby to change positions while sleeping if her face is against a blanket or other suffocation hazard. Re-breathed air is definitely a hazard and, as we mentioned, having a fan circulating air in baby's room can reduce the risk considerably.

One study found that SIDS babies had different heart rates than those not at risk. It has also been found that babies at risk of SIDS move the muscles of their upper airways in a different way than normal babies. They also have lower levels of the brain chemical serotonin.

Some babies, especially if they were premature or small for gestational age, may have *sleep apnea*, which causes them to stop breathing for a while during sleep and then snort themselves awake again. Even healthy, full-term babies can stop breathing for 15 to 20 seconds with no harm done.

There is no sure way to protect your baby from SIDS, but you can reduce the risk by:

- Positioning a baby to sleep on his back, rather than facedown on his stomach
- Keeping air moving with a fan in baby's room
- Keeping soft quilts, crib bumpers, stuffed toys, and pillows out of your baby's bed
- Picking up your baby when he cries. Being overtired from extended crying is a risk factor
- Not sharing sleeping space if you or anyone else in bed is a smoker, and never smoking around your baby or allowing smoking in your home
- Breastfeeding
- Never putting your baby down on a beanbag chair, sofa, waterbed, or couch for sleep

Why Babies Cry

Babies cry because they don't have any other way to communicate yet, and they cry for different reasons at different times: they want to be held, they're hungry, they're pooping, they're too cold or hot, they're having growing pains, or they're going through a developmental phase.

Researchers have even found that newborn babies' sound patterns will vary depending on the language spoken by his parents, with French babies crying in one "cry melody" and German babies in another, which suggests babies pick up language patterns in the womb.

And, as you'll soon find out, a baby's cry can also range in intensity from a mellow fussy sound for mild discomfort to a shrill, piercing shriek that can drown out everything else in the world and scramble your brain to the point that it's downright impossible to focus on anything else.

When your baby hits those intense tones, it can make your heart race, your blood pressure go up, your palms sweat, and your milk start leaking. If you're driving in the car with your baby and your baby starts to wail, pull over to a safe parking place: the distraction can be dangerous.

Naturally, you want to prevent the fussy sounds from turning into the shrieky ones, and the two ways to best do this are:

1. Feed your baby as soon as you see any signs of hunger, such as rooting (turning her head from side to side).

2. Keep your baby in close physical contact with you or another caregiver almost all of the time.

There's no need to worry that you will spoil your baby by too much physical contact, nursing, or attempts to soothe his cries. Research has shown that the faster parents respond to their baby's cries, the more easily and rapidly the baby can be quieted. You don't want to put a newborn on a feeding schedule, which can also decrease your milk supply. When you're establishing breastfeeding, you can't feed too often, but milk production can be slowed from feeding too infrequently.

You also don't want to try to set up a sleep schedule where you let the baby "cry it out" until at least 6 months of age (if ever). Young babies won't cry it out; because of their short sleep cycles, a baby who's hungry or distressed will just drop off to sleep for a short stretch out of exhaustion, and then wake right back up crying 20 or 40 minutes later.

That being said, it's also important to note that most, if not all, babies have periods when they cry for no discernible reason. If your newborn isn't hungry, but starts screaming, this can indicate an oncoming illness or ear infection, especially if she also feels warm or has a runny nose. Or it could be gas, uncomfortable clothing, pain from a new tooth emerging, or something may have set off her startle reflex. Or, your baby could just be nearing the

6-week crying peak, simply have had too much stimulation, or simply need to let off steam. So while you should respond to your baby's cries and try to identify and fix whatever problems you can, you also shouldn't take them personally.

For most babies, late-afternoon crying jags will ease up around week 12 to 16. In the meantime, there are some things you can do to help your baby's sleep-hormone cycles get in line:

- **Get outside.** After the sun comes up in the morning and after her afternoon nap, if weather permits and you feel up to it, take your baby outside to walk or play. A walk around the block can also help soothe late-afternoon crying fits, and exposure to the morning and afternoon sun will cue her sleep hormones to self-regulate. If weather doesn't permit or you don't feel up to going out, let her play by a sunny window. Babies sunburn quickly, so use caution between 10 a.m. and 3 p.m., when the sun's rays are the strongest.
- **Have lots of skin-to-skin contact.** Research has found that the more physical contact a baby has with caregivers, the fewer average minutes per day they cry. A soft carrier that lets you keep your baby close and your hands free is a great investment.
- **Put the baby down for a nap** in her crib at the same time every day. Young babies are ready for their first nap of the day about 2 hours after they wake up, and their second nap after lunch. Then put the baby down for a consistent early bedtime of about 7 p.m., and when she wakes up overnight, keep feedings restful. For babies, the deepest and heaviest sleep happens in the early evening, and lighter and shorter spells after the first deep stretch. (Interestingly, adults' sleep patterns trend the opposite way, with the deepest sleep cycles happening in the early morning hours around 3 or 4 a.m.) Use a nightlight so you can feed without turning on bright lights, and don't change her diaper unless there's poop. Most babies wake up very, very early—4:30 or 5 a.m. By about a year the two naps usually merge into one after-lunch nap, and your toddler may even let you sleep in until 6 or 7 a.m. (no promises).

- **If you can, heed the age-old advice to sleep** when your baby does, no matter the hour. If baby falls asleep in the car and you're not driving, put your seat back and take a nap yourself.

Understanding Colic

Rarely, there are babies who cry around the clock, which can be exhausting and even devastating for their parents, who spend their days and nights searching wildly for some special technique that can help their babies relax and go to sleep. Some babies cry so much that they earn the label of suffering from colic, an old British word for bad indigestion. The term is now used to describe inconsolable baby crying for long periods of time with no apparent cause.

Approximately 1 out of 5 babies earns the label of being colicky, or excessively fussy, as a result of their daily crying jags. The medical definition of colic is a condition of a healthy baby in which it shows periods of intense, unexplained fussing/crying lasting more than 3 hours a day, more than 3 days a week for more than 3 weeks.

Typically, baby-crying episodes start within the first 2 to 3 weeks and peak at around 6 weeks after birth. Most, but not all, cases of so-called colic resolve themselves on their own before the baby reaches his fourth month. The symptoms of colic—the distressed screaming, the wide-open mouth with lips that almost turn blue, the frowning brows, the flailing arms and legs, and the rock-tight belly—are identical to any expression of extreme baby pain, although the baby may or may not be in pain.

Some parents discover that what was labeled as colic was really an ear infection, an allergy to dairy products or baby vitamins, an immature and dysfunctional digestive system, or other physical problems, such as a hernia or an undetected physical condition. Sometimes sudden-onset crying can be caused by an oncoming illness, or something as simple as a string or hair wrapped around a baby's finger or toe.

If the crying doesn't go away and you're worried, it makes sense to have your baby thoroughly examined by his pediatric healthcare provider to try to uncover what's causing all the distress. Before you go, document a sample of your baby's crying episodes by keeping a journal about when it happens and how long it lasts. You might want to consider videotaping an episode so your pediatrician can actually see and hear your baby's behavior, since

babies have an uncanny way of being calm and sleepy when their appointments roll around. A blood sample may be needed as well as a urine sample. Bring along your baby's most recent poopy diaper too.

If your baby seems to have sieges of dire distress that you feel are not taken sufficiently seriously by your pediatrician, you may want to seek help from a baby specialist, such as a neonatal gastroenterologist.

It helps to keep reminding yourself that as overwhelming as your baby's crying may feel at the moment, the situation is temporary. Research has shown that colicky babies are more likely to turn out to be sweet and amenable toddlers, while passive, so-called good babies are much more likely to grow into demanding hellions after a year or so.

Other techniques to try when you're almost at your wit's end:

- Running the vacuum cleaner or dishwasher.
- Parking the bassinet next to a whirring window-unit air conditioner or fan.
- Putting the baby in a carrier on top of a running washing machine or dryer (don't leave baby alone).
- Taking the baby for a drive in the car while playing percussive, bass-heavy music, like hip-hop or military marches.
- Taking baby to a new climate, like an ice rink or arboretum, or just stepping outside if you're inside (or inside if you're outside).
- The one-arm hold. Drape your baby on your arm, facedown, with his head resting in your palm, and sway.
- Swaddle your baby tight, then

What to Do: Overwhelmed by Baby Crying

Intense, unrelenting baby crying can sometimes provoke parents toward roughness with a baby. There's a particular danger for special-needs babies, because their cries may be more shrill, and for parents who are isolated and don't get enough support or rest.

If you have the urge to shake or be rough with your baby, put him or her down safely in the crib and leave the room. Get out of range of the crying sound, take a deep breath, and call to find someone who can watch the baby while you take a mental-health break outside of the house. Call **800-4-A-CHILD**, a free, anonymous, 24/7 hotline staffed by professional counselors who can offer emotional support and strategies to help you deal with the crying and stress.

Sleep deprivation, baby crying, postpartum hormonal shifts, and little to no time to take care of your own needs can all conspire to make even the most together of new moms feel pushed to the edge of sanity. Don't try to pull long stretches of baby care duty alone without any time to take care of your own needs.

---

shush your baby loudly in his ear while moving him rhythmically.

- Chest rest. This is a good one for your partner to try. Lie on your back on the sofa, in a recliner, or in the bed, and place your bare or diapered baby facedown on your chest. Rest your hands on baby's back. Cover your baby's back and your arm with a sheet or blanket.

Safety Warning: Shaken Baby Syndrome

A baby's head is large and heavy in relation to his body, and babies' neck muscles are weak. Every year, thousands of babies and young children are seriously injured when they are violently shaken. Shaking a baby without supporting the head and neck can cause brain damage leading to permanent injuries and possibly death. Always support your baby's heavy head and vulnerable spine, and if baby crying is overwhelming you, put the baby down in the crib and step outside

and away from the sound until you feel calm again.

BABY SYMPTOMS YOU SHOULDN'T IGNORE

- **Excessive crying.** It's normal for a newborn to cry when he is hungry, needs to be burped, is cold, poops, or needs a clean diaper, and for a spell in the early evening, especially around the 6-week crying peak. But if your baby's cry sounds different and more high-pitched than normal and goes on literally for hours, then it could be a signal that something is wrong.
- **Fever.** Make an emergency call to your pediatrician if your baby is less than 8 weeks old and develops a fever of more than 100.4°F (rectally), or if he's 8 weeks or older with a fever above 104°F.

- **Jaundice.** More than half of full-term babies and about 80 percent of premature babies who are otherwise healthy develop a yellowish discoloration of their skin and the whites of their eyes soon after birth called jaundice or neonatal jaundice. Jaundice is not a disease, but a symptom that usually signals that a baby's liver simply isn't mature enough to process a substance called *bilirubin*, which is created as the body recycles old or damaged red blood cells. It isn't painful or dangerous and usually disappears in 1 to 2 weeks. Exposure to sunlight or artificial light can help jaundice, and your healthcare practitioner will probably want to monitor your baby and may recommend exposing your baby to special treatment lights.

- **Signs of constipation and/ or dehydration.** If your baby is formula-fed, it's possible for him to develop constipation. Stools may be hard and resemble small pellets. If your baby is breastfed, it's impossible for him to be constipated, but lack of stools in the first week could mean that he isn't getting enough milk, so be sure to tell your pediatrician if your newborn doesn't poop at least once per day in the first week. Dark urine or dryer-than-usual diapers may also be signs that your baby isn't eating enough, or is becoming dehydrated.

- **Sluggishness.** It's normal for a newborn to spend a lot of time sleeping, but if your baby is rarely alert and doesn't wake up for feedings, or seems too listless to want to eat, contact your pediatrician right away.

- **Infected umbilical cord.** If the stump from your baby's umbilical (belly button) cord gets pus-filled or red, swollen skin at the base or if your baby cries as though in pain when you touch the cord or skin, the site may be infected and you should contact your healthcare provider.

- **Infected circumcision site.** Call your doctor if your son's penis isn't healing or bleeds; the tip of your baby's penis is red, swollen, oozy, or foul-smelling; or scar tissue is forming lumps and/or adhering to the shaft.

Feeding Your Baby

BREASTFEEDING

Human breastmilk is more than food—it's living tissue that will build your baby's brain and help to protect the baby from disease. The American Academy of Pediatrics recommends babies be breastfed for at least 12 months. If you aren't able to pull that off, every day, week, and month that you do breastfeed adds to your baby's health.

Mother's milk is powerful enough to build a lifetime buffer zone to help protect your baby from diseases. There is strong evidence that breastfed babies have fewer cases of severe diarrhea. They have fewer colds and flu bouts and fewer ear and urinary tract infections. Human milk helps to protect babies from SIDS, juvenile diabetes, some childhood cancers, obesity, allergies, and chronic digestive diseases. As an extra bonus, children who are breastfed appear to have higher intelligence scores (about three to five IQ points) on the average than bottle-fed children. Breastfeeding isn't just healthy for babies; it also has benefits for moms. Immediately after birth, breastfeeding increases the level of oxytocin in a mother's body, which helps to stop blood loss and increase the tone of the uterus. It can also offer temporary protection from getting pregnant again, as long as you're still feeding overnight and don't supplement with formula (although you shouldn't rely on this). Some studies also appear to show that breastfeeding reduces a mom's risk of breast and ovarian cancer.

Breastfeeding pros:
- Human milk provides immunities to illness.
- It's portable: always there and ready to go.
- You don't have to mix it, heat it, refrigerate it, or sterilize it.
- It's free; you don't have to buy formula, bottles, or nipples.
- It helps you and your baby to bond.
- You don't have to get out of bed do it.
- Breastfed baby poop is less smelly.

Breastfeeding cons:
- It can be painful at first. Even if you've breastfed before and your baby's position is perfect, the first 1 to 5 days of breastfeeding can hurt. Acetaminophen (Tylenol) can help take the edge off. If the pain persists, let your healthcare provider and/or a lactation consultant know right away.

- It takes time. At first your baby may need to nurse for 20 minutes or more on each side, as frequently as every 90 minutes. So while yes, breastfeeding is free, it's only free if your time has no cost. After your milk is established, you can pump and store milk, which will give you a little more mobility. But pumping takes time, too.

"My nipples were so sore at first I had tears rolling down my cheeks. Fortunately, the pain went away after about 4 days, and after that there was no discomfort at all."

Getting Started with Breastfeeding

Your nipple and *areola*, the dark circle that goes around your nipple, are the perfect shape for fitting between the gums and into the mouth and palate of your baby when he nurses.

Your breasts have muscles that enable the nipple to stand up and harden when they're stimulated, so your baby can grasp on for nursing. When your milk begins to flow, you will discover that your nipple doesn't have just a single hole in the center but a series of five to ten pores that project the milk outward.

Six Tips for Breastfeeding Success

- Get help. Study a few good breastfeeding books in advance and/or attend La Leche League meetings while you're still pregnant to get advice. After birth, request the help of a lactation consultant or an experienced labor and delivery nurse if you have problems or discomfort.
- Start right away after birth. Breastfeed as soon as possible after birth, ideally immediately or within at least the first 2 hours.
- Keep your baby with you. Room in with your baby in the hospital. Get others to help you put your baby to your breast if your stitches are sore.
- Don't give your baby formula unless he shows signs of dehydration. Newborns sometimes have **nipple confusion**, which makes it hard for them to adapt to breastfeeding after they've been introduced to an artificial nipple and become used to nursing from a bottle.
- Feed your baby whenever he wants. Your baby will let you know when he needs to nurse. Don't try to schedule your baby's feedings.
- Breastfeed a lot and without time limits. Newborns need to nurse 8 to 12 times every 24 hours.

How you position yourself and your baby while you're nursing can make a big difference in your comfort and success with breastfeeding.

A newborn is a heavy weight to hold for long periods of nursing. Use every pillow you can find to

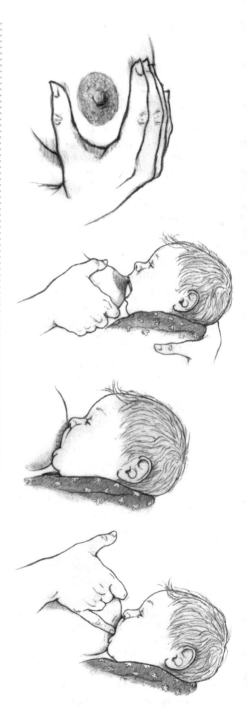

support your back, your arms, and even under your knees. A specialized breastfeeding pillow that wraps around your torso can be really useful.

Pay attention to how your baby is positioned as you get ready to nurse. Your baby's whole body should be aligned facing yours with his face and head aimed straight toward the breast, rather than tummy-up.

If you nurse lying down on your side, your baby should be on his side too, so his body is aligned chest-to-chest with you. Let the baby's head rest on the bed or on your arm. To change sides, pick up your baby, and hold him to your chest, and roll the two of you over together.

There are a few tricks of the trade. Help your baby get your entire nipple in his mouth by cupping your fingers in a U shape around your breast with your thumb on the outside, forefinger on the inside. Keep your fingers off your areola, and squeeze your fingers toward each other so your breast gets longer. Pressing backward toward your chest with your fingers will make your nipple stick out even further.

Once you've mastered the hand tricks, tuck your baby in your arm so his head is above the crease in your elbow. Face his body and head toward you. Using your opposite hand, squeeze your breast into a cone shape, and move your fingers back and forth so your nipple tickles your baby's lips. Wait for your baby to open his mouth wide. Then, bring your baby toward your chin first rather than nose first, so his mouth is at nipple level.

If you're having problems getting your baby interested in nursing, try spreading a little colostrum, the fluid that is secreted by a new mother's breast, on the tip of your nipple. A baby bonds to the smell of his own mother's breast, so don't put creams, lotions, or other scented products on or around your chest until breastfeeding is well established.

When you bring your baby in for nursing, his head should be slightly tilted backward with his chin pressed into your breast tissue.

The concept is to have your baby take in as much of your areola as he can. There should be more areola in his bottom jaw area than in the top of his mouth. If your baby's chin is tilted too far downward, it will make his tonguing action and swallowing harder.

Allow your baby to complete nursing on one side before moving him to the other. You'll know when he's had enough because his sucking will slow down and he'll relax and start to snooze.

You may be surprised at what a strong vacuum hold your baby has on your breast. To take your baby off of a nipple, always break the seal first: press down on the areola part that's near your baby's mouth, pull down on your baby's chin, or insert your pinky finger in the corner of the baby's mouth. Don't attempt to pull the baby off your breast without breaking the suction seal.

Alternate breasts with each feeding so one breast won't become larger than the other, and don't try to change breasts midstream in the hope that it will keep your nipples from being sore. It won't. Waiting to change breasts until your baby has totally nursed all he can from the starting side will ensure he's getting the important milk fat, which is more plentiful after you have been feeding for a while.

A football hold is a good alternative way of holding your baby if you've had a cesarean and your lower belly hurts. Tuck the baby underneath your arm on one side, so his body goes around the side of your rib cage. Support your baby at breast height with your hand holding up the base of your baby's head.

This position allows you to watch the baby carefully and to control his position better than other positions.

As you get into a nursing routine, you may notice that your baby is more likely to nurse in the evening and into the wee hours of the morning and less likely to nurse in the middle of the night and early morning. Feedings will be sporadic throughout the day.

It usually takes 3 to 4 days after birth for your milk to come in. When it does come in, it may feel like a warm rush of fluid that fills up your breast.

Until your milk arrives, your baby won't be drinking milk but small amounts of colostrum, a nutrient-rich liquid that is yellow or golden in color. It has high concentrations of protein, nutrients, and immune agents to protect your baby from infection.

The most important way to get your milk copiously flowing is to allow your baby to nurse a lot starting right away after birth, preferably within 2 hours, and then,

once your milk comes in, to let your baby stay latched onto your breast long enough so it gets completely emptied.

When your breasts are emptied of milk, your body gets the signal to produce more, so removing milk from the breast early and often is the key to kick-starting milk production after birth.

Sometimes your baby's experiences during labor and afterward can make establishing breastfeeding a little bit harder, too. Certain pain relievers can also affect a baby's nursing behavior. For example, meperidine (**Demerol**) used for labor pain has been found to delay and depress a baby's skill at rooting and sucking if it's given to a mother near the time of delivery. If you've had a c-section or a long and difficult labor, or if your baby has undergone painful procedures, such as circumcision or vigorous suctioning at birth, he may be sluggish and boycott nursing for a few hours.

Though it's the best-case scenario that you and baby establish breastfeeding soon after birth, it's also not the end of your breastfeeding career should concerns about the baby's hydration or weight loss, a hospital error, or your sanity mean that the baby gets a feeding or two of formula in the hospital. If your baby is dehydrated, or hospital staff is worried that the baby has lost too much weight since birth, or you're simply at the end of your rope, let the nurses give the baby a bottle, get some rest, and try again at the next feeding.

Help for Sore Nipples

The friction of your baby's nursing may cause your nipples to feel sunburned.

Sometimes nipple soreness may get even more painful than that, and your nipples may develop scabs or bleed slightly. There are several things you can do:

- **Check your position.** Your baby should be well supported at breast height with the baby's whole body against your stomach and chest. His head should be cocked upward, with his nose turned upward so his lower lips and chin are the first parts to contact your breast. Most of the dark ring around your nipple should be stuffed into his mouth with his chin pressed upward against your breast. (See positioning suggestions on page 241.)
- **Protect against infection.** Apply a thin layer of antibiotic ointment, such as Polysporin, after each feeding to help reduce infection.
- **Start the milk early.** Once your milk has come in, wash your hands, try to relax, and express some milk so that your milk is already flowing when the baby latches on.
- **Avoid harsh cleaning.** Use only water, not soap, to clean your nipples.
- **Cure with breastmilk.** Apply your own milk to your nipples after nursing, and allow them to air dry. Human milk has antibacterial properties that can help your nipples to heal.
- **Use a lubricant.** Apply USP-modified lanolin, such as Lansinoh, to soothe your nipples between feedings.

- **Wear absorbent materials.** Avoid bras or breast pads with synthetic fabrics or plastic liners.
- **Try tea.** Apply warm, wet black tea bags as a compress. They contain tannin, which soothes the skin.
- **Get help.** Persistent or toe-curling pain may mean trouble. If your nipples are cherry red, you may have *thrush*, a yeast infection that causes sore, cracked nipples. If breastfeeding pain persists beyond a few days, let your healthcare provider know.

Pumping and Storing Breastmilk

After the first 3 or 4 weeks or so, when your milk supply is well established and your baby has bonded to your breast, you can start to hand-express or pump extra bottles of milk from the opposite breast while your baby nurses on the other side. Having extra pumped milk will let your partner have a chance to feed the baby, and finally you'll have a chance to rest or run an errand during a feeding time. Each pumped feeding will earn you about 60 to 90 minutes of furlough.

Human milk has built-in antibacterial properties that make it keep well. One study even found that after 8 days of storage in the refrigerator, some milk samples had fewer bacteria than the day they were expressed.

Breastmilk can be stored at room temperature of 60°F for 24 hours, from 66°F to 72°F for 10 hours, or in a 32°F to 39°F refrigerator for 8 days. If your refrigerator has a separate freezer section, milk can be stored safely for 3 to 4 months. It will last for 6 months or longer in a deep freeze that can hold the temperature at a constant 0°F.

When you're gathering milk to be stored, make sure that your hands are clean and, if you use a breast pump, that the components and bottles have been washed in hot, soapy water and allowed to air dry.

Milk can be stored in a plastic or glass bottle with the top sealed and screwed on tight, or you can purchase freezer bags designed specifically for milk storage. You can add fresh milk to frozen milk as long as there is less fresh than frozen.

Remember that the milk will expand when it freezes, so allow adequate space. Date the bottles or bags by writing on masking tape with a marker or ballpoint pen.

Defrost the milk under warm running water.

MEDICATIONS AND BREASTMILK

Most drugs taken by mothers pass to their babies through their milk, but usually it is in very small doses, less than 1 percent of what the mothers take. Most pain medications are safe to take, and it is usually considered safe to continue breastfeeding when taking most common medications.

After birth, let your healthcare provider know that you are breastfeeding. Many drugs have never been licensed for use during lactation. That means manufacturers have not undertaken research to confirm whether or not their drugs are safe for nursing babies.

Data may be available on the amount that gets into breastmilk. Simply because trace amounts of a drug show up in a mother's milk does not mean the baby is being harmed.

If there is not enough information on the safety of a specific drug, your caregiver may be able to substitute another drug that will work equally as well. Your baby's age may be an important factor. A premature baby, for example, may be more vulnerable to even trace amounts of drugs in breastmilk, while an older baby or toddler will have a mature elimination system able to detoxify and get rid of drugs.

The definitive book on medications and breastmilk is Thomas W. Hale's manual, *Medications and Mother's Milk*. Most pediatric healthcare providers' offices have a copy and can look up information about the safety of specific medications for you, or you can buy or borrow your own.

Smoking and Breastfeeding

It's definitely better if you don't smoke if you're a breastfeeding mom, because your baby will be exposed to nicotine in your milk.

Breastfed babies whose mothers smoke are less likely to have acute respiratory illnesses and a lower risk of dying from SIDS than babies whose mothers smoke and feed their babies formula. But if you smoke, don't stop breastfeeding in the belief that formula feeding is safer for your baby.

If you are unable to give up smoking, but still want to breastfeed your baby, here are some hints for how to do that:

- Smoke for shorter times and less often. Your baby is very vulnerable to passive, secondhand smoke, and amazingly there's even evidence that third-hand smoke fumes that linger on your clothes and exhaled breath increase the risks of SIDS. If you must smoke, step outside, snuff out the cigarette after an inch or less, and cut down on the number of cigarettes you smoke each day. If you or your partner smoke, don't share a sleep area with your baby.
- Smoke after feeding. It takes approximately an hour and 15 minutes for nicotine to clear from your body, so try to limit your smoking to immediately following a feeding to allow as much time as you can in between smoking and nursing.
- Use iodized salt on your food. Recent research appears to show that smoking reduces the transport of iodine through breastmilk. Iodine is critical for a baby's thyroid hormone formation during pregnancy and the first years of life, and insufficient iodine has been associated with developmental brain damage. Using iodized salt on your food and eating iodine-rich foods like fish may help. (See our practical ideas for giving up your smoking habit on page 144.)
- If you're trying to stop by using a nicotine skin patch, your baby will get less nicotine than if you smoke. Wear the patch during the day and remove the patch at night when you need it least so your baby will get less nicotine during night feedings.

Weaning

As we mentioned earlier, the American Academy of Pediatrics and every major healthcare organization in the world recommends breastfeeding at least for the first year, which can confer huge health benefits on your baby (and many organizations recommend 2 years). While that can seem daunting during the newborn stage when the baby is nursing every couple of hours around the clock, it gets easier as time goes on. Your baby will get more efficient at nursing and your body will get more efficient at making milk. You'll hopefully be able to pump milk so you'll have breaks from being attached to the baby. And as baby's hormones shift and his stomach capacity expands he'll be able to sleep for longer stretches at night. After the baby starts solids at about 6 months he'll replace a few feedings a day with solid food, and by 9 months your baby may be nursing just a few times a day. By a year you may find that your only feeding is just before bedtime or if your toddler needs comfort.

Experts agree that the best strategy for weaning before 6 months is gradually and gently. Stopping abruptly can cause you to experience painful engorgement for a few days.

If you want or need to introduce formula, eliminate one daytime feeding at a time while maintaining the early morning and go-to-sleep feeds in the evening. Then drop the morning feed and finally the last feed of the evening.

If you're formula feeding, still ensure that your baby is held and gets eye contact, so your baby still gets closeness and **bonding**.

How to Turn the Milk Off

If you choose not to nurse your baby after birth, or if you nurse for a while and then decide to stop, expect that you're going to have some pain at first. The best advice is to take it easy and wean slowly. Your breasts will become swollen and hard for 2 to 4 days, and you may run a slight fever. The official name for this tightness and congestion is engorgement, and it can be unpleasant, if not painful. Here's how to help ease your discomfort:

• Bind your breasts for 24 to 48 hours. Use an extra-wide elastic (ACE) bandage. Wrap it tightly around your breasts three or four times, and pin it in place. This will compress your breasts and slow down milk-making.

• Apply ice packs. Or use a towel-wrapped bag of frozen vegetables for 15 minutes on and 45 minutes off. (If you leave the ice pack on for longer than 15 minutes, it may cause your breasts to swell even more.)

• Wear a bra. Wear a supportive bra at all times. A snug sports bra is best, and an underwire is the worst. Avoid extra pressure anywhere on your breast.

• Don't take a drug to stop the milk. If you're offered any drug to suppress lactation, refuse it. No drug is approved by the FDA to suppress lactation.

• Keep warmth away from your breasts. Stand with your back to the shower.

• Apply cabbage leaves. An often-used home remedy for breast swelling is to place raw cabbage leaves under the ice pack. Cabbage is thought to have anti-inflammatory properties.

• Don't express milk. Though it will relieve the pain temporarily, it'll encourage more milk production.

BOTTLE FEEDING

Baby formulas continue to improve every year as more is learned about the components of human milk. Modern-day formulas could be called artificial human milk. They're created from homogenized vegetable and animal fats, oils, and skim milk to closely imitate the fatty-acid content of human milk.

Liquid formulas may also contain thickening and stabilizing agents for uniform consistency.

Most formulas come in three versions: powdered, ready-to-feed bottles, and concentrated liquid. Powdered is the least expensive, and ready-to-feed bottles are the most expensive. Because all baby formulas must meet stringent federal nutrition and hygiene standards, there's no essential difference between generic and brand-name formulas, though some brand names may offer additional ingredients or specific formulations, such as extra DHA or specially processed "comfort proteins."

Make sure that the formula is fortified with iron. Be careful to follow the formula manufacturer's instructions to the letter when you mix formula. Formula that's too concentrated can put a strain on baby's kidneys. Formula that's too diluted with water can keep your baby from getting critical nutrients.

Only prepare formula in small batches, so that you're sure it's fresh. Keep it refrigerated, or use an ice pack in your diaper bag if you'll be out for more than an hour. Discard leftover formula rather than serving it a second time. Baby's mouth and saliva can cause the formula to become contaminated with bacteria.

There's no medical reason to heat formula, but some babies appear to prefer it served at body temperature. You can take the chill off of fresh formula by running the bottle under warm faucet water for a few minutes, or floating it with a cap on in a bowl of warm water.

You can also buy bottle warmers for the same purpose. (Note: Adult fingers and hands aren't sensitive enough to sense heat differences. Always test a sprinkle of the milk on your wrist just to make sure it's not too hot.)

There's no need to use boiled, purified, or "nursery" water for formula, though if you use powdered formula and your tap water comes from a well, be sure to have the water tested periodically, especially during hot weather, for the presence of *E. coli* bacteria and other contaminants.

If you want to save money on formula, it can help to let formula companies know that you'd like to be put on their mailing list for samples and coupons. You can do this by calling their toll-free customer service numbers. Another way to save on formula is to buy it by the carton from baby-discount stores. Just be careful to examine the labels on the cans to be sure that the formula's fresh and the use-by date won't expire before your baby's able to consume all the cans.

In rare instances, a baby may have an allergic reaction to the proteins or sugars in the cow's milk portion of a formula. Rarely, a baby's allergic reaction to formula can be serious—life-threatening vomiting, hives, bloody diapers, poor weight gain, and/or breathing problems. If a baby is allergic to formula proteins, there are alternative formulas made with soy protein (not the soy milk found in health food stores) and more refined, predigested formulas, called protein hydrolysates.

Your baby's healthcare provider should prescribe one of these alternative formulas if your baby shows symptoms of being allergic to regular formulas. Ask about recent research that links soy formulas with an increase in vulnerability to peanut allergies and the way soy could affect your baby's processing of certain minerals.

Bottle-Feeding Supplies

Baby bottles can be found in a variety of shapes and designs. Whatever you opt for, pick one shape and stick to it, because having a drawer of different bottle and nipple sizes to be matched up can drive a parent crazy.

When it comes to cleaning, the simpler the bottle shape, the better.

Bottles should be dishwasher safe and BPA-free, and come with easy-to-read ounce markings on the side for measuring.

The more transparent the bottle, the easier it is to make sure they're clean. Glass bottles are the easiest to get squeaky clean, but of course they're also breakable. If you decide to use them, never let your toddler walk around with one (and tether them to the high chair).

Angle-necked bottles are the latest in baby-bottle inventions, they're designed to keep baby from swallowing too much air. Angled bottles are more comfortable for parents to hold, especially when a baby's trying to suck out the last dregs of formula. They help by collecting the last of the formula in the nipple so baby isn't sucking half air and half liquid.

Bottles with built-in straws are a bad buy because it's next to impossible to scrub the entire milk residue from the inside of the straw. Also beware of bottles in cute shapes like doughnuts, bears, animals, soda bottles, or sports equipment. Spoiled milk residues stuck in hard-to-reach nooks could pose a health hazard.

Using a disposable bottle system is another alternative. Usually, you can buy a starter kit in one box, with bottle-size plastic rings for holding throwaway liners that resemble plastic sandwich bags and special nipples or nipples and plastic rings for securing the liners inside the holders. Once you've used up all the liners in the initial box, you'll have to buy replacements that come in a roll. While the system saves dishwashing hassles, it will be more expensive in the long term than reusable bottles, and there's always the problem of running out of liners.

All in all, standard reusable bottles are still the best and most economical solution. You'll also want to buy a baby-bottle brush and a small plastic cage for holding nipples in the dishwasher, or a drying rack for the bottles if you plan to hand wash them.

> *"I'm really proud of myself for breastfeeding for 3 months, because honestly I found it very challenging. I felt a lot of pressure from everyone to do it. For myself, I was relieved when she finally went on the bottle."*

Nipple Know-How

Babies seem to have their own preferences when it comes to the shape and feel of the bottle's nipple. Nipples, like bottles, come in a variety of shapes and materials. In addition to the standard nipple, other models are designed for special uses: for premature babies with sucking problems, for pulpy juices, or for feeding toddlers formula thickened with cereal.

So-called orthodontic nipples are elongated, almost hourglass-shaped. Advertisers claim they're better for baby's jaw development, but the center of the nipple is hard to get clean, and if it's made of latex, it may rot over time, causing it to become sticky and interfering with milk flow.

Start first with a standard, newborn-size nipple, and then experiment with other versions if your baby seems confused at feeding time.

Be sure to read the directions for the nipples after you get them home.

Some nipples come with special breathing holes on the base to help adjust the amount of milk flow according to how tightly you screw on the plastic bottle ring. All nipples should be boiled about 5 minutes before using them for the first time to be sure that dust and chemical residues are removed. Note: There is no need to boil or sterilize nipples after the first time.

Most nipples are molded from latex, a form of rubber, or from silicone. Silicone nipples are made from a clear material used widely in the medical world. It's durable and isn't likely to cause allergic reactions. Latex, on the other hand, can cause allergy problems in babies. Latex nipples also tend to rot over time from exposure to saliva and the acids in milk. On the other hand, silicone nipples can rupture and tear if a toddler chews on them, and they're slippery, which may cause difficulty for young babies. Whatever kind you choose, inspect nipples closely every few days for tears or abnormalities, and replace old nipples with new ones every 3 months or so.

Bottle Safety Notes

Never heat baby's formula in a bottle using a microwave oven. The formula will heat unevenly and develop hot spots, which can burn baby's mouth. This can also cause disposable bottles to rupture. Instead, use a bottle warmer or immerse the bottle in a bowl of warm water. Don't prop a bottle up to stay in baby's mouth. Every year in America, someone invents a contraption for holding a bottle in a baby's mouth so parents don't have to do it, but not only do these less-than-loving contraptions rarely work, they can be dangerous if your baby begins to spit up or choke on formula.

Burping

While breastfed babies usually don't need burping, bottle-fed babies often swallow air and stop drinking temporarily.

If your baby abruptly stops feeding, remove the bottle from your baby's mouth and sit him upright while patting him gently on the back.

Usually that will bring up a big burp along with some milk, and baby will be happy to settle back to drinking.

Another way to bring up air is to place baby up on your shoulder. (Be sure to cover your shoulder with a diaper or towel first.) After a few pats, air usually comes up.

Spitting Up versus Vomiting

All babies spit up from time to time. Babies have very immature muscles inside their throat, which makes it difficult to hold milk inside.

Spitting up is made worse by a baby's being upset and crying hard before getting fed, eating too fast, or from swallowing air while feeding.

Milk sometimes comes up with an air bubble when a baby burps, and sometimes milk may come out his nose too. Most spitting up usually resolves itself by the fourth to sixth month.

If your baby arches his back and starts to cry before he spits up, or if he seems to be in pain when it happens or when you lay him down after a feeding, he may have GERD (which stands for gastroesophageal reflux disease). The milk the baby swallows gets mixed with stomach acids, causing a burning sensation in the baby's throat when the milk comes back up.

If your baby has GERD, you can help him to be more comfortable by keeping him upright for 10 to 15 minutes after eating. Sometimes an infant-only car seat can provide the best angle for the baby.

Just be sure to stay with your baby to make sure the seat isn't tipped over by a pet or sibling. Feeding your baby smaller amounts but more often may help to reduce his discomfort, too.

Most problems with spitting up will resolve themselves as your baby matures, but in the meantime, you will need to make sure that your baby doesn't become dehydrated from the loss of fluids. Dry lips are a common sign of dehydration. If it worsens, the inside of the baby's mouth will also become dry, his urine will become stronger and darker, and he will become sluggish with sunken eyes. Your baby's healthcare provider may suggest a way to thicken your baby's formula to make it stay down better and may explore whether your baby is having an allergic reaction to his formula. If

so, a predigested version that will be easier for his body to absorb may be suggested. There are also a variety of medications that can be used to make your baby more comfortable by treating the acid in his stomach, speeding up the emptying of his stomach, and easing throat discomfort. Projectile vomiting is when large amounts of milk shoot out of your baby's mouth and travel 2 or 3 feet or even more for two or more feedings, and your baby seems ill. Contact your baby's healthcare provider right away if your baby is vomiting repeatedly and/or the vomit is red, dark brown, black, or green from bile.

Baby Bottle Mouth

Never put your baby to bed with a bottle. Babies can get an extreme form of tooth decay from being put to bed with a bottle. The acid and sugars in formula and juices pool in the sleeping baby's mouth and begin to erode tooth surfaces. The problem is usually difficult to detect, because it starts with chalky spots on the inside of baby's front teeth where you're not easily able to see. The teeth eventually begin to break down and crumble.

While children will lose their baby teeth anyway, dentists warn that a baby's jaw development and the angle at which permanent teeth emerge can be affected by the premature loss of baby teeth.

If your baby can't stand to go to bed without a bottle, try a small bottle of water.

Pacifiers

Babies have an instinct to suck, even when they've had enough to drink. Pacifiers have both good and bad points. On the plus side, a recent study appears to show a connection between the regular use of a pacifier and the reduced chance of a baby dying from SIDS. And if you're breastfeeding, it's just not possible to be a human pacifier day and night.

On the downside, prolonged pacifier use in childhood has been associated with jaw deformities and may contribute to speech impediments.

Just as with bottle nipples, pacifiers come in a variety of materials and shapes. You may want to buy several types to try with your baby. Again, boil them for 5 minutes before first letting your baby suck on one. If a pacifier drops on the floor, don't put it in your mouth to clean it. Bacteria from your mouth can spread

to your baby's and cause tooth decay. When it comes to a dropped pacifier, take into account where it drops—would you feel safe letting the baby lick that spot? If it's your living-room carpet it's probably fine; if it's the floor of the grocery store you'll want to wash the pacifier with hot water and soap before you give it back to your baby. If your baby is very attached to her pacifier, use a pacifier clip and/or carry a few spares when you go out.

One important warning: Never tie a pacifier around your baby's neck using a ribbon or string. Your baby could strangle if the string gets caught on something. Also always inspect pacifiers frequently to be sure the shield hasn't cracked and the nipple hasn't started to pull loose.

Bathing Basics

New babies really don't need baths—they don't sweat, eat solids, or crawl around and just don't get very dirty (except in the neck fold). A warm damp washcloth is usually all it takes. Bathing can also be hard on a baby: anyone who claims that giving a new baby a bath is "fun for you and baby" either never had a baby or forgot how new babies tend to hate being undressed and messed with. Temperature changes, such as those caused by the cooling of water as it evaporates off their wet skin, usually will arouse screams of protest. Too much rigorous cleaning can also deplete your baby's natural skin oils and cause dryness.

It will be easier on both of you if you hold off an immersion in a bath for as long as possible, and definitely until after the circumcision and umbilical cord sites have healed. Even then, your newborn won't need a daily bath—once a week is plenty.

There are ways to keep your baby clean during the pre-bath days. Brush his hair from back to front with a soft brush to stimulate the scalp and help prevent *cradle cap*, and clean up after bowel movements using a damp, lukewarm washcloth, a pre-moistened baby wipe, or a spray bottle filled with warm water. Rubbing a newborn's tender skin with a regular washcloth is too harsh—wipe gently with a soft, knit baby washcloth instead.

The best timing for your baby's bath is when he is alert but not hungry. Go slowly. Babies react to being lowered quickly and to sudden changes in temperature—especially when you undress them, and they feel bare and cold. The trick for those early days is to keep your baby wrapped loosely in a warm towel or blanket while you gently wipe down his body and folds with a warm, soft washcloth.

There are a variety of products to help you with bathing. A hooded towel and several baby washcloths will come in handy. You can also purchase a baby bathtub or a bathing insert that looks like a small hammock seat lined in terry cloth or other absorbent materials to prop in a sink or the big bathtub. Large, thick, baby-shaped bathing sponges are inexpensive and help to cushion baby's back and bottom in a tub or sink. (We discuss how to choose a baby bathtub in Chapter 6.)

Many parents opt to use the kitchen sink, with extra cushioning for baby's first bath. To prop up baby, simply fold a thick bath towel and line the bottom of the sink with it. Then add a few inches of warm water. Keep a measuring cup full of warm water within reach for pouring over your baby's body to rinse off soap.

Another practical bathing option to consider is taking your baby in the tub with you. Sit yourself down in waist deep, mildly warm water in the bathtub and let your partner hand the baby over to you. (Don't try to do this on your own—you could slip and hurt both of you.)

In the seated position, bring your knees up to support the baby, so his buttocks are resting against your belly with his head aimed toward your knees. Then soap, and rinse.

Have your partner take the baby and wrap him in a big, warm towel while you finish bathing and getting out of the tub. The advantage to this whole-body approach to baby bathing is that most babies are soothed by skin-to-skin contact, and you can nurse him if he gets upset.

When your baby's healed and ready for the first real bath, make sure the room's toasty warm. Your hands aren't good thermostats when it comes to judging the hotness of your baby's bathwater. Use the underside of your wrist instead. And before you take hold of your baby, wash your hands to remove any germs.

Gather together everything you'll need so it's within arm's reach. On the list are a clean gown or T-shirt; a fresh diaper; a gentle, non-perfumed soap such as Aveeno or unscented Dove; a soft baby hairbrush; a plastic measuring cup to hold warm rinse water; a baby washcloth; and a big, soft towel. Babies are as slippery as eels when they're wet. Hold your baby so his head is supported on the wrist of one hand with the fingers of that same hand holding baby's arm. Remember, never take your hands off your baby or leave him unattended—even if the telephone rings or someone comes to the door. Babies can drown in less than an inch of water in only a minute or so.

It really doesn't matter where on

your baby's body you begin the job; just be gentle about it, or simply use your fingertips and palms to do the job. While some advice books suggest you wash the baby from the top downward, we suggest doing his body first. That's because his head is more vulnerable to heat loss from evaporating water, and most babies and young children hate having their faces washed.

Be careful not to cover your baby's nose or mouth with a washcloth, and clean just one side of the face at a time. Remember to keep soap away from his eyes. Once you've cleaned and rinsed all parts except your baby's scalp, you may want to pick baby up and wrap him in a towel with just his head uncovered. Then put him in a football hold, and gently lather his scalp using a few drops of tearless baby shampoo. Hold his head in a downward direction and use the measuring cup filled with warm water to rinse so the water flows to the back of his head and away from his forehead and eyes.

After you're done, use an edge of the towel to gently pat his head dry. Then it's time to put on a fresh diaper and clean clothes.

If your baby screams and protests being bathed the traditional way, try keeping him wrapped in a warm, soft blanket or towel and damp-mopping his body, one part at a time, with a warm washcloth. You can also do this cleaning while holding your baby in your lap.

Later, after a few baths this way, you can try lowering your baby— blanket or towel and all—down into the warm water of the baby tub before starting the unwrapping and washing process.

EYE CLEANING

You may notice a white, yellow, or greenish discharge that collects in the sides of your baby's eyes on the side nearest the nose. This usually means that the baby's tear ducts are still too small to handle the pool of tears. You can gently clean away the mucus by wiping from the corner of eye, starting near the nose, toward the outer edge of the eye. Use a damp cotton ball dipped in warm water, but inspect the wet end of the ball first to make sure there are no loose cotton fibers that could be irritating.

If the discharge doesn't go away after a few days of gentle cleaning, or your baby's eyes look bloodshot, you may want to contact your healthcare provider.

SKIN RASHES

Most babies develop odd rashes from time to time, and there are hundreds of different varieties.

Everyday rashes are caused by a baby's sweat and oil glands not functioning normally for the first few weeks after birth. You may see little whiteheads (known as milia) on his face, or tiny pimples on his face between the third and sixth weeks. The bumps will disappear on their own and require no special care. Don't pick at them, as doing so may cause infection. Also keep baby's nails short to prevent scratching, which may also lead to infection.

Sometimes rashes are caused by the baby coming into contact with harsh chemical and perfumes in their clothing or in sheets. We suggest laundering all of the fabrics that come in contact with your baby in an unscented detergent and not using a fabric softener or perfumed softening sheets in the dryer.

Heat rash, sometimes called prickly heat (its medical name is miliaria rubia), is an itchy, red rash with small bumps or fluid-filled blisters that is caused by plugged sweat glands. It usually shows up in hot, humid weather, but sometimes babies get it in the winter, particularly if they are overdressed. You'll usually find it in the creases or skin folds around a baby's neck, on his back, in his armpits, or in the diaper area.

You can help to prevent heat rash by keeping your baby in the shade or indoors during the hottest part of the day, giving frequent lukewarm baths, using clothing made of absorbent cotton, and avoiding greasy ointments or skin lotions that hold your baby's sweat in. If your baby seems ill and cranky or has a fever, or if the rash spreads to other parts of the body, contact your baby's pediatrician.

Cradle cap (medical name seborrhoeic dermatitis) is a harmless, scaly, crusty area, usually on a baby's scalp but sometimes at the hairline or on the nose, behind the ears, or in the eyebrows. It is not an allergy, and it isn't caused by a lack of bathing. The patches of cradle cap can be yellow, pink, or brownish in color and usually show up in the first few weeks of life and disappear after a few months. The condition is very common and affects 1 out of 2 newborns.

It's not clear what causes cradle cap, but it's probably related to your baby's oil glands, which aren't yet fully developed. The condition will usually disappear without needing treatment. Swaddle your baby with just his head out, and then gently rinse his scalp with lukewarm water using the kitchen sink and a watering can or a measuring cup. Shampoo with a gentle baby shampoo (or mild dandruff shampoo, if your baby's healthcare provider approves), then rinse thoroughly. Contact your baby's healthcare provider if the rash spreads to other parts of your baby's body, if it bleeds, or if it appears red, swollen, or infected.

Eczema is a broad term for dry, itchy, inflamed skin. The first signs usually develop in the first 3 months of life. The baby with eczema will have red, scaly skin, and there may be red patches on his cheeks, followed by an inflammation of his scalp, arms, and legs. The patches will be itchy, which may make your baby restless and cranky. Babies and children with dry, very sensitive skin are more vulnerable to it, but allergies, such as to formula ingredients, pollens, or house dust, can cause an outbreak or make it worse. Heat, excess humidity, chafing, and soaps, or the strong chemicals and perfumes in detergents and fabric softeners can also aggravate it. The causes of eczema are not completely understood but are probably genetic. Notify your baby's healthcare provider, who may prescribe medications to help with the itching and a moisturizer to make your baby more comfortable. Also, protect your baby from those who have active cold sores caused by herpes, which might cause serious complications if your baby becomes infected.

Your Baby's Healthcare

It's important to choose your baby's pediatrician before giving birth. This lets your baby get personalized care from the very beginning; plus, most health insurance policies will pay for your baby's first exam in the hospital. (For help in choosing a healthcare provider for your baby, see page 7.)

The first checkup can be as soon as within 48 hours of discharge from the hospital if the mother is breastfeeding, had an early discharge from the hospital, or if there are other complications that need to be monitored. The American Academy of Pediatrics recommends well-baby checkups at the following ages: 2 weeks old and 1, 2, 4, 6, 9, 12, 15, 18, and 24 months.

If this is your first visit with your baby, you may need to fill out forms and present your insurance card. Your healthcare provider may provide a waiting room for healthy children separated from the one for sick kids, but sanitize you and your baby's hands on the way in and out anyway.

Once you're in an exam room, your baby will be measured and weighed and then have a complete physical exam. You will be asked a series of questions about your baby's feeding, wetting, and sleeping patterns, and you may be asked about how you and your family are coping with your new arrival. Your baby may remain calm during the process, or he could protest loudly at the change in temperature or the pain from an immunization.

If you're nursing, ask your provider if you can nurse your baby through the experience, or immediately afterward to help distract him from any discomfort. If you're bottle-feeding, carry along a comforting pacifier or bottle of formula. A bit of sugar water is also effective pain relief for a baby. Ask your healthcare provider if the office has any on hand.

Rather than trying to race home if your baby's upset, ask your healthcare provider if there is an available room where you can sit quietly and feed your baby until the two of you are calm again before trying to put him in his car seat to drive home.

STATE-MANDATED NEWBORN SCREENING TESTS

The uniform screening of newborn babies mandated by states began in 1962, with blood tests to identify babies with phenylketonuria (PKU). Since then the program has expanded to test for a variety of potentially serious diseases. These tests vary from state to state. Now, more than 4 million newborns a year are tested, which helps to identify about 3,000 babies with serious diseases that can usually be treated early, even before symptoms develop. If your state requires testing, your baby will have blood drawn before going home from the hospital, usually using a **heel stick**, and the blood specimen will be placed on a special filter paper that is sent to a centralized lab for testing.

A repeat or second newborn screen may be required, often after your baby's first checkup, especially if the first test was done in the baby's first 24 hours of life. Some states, such as Texas, mandate by law that two screens be done.

Phenylketonuria (PKU) and congenital adrenal hyperplasia (CAH) are screened for in all states, and other states require tests for other diseases as well. Six states, for example, test for cystic fibrosis, and New York tests for HIV.

If you would like to know more about the tests, ask your baby's pediatrician what your baby will be screened for, when, and how.

IMMUNIZATIONS

Your pediatrician will recommend an immunization schedule for your baby. Prior to starting your baby's routine immunizations, you may want to ask the doctor for information about the potential mild and rarer serious side effects of vaccines, the best timing for them, and the prevalence and dangers of the diseases from which the immunizations provide protection. Some, but not all, immunizations cause mild,

temporary after-effects, such as fever and irritability for a few hours afterward. In rare instances, immunizations can have more serious consequences. Ask your provider what to expect and if there are any medications to help your baby's symptoms. Also ask how to tell if symptoms are serious enough to warrant a call to the office.

Most likely your baby will be given three separate hepatitis B immunization shots, including one in the hospital, especially if tests show you to be hepatitis B positive.

Your provider will also recommend the DTaP (diptheria, tetanus, and pertussis—whooping cough), MMR (measles, mumps, and rubella—another form of measles), varicella (chicken pox), HIB (haemophilus influenza B), and PCV-7 (pneumococcus). The smallpox vaccine has been discontinued.

BABY ILLNESS

It's likely that your baby will get sick at some point, though if you're breastfeeding, your baby will be just as immune to germs as you are. Still, help prevent illness by making sure that all visitors who hold the baby wash their hands, and politely ask anyone with a cold to delay their visit until they're well again. Most common illnesses are caused by invisible bacteria and viruses transmitted from one person to another. Coughing, kissing, or hand contact can transmit illness. In rare cases, signs of sickness, such as a fever, sluggishness, rashes, or a runny nose can be the start of something serious, but, in most instances, it just means your baby's caught a more common bug, like a cold. Any time you suspect your baby has a temperature, it's important to contact your baby's pediatrician immediately. That's because your baby's body is only beginning to develop antibodies to illness, so sickness can be much more serious than it would be later on when your baby's internal defenses have become stronger. Sometimes, serious problems may at first look like an oncoming cold but then quickly worsen.

A baby's symptoms may take hours or days to develop after germs have been passed on. Symptoms of oncoming illness can include demanding to nurse more often or less often than usual, or the opposite, refusing to eat; a fever of greater than 100.4° F; crankiness or excessive sluggishness; and vomiting or diarrhea.

Taking Your Baby's Temperature

A fever is a sign that your baby may have an infection. A fever in a baby under 2 months of age may be especially significant and should be reported to your baby's healthcare provider right away. The easiest way to tell if your baby's running a fever is to kiss his forehead to find out if it feels hotter than normal. A normal temperature for a baby is between 97°F and 100.4°F (36°C to 38°C). A rectal temperature higher than 100.4°F in a baby under 2 months of age should be reported to your baby's healthcare provider. The American Academy

of Pediatrics (AAP) recommends that pediatricians and parents no longer purchase and use glass thermometers that contain mercury; instead, purchase an easy-to-read digital thermometer from a pharmacy or on the Web. Most cost less than $10. Ear thermometers cost more and may not be as accurate. Don't try to get your baby's temperature by mouth; it probably won't work and you might injure his delicate tissues. Your best two choices are by placing the sensitive part of the thermometer in your baby's *rectum*, or putting it directly beneath his armpit and gently holding his arm down. The armpit method, called axillary temperature, is about 2° cooler than a rectal temperature.

A rectal temperature is usually more accurate and not as uncomfortable as it may sound, for the baby, anyway. If your pediatrician asks you to take your baby's temperature rectally, you can take it while diaper changing by holding your baby's ankles, spreading his buttocks, and grasping the thermometer between your middle and index finger with your other hand. Gently insert it in about 1 inch. Don't use a digital thermometer if it has a sharp, pointed probe that could injure your baby's rectal area.

A second way is to place your baby facedown on your lap with his legs dangling from your thigh. Support the thermometer with your cupped hand so that it sticks out from the base of your fingers. Either way, the thermometer should be lubricated with petroleum jelly. Newer thermometers with flexible tips are safest. The thermometer will beep when it's ready. (Have tissue on hand: Your baby may poop when the thermometer's on the way out.)

Write down your reading and the date and time you took it. When you call your pediatrician, make sure he or she knows the method you used to get your baby's temperature reading.

You'll find these items, all of which are available in a pharmacy, helpful when your baby gets sick:

- A medicine spoon or dropper. It should have easy-to-read markings on the side to help measuring doses.
- Saline nose drops or sprays. These drops in baby strength will help to break up stuffy noses for babies.
- A bulb syringe (nose bulb). It will have a bulb such as on a bicycle horn on one end and a rounded suction tip on the other. It's for suctioning out baby's nasal mucus.
- Thermometer. Ask your baby's healthcare provider what type of thermometer to use and the recommended way of taking the baby's temperature.
- Baby-strength acetaminophen. Use Tylenol (or another brand) for treating your baby's fever in concentrated drops if your baby is over 8 weeks old. Consult with your physician before administering acetaminophen; too much acetaminophen can hurt your baby's liver. Note the date, the time, and how much of any medication you've given your baby to share over the telephone with your doctor.
- Petroleum jelly. Use it for lubricating the thermometer if your doctor wants a rectal reading.
- Diaper rash cream or kaolin clay powder. For when baby's bottom gets red and looks raw.

Fever: Treat or Not

During an illness, babies and toddlers can suddenly spike a high fever that would seem very dangerous for adults, and some babies may even go into a convulsion when a fever rapidly rises over 101°F. While conventional wisdom used to be that fevers should be brought down right away, more recent research suggests that fevers serve a purpose. Contact your baby's caregiver immediately if your baby gets a (rectal) temperature higher than 100.4°F. If your baby does have a fever or a seizure, it's important to contact your doctor immediately to get instructions about what to do next. In the meantime, try to cool your baby by undressing him to his diaper and gently wiping him off with lukewarm water.

If your baby has a convulsion, it will look like odd, spastic movements in his body for a very brief time, and then he may fall into a deep sleep. Your job is to simply protect the baby from hitting his head or limbs on anything. Don't try to put anything in his mouth; it could cause injury. Your doctor may recommend a fever-reducing medication, such as acetaminophen (e.g., Tylenol) for babies. It will be a concentrated liquid that comes with its own dropper. It's critical to give the exact dosage as recommended! Administering too much medication is a common mistake that parents make because the gradations are so tiny when you're using a small dropper. Measure the liquid in a bright light, so you can see what you're doing.

Ibuprofrin (Motrin) is not approved for babies younger than 6 months of age. Aspirin is also not recommended for babies and young children with flu-like symptoms of illness because it has been linked to a rare but serious disease called Reye's syndrome that most often affects children between the ages of 3 and 12.

Colds and Infections

Colds are especially hard on young babies. They can only breathe through their noses when they nurse and not through their mouths like children and adults can. The colds begin with irritability and eating changes, clear fluid running from the nose, sneezing, and possibly a low fever.

Our grandmothers used to say: "You can treat a cold, and it will be over in a week, or you can do nothing, and it will end in 7 days." There's some truth to that. But sometimes colds can develop into something more serious.

RSV stands for respiratory syncytial virus (pronounced sin-SISH-al), one of the most common sources for serious pneumonia and other infections of baby's nose, throat, and lungs. Every year, 90,000 babies are hospitalized with RSV-related illnesses.

It's estimated that nearly half of all babies catch some type of RSV every year, usually in winter. Its symptoms are like a cold: stuffy, runny nose; a low-temperature fever; and a cough. Sometimes bacteria come along to cause an

inner-ear infection at the same time.

Preemies and babies with serious diseases, such as HIV, congenital heart disease, or lung conditions, are more vulnerable to the serious side of RSV. It may begin as a simple cold and then become more serious. Symptoms include a fever higher than 100.4°F for a baby under 3 months of age, or higher than 102°F for older babies and toddlers. Other serious symptoms include fast breathing or difficulty getting breaths, a whistling noise in the chest when breathing out (wheezing), a deep or frequent cough, disinterest in nursing, and listlessness or unusual irritability. Contact your baby's pediatrician for instructions about what to do.

Ear Infections

Next to colds, inner-ear infections (*otitis media*) are the most common reason parents take a baby to the pediatrician. As many as three out of four babies have some form of ear infection by age 3. Typically, the infection will set in a few days after a cold has started. You can't see that the baby has the infection; it's on the other side of the eardrum. If your baby has an ear infection, he's likely to be cranky (you'll think it's colic), he may bat at his ear, or he may temporarily lose some hearing and scream in extreme pain.

Your doctor will want to examine your baby's ears and may suggest a painkiller such as acetaminophen or ibuprofen, along with a course of antibiotics if a bacterial infection is suspected.

In the meantime, you might try

keeping your baby in a semi-upright position, such as in a car seat, high chair, or swing. It might also help to apply a mildly warm, moist towel to your baby's jawline under the ears. Usually, these infections get better after several days of treatment.

Diarrhea

Diarrhea can be dangerous for babies during the first 4 months of life.

It can be brought on by an illness, a change in formula or vitamins, and/or taking antibiotics. Although a baby's normal stools may resemble diarrheal disease, it is rare in babies fed only breastmilk. A baby's having more stools that are liquid and sometimes foul-smelling signals true diarrhea. You may see solids sitting on top of the diaper core with a ring of staining where the semi-liquid part of the diarrhea has soaked in. The risk of diarrhea is that it can quickly deplete your baby's fluid stores, leading to dehydration—a serious threat to young infants. A dehydrated baby may be more sluggish than usual and harder to rouse, may have a dry mouth, and may go for hours without wetting a diaper. If your baby is getting dehydrated or you see blood in the stool, you should contact your healthcare provider immediately.

Thrush

If your baby's tongue and cheeks stay coated in white patches that won't wipe away, he may have thrush, a fungus-caused problem. This yeast infection grows in moist places, and it may also appear as red, irritated patches in the folds of your baby's skin, such as on the neck or in the armpits and thighs. Sometimes a cherry-red diaper rash that doesn't clear up easily can also be caused by yeast. If you also have red, itchy, cracked nipples, sometimes with white patches, this may also be yeast-related. Both a mother and baby may need to be treated to prevent re-infecting one another. Your healthcare provider will suggest medication to treat it.

EMERGENCY BABY LIFE SUPPORT

Baby life support is emergency measures to keep your baby alive and breathing until help comes. It is rare for a baby to need emergency resuscitation, but it's a very good idea to take a course in life support or CPR through your local American Red Cross chapter or the American Heart Association.

In the meantime, here are some basic instructions to rehearse: CPR stands for cardiopulmonary resuscitation. This is the lifesaving measure you can take to save your baby if she shows no signs of life (breathing or movement). CPR uses chest compressions and rescue breaths to circulate blood that contains oxygen to the brain and other vital organs until emergency medical personnel arrive.

STEP 1: CHECK YOUR BABY'S CONDITION.

Is your baby conscious? Flick her foot or gently tap on her shoulder and call out. If she doesn't respond, have someone call 911 or the local emergency number. (If you're alone with your baby, give 2 minutes of care as described below, then call 911 yourself.)

Swiftly but gently place your baby on her back on a firm surface.

Make sure she isn't bleeding severely. If she is, take measures to stop the bleeding by applying pressure to the area. Do not administer CPR until any bleeding is under control.

STEP 2: OPEN YOUR BABY'S AIRWAY.

Tilt your baby's head back slightly with one hand and lift her chin slightly with the other.

Check for signs of life (movement and breathing) for no more than 10 seconds.

To check for your baby's breath, put your head down next to her mouth, looking toward her feet. Look to see whether her chest is rising and listen for breathing sounds. If she's breathing, you should be able to feel her breath on your cheek.

STEP 3: GIVE HER 2 GENTLE BREATHS.

If your baby isn't breathing, give her two little breaths, each lasting just 1 second. Cover your baby's nose and mouth with your mouth and gently exhale into her lungs only until you see her chest rise.

Remember that a baby's lungs are much smaller than yours, so it takes much less than a full adult breath to fill them. Breathing too hard or too fast can force air into the infant's stomach or damage her lungs.

If her chest doesn't rise, her airway is blocked. Give her first aid for choking. (See *www.heart.org.*)

If the breaths go in, give your baby two breaths in a row, pausing

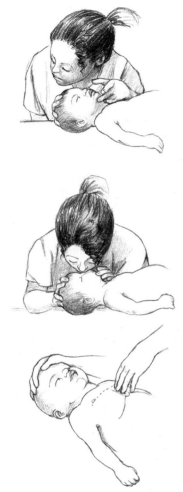

between rescue breaths to let the air flow back out.

STEP 4: GIVE HER 30 CHEST COMPRESSIONS.

With your baby still lying on her back, place the pads of two or three fingers just below an imaginary line running between your baby's nipples.

With the pads of these fingers on that spot, compress the chest ½ inch to 1 inch. Push straight down.

Compressions should be smooth, not jerky.

Give her 30 chest compressions at the rate of 100 per minute. When you complete 30 compressions, give 2 rescue breaths (step 3, above).

STEP 5: REPEAT COMPRESSIONS AND BREATHS.

Repeat the cycle of thirty compressions and two breaths. If you're alone with your baby, call 911 or the local emergency number after 2 minutes of care. Continue the cycle of compressions and breaths until help arrives.

Even if your baby seems fine by the time help arrives, you'll want to have her checked by a doctor to make sure that her airway is completely clear and that she hasn't sustained any internal injuries.

Finding Childcare

Finding a responsible caregiver for your baby is an important job. Babysitters, babysitting co-ops, day care centers, home day care settings, nannies, and au pairs— there are a huge variety of ways to find help in caring for your child. The important thing is that your child receives loving, responsive care that is stimulating and offers opportunities for learning and growth. Below are your options for finding child care.

HIRING A BABYSITTER

Babysitters are for occasional childcare needs. You can use members of your family, hire an adult neighbor or teen, or go through a formal agency that provides professional babysitters for a fee.

What's needed is a responsible person who is mature enough to think clearly in emergency situations, who can follow your directions to the letter, and who will show up as promised. When it comes to caring for a baby, kindness and gentleness are to be preferred over a rigid, disciplinary approach.

Your local chapter of the American Red Cross may offer "Babysitters Training," a special course for kids 11 to 15 that teaches basic first aid, feeding, diapering, and other useful skills. You can find your local chapter, where you can call for information on qualified babysitters, online at *www. redcross.org*. Guidance counselors in junior highs and high schools can sometimes offer help in finding just the right young person for your needs.

It's important to have the sitter visit you at home with your baby before leaving your baby at home alone with her. That's when you can teach the sitter your basic routines and rules. Diapering, feeding, and sleeping routines should be demonstrated, even though a sitter may claim to be familiar with all of these skills. Formula preparation for your baby may require careful directions plus written instructions.

You'll want to come to an advance agreement about payment, transportation, and hours needed for the job. Some teens, for example, may not be able to stay out past 11 on school nights.

Before you go out, be sure to post important telephone numbers: how to reach you in an emergency, a nearby relative or neighbor who can be called upon if there's a problem, the number to call for emergencies (911), and the number of your baby's doctor.

USING BABYSITTING CO-OPS

If you're only seeking occasional babysitting, you may want to join with other parents in forming a babysitting cooperative. Usually, a co-op consists of four to five families who agree to exchange babysitting duties with each other in exchange for points instead of money. Co-ops that have been around a long time can grow to be much larger—fifty or more families. Running a successful co-op requires good organizing skills. The larger the group, the more organizing that will be required. During the initial planning stage, you'll want to decide together to limit the number of families that can participate and, perhaps, make a list of the values or qualities of the families you want to have as members; otherwise, you may find members you don't wish to use. You'll need a chairperson to oversee the running of the co-op and a secretary whose job is keeping records of people's points. You can either give your officers

extra credit for their duties, or you can rotate responsibilities, but organizational and follow-through abilities are important qualities for your leaders. The chairperson's job is to oversee the running of the co-op, to plan regular co-op meetings so everything runs smoothly, to help in setting up basic rules (such as delivery and pickup of children, not sitting sick children, and a point scale), and to intervene in conflicts between members (e.g., when a member fails to carry out his babysitting duties).

HIRING IN-HOME CARE

If parents can afford it, most would rather have their babies kept in their own homes, rather than having them watched in some other setting. The advantages of keeping your baby at home are the additional security for your child of being in a familiar setting and the lessening of exposure to childhood illnesses, including colds and chronic ear infections.

To achieve in-home care, you may want to consider having (or hiring) a relative, such as your baby's grandmother, to care for your child or using a worker who provides childcare or childcare plus housekeeping for a living.

A more costly option is to hire a nanny or au pair using a professional agency that subcontracts with a person, paying them to work for you. Most agencies handle recruitment, hiring, and the financial aspects of salaries and health insurance. These agencies often charge top dollar for their services, and those whom they hire may only be available for limited spans of time, but some families with the resources find that nannies are a wonderful solution for in-home childcare. If you aren't able to manage the costs of having your child cared for in your own home, you may want to consider finding a mother or older person who would be willing to care for your baby in their home. The best solution is usually an at-home mom who wants to supplement her income by caring for one or two other children besides her own.

The closer to your home, the better.

Look for a neat, orderly house, safe baby equipment, plenty of baby toys, and a person who seems to genuinely enjoy talking and playing with babies and tots. Too many kids in one house can mean that your baby has to cry for attention, and he may be vulnerable.

FIND A COMMERCIAL CHILDCARE CENTER

Not all childcare centers will accept infants. For that reason, centers that care for babies are in high demand, often have long waiting lists, and charge premium prices.

Providing quality care for babies requires an intense relationship between babies and caregivers, and the best centers have a low ratio of staff members to babies (3 to 1 or better).

Also remember that staff members can call in sick—so a large baby-to-staff-member ratio means your baby may end up with less attention on some days, simply because there aren't enough people on hand to care for everyone.

The number one quality to look for in a center that cares for babies is an atmosphere of warmth and affection. Good caregivers genuinely love babies and relate to them as people, not simply charges to be routinely fed and then put to sleep. Observe how the staff relates to individual babies, especially babies who are unhappy. Staff training is important too. Teachers and aides should have degrees in early childhood education or other infancy areas or, at a minimum, a year of specialized training in caring for babies. Ask about ongoing staff training as well.

Visiting a center more than once is an important way of determining how well babies are cared for. The center should have open doors when it comes to parents' visits, and you should be welcomed to visit the center and your baby whenever you wish. The facility should be brightly lit and immaculately clean, and offer safe equipment and a variety of playthings for babies.

QUALITIES OF A GOOD CAREGIVER

There are very special characteristics that make for a good caregiver. She should genuinely love children. The ideal person is self-confident, affectionate, and positive in the way that she interacts with children.

Not all caregivers are suited for caring for babies. While a firm disciplinarian might be suitable for an active, unruly preschooler, babies thrive in a flexible, responsive environment where a baby's needs are more important than a list of rules.

Consistency is important. In interviewing potential homecare providers, try to determine the stability of the person and the situation. High turnover in sitters can cause a child distress and affect his security. At the same time, don't be afraid to change caregivers at any point if you find yourself feeling uncomfortable.

Sanitation and infection control are critical issues, so it's important to take a look at how babies are being diapered, since feces and saliva are two ways that serious infections can be passed from one baby to another. Observe staff hand washing and food handling, and ask about the sanitizing of toys. A good center will routinely sanitize baby playthings that have been mouthed and touched by a baby.

What are the center's sick baby policies? Will you need to keep your baby at home, or is there a sick bay where sick babies can be cared for without spreading germs to other babies? Remember, if the center lets sick babies come, then your baby will be exposed to illnesses too.

Look for daily educational and exploration activities that are suitable and safe for infants. Your baby should have a chance to play with a variety of materials with baby-conscious outdoor opportunities as well. Toddlers and babies should play in separate spaces. (See Resources on page 338 for Web sites with lots of information on childcare issues.)

Some state-of-the art centers allow special cameras so you can check in on your baby at any time during the day using your computer and a Web cam. Some businesses also offer mini-cams for hidden, at-home use, so you can virtually look in on your child during the day. Those are very costly options, but if you can afford it and the monitoring gives you more peace of mind, you may decide doing so is worth the price.

Travel with Baby

A special event is coming up for your family, or the holidays, or your mother's birthday, or a sister's wedding, and you're duty bound to board an airplane or drive a car to get there. Here are our suggestions to help you and your baby survive the travel stress.

It's amazing how much stuff you'll end up packing to cover your baby's travel needs! And most of your baby gear should be carry-on luggage and not checked ahead of time. If you're planning to fly with your baby, book your flights for the least crowded times of day. You may want to fly a day or two early if you're coming up on a holiday when there will be heavy crowds in the airport.

Try to get the bulkhead seats if you can—it will give you more legroom, and your tot will have squirm room. Plan to arrive at the airport 2½ hours early, instead of just 1. That gives you plenty of time for diapering and feeding your baby and keeps you from experiencing last-minute panic when cabs don't show up, parking is a hassle, or long lines slow down your check-in process. Most airlines will allow you to carry your baby's car seat onto the airline if it's been approved by the Federal Aviation Administration (FAA). If it has been, there will be a sticker on the seat that says it. (Note: Most booster seats are not FAA approved.) The only problem with fastening your baby down during the flight is that the airlines will probably expect you to purchase an extra ticket for your baby. Talk with the airline representative in advance.

Although in-flight injuries to babies and toddlers are rare, they do happen. Usually, they're injured when a plane hits turbulence and the baby flies out of his parent's arms, striking seat backs or luggage compartments.

The easiest way to install your baby's car seat in the airplane seat is to push the rear seat back as far as you can first. That gives you more leeway for fiddling with the belts.

Most babies cry during takeoff and landing. There's a simple explanation: Babies have huge middle ear canals on the inside of their eardrums that allow air to expand as pressure builds, causing pain. Letting your baby nurse or drink formula may help, but don't overfeed your baby! That can cause vomiting. Be prepared for that, or for getting your lap soaked, by bringing along a lightweight change of clothes for both your baby and you.

When the "fasten seatbelts" sign is turned off, consider taking your baby for a brief walk or two in the aisle if the refreshment cart isn't too near. You may need to change your baby's diapers on the closed lid of the toilet seat. Bring your own changing pad for sanitation. A flight attendant may let you use her fold-down seat at the rear of the plane for the job.

When you arrive at your destination, the car rental company will insist that your baby ride in a car seat. Most will promise you a rental seat when you call to make your reservation, but if you're traveling during peak vacation and holiday periods, you may find yourself at the airport with no seat for baby, and thus no car. Play it safe by bringing your own. (Some of the big baby equipment stores sell zippered car seat carry cases.)

What to Pack

- **Your doctor's telephone number.** Make sure you have it at all times in case your baby gets sick and you need medical advice. (And don't forget your medical insurance card.)
- **Car seat.** You can use it on the airplane if it is approved by the FAA. Rental car companies require that you use a car seat, but sometimes, especially during holidays, they run short. Just bring your own.
- **Sun shield.** Use a suctioned shade for the window nearest baby to prevent glare and sunburn.
- **Heat protection.** Take a thick blanket or beach towel to cover your baby's seat when your car's parked. Babies are far more vulnerable to heatstroke than children or adults, and they can die from it. Don't ever leave your baby inside the car without the air conditioning running and an adult present during the summer.

Interior temperatures soar to 120°F and higher!

- **Diapers.** Newborns wet the most of babies at any age. They use up a minimum of 10 diapers in 24 hours. Plan ahead just in case you end up stranded with car trouble, or sitting in an airport because a flight's been canceled.
- **Formula.** If you're not breastfeeding, the same goes for premeasured, powdered formula and bottles.
- **Clothing.** You'll need a collection of baby T-shirts or gowns to make sure you're covered for all the wetting and spit-ups that babies routinely do.
- **Pacifier.** If your baby uses a pacifier, then pack three or four new ones that you've boiled for at least 5 minutes to remove chemical residues. A pacifier can help to balance air pressure changes in plane cabins.
- **Cloth diapers.** A handful of cloth diapers make great milksops on airplanes and for burping baby.
- **Sealable plastic bags.** Carry along three or four zippered plastic bags in the two-gallon size if you can find them for storing wet diapers and soiled clothing until you can get to a washing machine. Also carry smaller, sandwich-size bags for odds and ends.
- **Wipes or washcloths.** Put several folded, damp washcloths (or disposable baby wipes) for damp mopping jobs in one of the sealable plastic bags.
- **Clothes for the weather.** If it's winter, you'll need to pack a soft, warm blanket for carrying baby outside, and a knitted hat and booties for extra warmth. If you're going into warm weather,

baby will need a brimmed hat.
- **Skin protection.** A tube of *zinc oxide* or a jar of petroleum jelly may come in handy as bottom protection if a rash shows up.
- **Medications.** Baby-strength Tylenol and a thermometer will be useful if baby spikes a fever. But don't use any medication without your healthcare provider's approval.
- **Stroller or front carrier.** A lightweight, easy-to-fold stroller with a good canopy, or a clip-on gooseneck umbrella will come in handy for sightseeing and strolls; however, these types of strollers are not recommended for newborns younger than 4 months old (see Chapter 6). But if you're flying, be careful about checking your naked stroller as a piece of luggage! The frame may get bent unless you secure it into a protective box like those used for golf bags.
- **Sleeping options.** If you're driving and have to bring your own baby bed, then consider purchasing an easy-to-fold travel play yard. It should have a firm mattress pad that's fastened down well. Don't waste your money on models with bassinets or diaper-changing add-ons—those features aren't worth it, and they may be unsafe if there's a chance baby could roll overboard or get caught between the tubular components. (See Chapter 6.) Your other option is to rent a crib at your destination from a local rental service store. Inspect the crib when it arrives to make sure it's in good working order with no loose hardware or missing bars—both can cause deadly strangulation accidents.

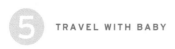

Plan to bring your own mattress protector, blankets, and fitted sheets.

Don't be surprised if you find yourself more tired when you get back home than before you left! Many parents say they return home feeling like they need a vacation after their vacation. One solution is to purposely plan an in-home family retreat for a few days after you get back home—carry-in dinners in the bedroom in front of the TV, leisurely walks in the park or nearby woods, hiring a neighborhood teenager to wash the dirty clothes. Downtime is critical before day-to-day work pressures inundate you again.

6

Baby Gear Primer

Surprise! Equipping, feeding, and outfitting your tiny offspring is likely to cost between $5,000 and $8,000 during your pregnancy and the first year of your baby's life. Our guide is designed to help you figure out what to buy immediately, what you can buy used, which items you can wait to purchase until later, and what you may not need to buy at all. And always keep in mind your newborn couldn't care less what brand names or cute designs are on her gear or how much you spend. Your baby's primary motivation will be to get held, keep warm, get fed, be rocked, and have wet diapers changed, over and over again.

Two-Minute Money-Saving Baby Gear Roundup

Many novice parents (and grandparents) make the mistake of assuming that by paying a huge price for designer baby gear, they're getting better quality and safety. That's simply not the case. Middle-of-the-line products often hold up equally well, and sometimes they perform even better than pricey top-of-the-line models.

If you buy the highest-priced stroller, for example, you're most likely paying for a larger frame, thicker padding, and more accessories—all of which make the stroller heavier, bulkier, and less portable.

Sometimes manufacturers rent well-known logos and brand names from other companies just to sell products. But if you buy a car seats or stroller labeled, say, "Eddie Bauer" or "Jeep," it doesn't mean the products are any less vulnerable to flaws and/or safety *recalls*. Research pays, and you can save thousands—and maybe your baby's life—by just checking product reviews and recall lists on consumer sites.

Here's a quick list on how to save more than $2,000 in baby gear costs:

• **Window shop first.** Don't buy any big-ticket item without comparison shopping. Troubleshoot for potential problems by pulling floor models down from the shelves. If it folds, fold it. If there are removable items, remove them. Write down model names, numbers, and prices so you can compare prices with online retailers (but remember to include shipping costs when you comparison shop).

• **Ask other parents.** Your friends who have kids will be good for opinions, and so are Internet sites featuring parents' product reviews, like *www.amazon.com* or *www.consumerreports.org*.

• **Don't buy anything until after the baby showers are over.** People love buying for babies. Spread the joy (and expense) by giving your relatives, friends, and grandparents a chance to outfit you with what you need. And, of course, save gift slips and tags, so you can return or consign what you don't need. An added bonus of this is the less time you spend in stores, the fewer opportunities to impulse buy.

• **Don't bother with toys.** It sounds cruel and unusual to deny a baby toys, but the truth is that newborns couldn't care less about stuffed animals, mobiles,

and so on. Babies are interested in human faces and the things big people show interest in, like your keys and cell phone, remote controls, and kitchen paraphernalia. Wait until you meet your baby and know what his or her interests are before you stock up on toys—for instance, if she's crazy about your keys or phone, then you'll want to get a mouthable toy version.

• **Find your local consignment shop, flea market, or thrift store with kids' clothes and stores.** Not only can you find great clothing and gear deals, but you may also be able to recycle your own kids' unwanted or unused stuff later.

• **Beware of salespeople.** No offense to the retail industry, but don't trust salespeople to be straight with you. When you're ready to start buying, remember that even mild, grandmotherly shop clerks are experts at subtly (or not so subtly) guiding you toward buying more than you need. Don't let them "upsell" you into high-margin items like a luxury mattresses, matching bedding sets, travel systems, or high-definition video baby monitors.

• **Shop the big guys.** Kmart, Wal-Mart, Target, and Costco sometimes offer great deals on house-brand no-frills baby products. Watch for sales and specials at the big megastores for babies too, such as Babies-R-Us and Baby Depot (sometimes found inside Burlington Coat Factory stores), but make sure you understand the return policy.

• **Know what you're looking**

for. Research online and then have your product picks down in writing before you enter a giant baby emporium, or you may find yourself overwhelmed. And keep in mind that the little doodads that you throw in at the last minute can really add up.

• **Buy a new, not used, crib and car seat.** New safety features hit the market all the time, as do product recalls for design flaws. A used car seat could have been in an accident and have invisible cracks in the frame that could compromise its ability to protect your baby, and all drop-side cribs have been recalled, which are the majority of cribs manufactured in the past several decades. Plastics and hardware also weaken and wear with age.

• **Buy a convertible car seat,** one that will be good for infants and kids from 6 to 30 pounds. These seats can ride facing backward or forward and will remain useful for 2 to 3 years. The American Academy of Pediatrics recommends that all children under the age of 2 ride rear-facing in the backseat. If possible, try to install the seat in the store's parking lot, so you can exchange it right away if it's difficult to use. To safely install the seat, refer to your car's owner's manual and the car seat's own directions. Then have your installation checked at your local fire or police station (many hospitals and police and fire stations offer free car seat check days periodically).

• **Buy a stroller and car seat separately.** You don't need the weighty stroller that comes with car seat/stroller package deals.

Instead, consider a strap-on, hands-free soft carrier such as the BabyBjörn for walks while your baby is small, keeping the car seat strapped in the car, and then later buying a separate, lightweight, maneuverable stroller with a reclining back once your baby's strong enough to sit up on her own (usually 4 to 6 months). While the "baby bucket" car-seat/carriers will be convenient should your baby fall asleep in the car, they're also unwieldy and responsible for many a mom's pulled shoulder and bruised thighs. They also have a very limited (6-month) life span and don't provide the stimulating natural motion that soft carriers provide.

• **Carefully pick your soft carrier.** A comfortable, easy-to-use soft front carrier is a must, since your baby may want to be attached to you at all times. Try on carriers to make sure they're easy to get on and off—if the store won't let you try them on be sure to save receipts. Avoid slings, which pose a suffocation hazard to babies and also can cause you back and neck strain.

• **Breastfeed your baby for as long as you can.** You can save your family about $1,000 a year given the cost of formula and bottles. Breastfeeding is also more convenient—you'll have less stuff to cram into your diaper bag, and you can go anywhere on a whim with your baby and have sterile milk at the ready, come what may. You can purchase a good breast pump for less than $250 and still save compared with the costs of formula feeding.

• **Use dark-colored washcloths instead of wipes.** Two to 3 years of using many disposable baby wipes a day will really add up. Plus, premoistened wipes may contain potentially harmful chemicals and irritants. For routine changes of wet diapers at home, a swipe with a damp washcloth will do.

• **Don't buy bedding sets.** They're generally overpriced, and fluffy comforters, pillows, and crib bumpers should be banned from your baby's sleeping space anyway. Just buy or register for single crib sheets and sleep sacks or pajamas for bedtime, and have your toddler help you pick out a comforter and pillow when it's time for a big-boy or -girl bed.

TIP

Manufacturers of baby products often offer free samples, money-saving coupons, and giveaways (such as free diaper bags). Some also underwrite free parenting magazines and Internet sites.

Baby Showers

Baby showers date back to ancient Greece, though before the 1950s, babies were welcomed with gifts after birth. Today, most new moms-to-be will have a shower between weeks 35 and 37, with guests invited electronically. Because showers are still basically about collecting gifts on behalf of an expectant mom, though, they're still never thrown by the woman herself and remain traditionally hosted by the woman's closest female friend.

In the 1950s, neighborhood moms would gather for cigarettes and martinis, bearing gifts of homemade diapers, hankies, booties, and blankets. These days showers have evolved into all kinds of permutations, like the family shower, the co-ed friends' backyard barbecue/shower, and/or a business power shower where co-workers and underlings are expected to pay tribute. There's even the virtual online shower, and the dad's baby-bachelor shower, where a dad-to-be's pals or co-workers give him silly gifts (gas mask and pee-pee tepee, anyone?) and take him out for lunch or a night of drinks and carousing.

Whether you're a guy, girl, or online avatar, if you're the recipient of a shower, you have four major duties:

• Expressing surprise and delight with every gift.
• Appointing someone to track who gives you what.
• Hand-writing and snail-mailing thank-you cards.
• Exchanging multiple or un-wanted gifts ASAP.

Shopping for Baby

It makes sense to postpone your shopping until you've had a baby shower (or two or three, as moms-to-be are sometimes treated to multiple showers). Not only are baby showers fun, but they can help you stockpile what you need for Junior.

You have a couple of choices about getting the word out about what you need so you won't be inundated with cute but not-so-useful stuff. Don't be shy about hinting—if you need something, say so! In fact, people will probably ask what you need and where you're registered.

Your baby-shower hostess will probably ask for your registry information to be enclosed baby-shower invites. Consider registering with an online service that lets you compile all of your information at a single site.

Another way to make your baby needs known is by using a baby registry at a major store. Similar to bridal registries, baby registries are wish lists for expectant parents, created by filling out forms and walking around the store and making choices with a sales associate or bar-code scanner.

With large national chains, you will be given a computerized wand so you can wander through the store zapping the product code for anything that strikes your fancy. Your gift selections will then be downloaded into a gigantic database that can be accessed online nationwide or in store kiosks by anyone who walks in and wants to buy you a gift.

One advantage of a registry is that it will let gift buyers know what's already been bought, which helps to keep you from getting duplicate gifts.

Essential Products for Before Baby Arrives

PRODUCT	OUR RECOMMENDATION	IMPORTANT FEATURES
BOTTLES & NIPPLES	Four, 4-ounce size for storing breastmilk or formula	Opt for BPA-free plastic with easy-to-read measurement lines and a set of silicone nipples
CAR SEAT	A "convertible" seat designed to face rearward for the 2 years with a high upper weight limit	A 5-point harness system with an easy-to-use buckle

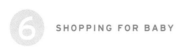

ESSENTIAL PRODUCTS FOR BEFORE BABY ARRIVES, *CONTINUED*

CRIB & CRIB MATTRESS	A new, mid-priced, JPMA-certified crib with a quality wood finish to match your home décor and a firm mattress	Smooth, splinter-free wood with well-attached bars and firmly attached sides with no drop side; a mattress with thick upholstery (ticking) and double-stitched edging
DIAPERS & CLOTHING	(See list on pages 299–302.)	(See list on pages 299–302.)
DIAPER WIPES	One carton.	Any brand, unscented; a wipe dispenser or warmer is optional
SHEETS & BEDDING	Three or four fitted bottom sheets and at least three to four sleep sacks or sets of footie pajamas instead of blankets	Don't put crib bumpers, blankets, puffy quilts, or stuffed animals in your baby's crib

Optional Products for Before Baby Arrives

PRODUCT	OUR RECOMMENDATION	IMPORTANT FEATURES
BREAST PUMP	One double electric	Adjustable speed and suction, battery pack
CRIB MOBILE	One	Windup or battery operated
HIGH CHAIR	One adjustable-height	JPMA-certified, one-hand tray release, sturdy belt, easy-to-clean upholstery
NURSING PILLOW	One	A firm doughnut shape for supporting baby during feeding
MONITOR	One	To listen for baby sounds, 900 MHz with rechargeable batteries, video optional
PACIFIERS	One	Note that while some babies adore pacifiers, others just aren't interested in them
ROCKER & FOOTSTOOL	One each	Comfortable with moisture-resistant washable upholstery

OPTIONAL PRODUCTS FOR BEFORE BABY ARRIVES, *CONTINUED*

SAFETY GATE	As many as needed when baby begins to crawl; one for top and one for bottom of each staircase	Easy to open and close with one hand, wall-mounted with hardware
SOFT CARRIER	One	Washable, comfortable, simple to put on, sturdy buckles, snaps, and straps
STATIONARY EXERCISER	One	Removable, machine-washable, height-adjustable seat, bouncy action, and fun toys for 6- to 12-month-old baby
STROLLER	One mid-weight	Sturdy, easy to fold, reclining seat, ample storage bin
SWING	One	Portable, easy to store, un-annoying music with volume control
TOYS	One or two rattlers or teethers	Bright colors, sized for tiny fists, recommended for age 3 and under

WHERE TO SHOP FOR THE BEST BARGAINS

- **Discount chains.** Huge discount chains like Wal-Mart, Kmart, Sam's Club, and Costco are great places for saving money on everything. Although their baby-product lines are frequently limited to rather basic, no-frills models, their prices are often better than you can find anywhere else; plus, you can buy disposable diapers in bulk at great savings.
- **Baby superstores.** Gigantic baby superstores are next in line for savings. The list includes Toys-R-Us, Babies-R-Us, Buy Buy Baby, and Baby Depot sections found inside Burlington Coat Factory stores. Most carry a huge inventory of products, with advertised models at a substantial savings.
- **Retail chains.** Mainline retail chains such as JCPenney and Sears carry limited stocks of mainstream baby products, such as cribs, strollers, and clothing items. Prices are generally reasonable. Occasionally, you may be able to grab a great bargain during special discount days, such as baby week, or with end-of-season or change-of-model markdowns. (New baby product models usually debut in late fall and the first of the year.)
- **Internet stores and manufacturers' sites.** Baby product sites on the Internet sometimes offer huge discounts,

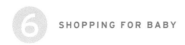

but e-tail outlets come and go quickly, so make sure you're dealing with a reputable, enduring firm. Don't agree to back order if the product is not presently in stock, or you may get stuck with long delays. Some manufacturers offer periodic warehouse sales through their Web sites. In both cases, don't forget to factor in shipping and handling costs when comparing prices.

• **Specialty baby stores.** Independent baby stores usually carry upscale products and accessories not available at huge discounters. You're likely to find excellent customer service there with managers willing to respond to every nagging product question. Price tags are usually higher, but so are service levels.

• **Baby product catalogs.** Direct mail catalogs carrying baby goods make for interesting browsing, but by the time you add shipping and handling costs, you probably haven't saved very much at all.

• **Yard sales and consignment shops**. Clothing and toys are great finds at yard sales, but cribs and car seats aren't. Ever-changing federal regulations make each new generation of car seats and cribs safer than those manufactured even a year earlier.

FATAL PRODUCT FLAWS

Just because a product appears to be designed for use by babies, there is no guarantee it's going to be safe. Every year baby products injure tens of thousands of babies seriously enough to require hospital emergency room treatment. The three biggest causes of baby product–related injuries are poor design, misuse, and product deterioration after use.

The competition among baby product manufacturers is fierce. When an innovative product design makes a big profit in the marketplace, other manufacturers quickly follow with nearly identical clones. The only problem is that fatal flaws get copied and reproduced. Over the decades, products that might have once appeared to be wonderful contraptions for babies have only later been discovered to have serious, baby-threatening flaws. Sometimes parents misuse baby products by relying on them to serve as babysitters. Many babies have died when they were left alone in a device and got into trouble with no one to there to help them. They've fallen over in suctioned bathtub seats and drowned, gotten strangled in the frame strollers when they were supposed to be napping, or strangled when their necks got captured on the partially folded side of a playpen or a crib while their parents were somewhere else in the house.

Parents often fail to follow manufacturers' age and weight guidelines, unintentionally putting their babies at risk. A too-big baby could overload a car seat and could be killed, a toy meant for an older child could have small parts that a baby could chew off and choke on, a curious toddler could open the battery compartment of a kid's toy and choke on the batteries.

All baby products eventually break down from the wear and tear that parents and babies give them. Wheels fall off strollers, safety latches get bent and stop holding, seatbelts fray, buckles break—and sometimes these product failures can be a life-threatening hazard for a baby. The worst offenders are old, malfunctioning cribs with missing bars, broken hardware, or drop sides that are responsible for the deaths of nearly a hundred babies every year in the U.S. Most co-sleepers and sleep positioners have been recalled also.

WHAT "CERTIFIED" MEANS

All baby products have to meet minimal product safety standards set by the federal agencies listed in the next section. But some baby products display a certified seal on their frames. That means they have met voluntary safety guidelines overseen by manufacturers themselves, the JPMA (the Juvenile Products Manufacturers Association). When a product carries a certified sticker, it complies with certain safety guidelines, and the manufacturers' product line has passed rigorous tests for durability and safe design. Currently, the JPMA certification program includes the following baby product categories: bassinets and cradles, bath seats, booster seats, carriages and strollers, changing tables, children's folding chairs, framed infant carriers, full-size cribs, gates and enclosures, handheld infant carriers, high chairs, infant bath tubs, infant bouncers, infant swings, play yards and non-full-size cribs, portable

bed rails, portable hook-on chairs, soft infant carriers, stationary activity centers, toddler beds, and walkers.

But note: Not all baby products and baby product categories are certified. And manufacturers can choose not to participate in the voluntary sticker program, or its products can fail, so they will not have the sticker. Often, imported products, even though they may be perfectly safe, will not be certified. It's too bad baby products aren't required to be certified!

Protecting your baby from baby product dangers:

• **Shop carefully.** Make sure the product is right for your baby. Check out the manufacturers' recommended age and weight recommendations guidelines, and read all the warnings before you buy.

• **Follow the directions.** The manufacturer's directions contain information that is critical for your baby's safety and detail whom to contact when there's a problem. Put all your baby product receipts and literature in a single file so you can find them when you need them.

• **Mail the registration card.** Even though it may make you a target for junk mail, it's also the primary way that manufacturers locate customers who have bought bad products to inform them there's been a recall.

RECALL RECONNAISSANCE

Federal agencies have the power to recall baby products that pose dangers, and literally millions of baby products have been banned, pulled off shelves, or undergone corrective actions to retrofit the unsafe parts.

In spite of federal actions, product-related accidents and injuries continue to happen, sending more than 77,000 babies to emergency rooms for treatment and killing more than eighty babies every year.

New products introduce new baby dangers into the marketplace, old and worn-out products fail, and greedy importers ignore federal regulations by selling shoddy goods that fail federal standards.

Keep on top of recalls, and report baby product problems by frequently accessing these federal sites:

U.S. CONSUMER PRODUCT SAFETY COMMISSION (CPSC)

Washington, DC 20207-0001
800-638-2772
www.cpsc.gov
Regulates the safety of most baby products, clothing, bedding, and toys. (Car seat recalls generally come from the National Highway Traffic Safety Administration—see below.)

NATIONAL HIGHWAY TRAFFIC SAFETY ADMINISTRATION (NHTSA)

400 Seventh Street, SW
Washington, DC 20590
888-327-4236
www.nhtsa.dot.gov
Regulates and recalls children's car seats and rates their installation instructions.

FOOD AND DRUG ADMINISTRATION (FDA)

5600 Fishers Lane
Rockville, MD 20857
888-INFO-FDA (463-6332)
www.fda.gov
Regulates baby food, medicines, and cosmetics, such as bathing products and diaper rash creams.

PRODUCT
CRIBS
CAR SEATS
PORTABLE PLAY YARDS
STROLLERS
BEDDING

FATAL FLAW
Hardware could bend and break. Bars work loose. Decorative posts capture baby's clothing. Parents fail to follow directions: they place seats in the front seat of the car in front of killer air bags, seats are installed incorrectly, children aren't safely secured in the seat, or the child is put in the wrong seat for his weight. Sidebars may not click into place when they're set up, forming a loose V shape. Large leg holes or gaps in the frame might allow the baby to slide out. Sharp hardware could capture small hands and fingers, especially when the frame accidentally collapses. Puffy, soft surfaces on quilts, loose sheets, and stuffed crib toys could suffocate or strangle a baby.

WHAT HAPPENS
Babies' vulnerable necks get caught in gaps between the mattress support and the crib, between the bars, or when drop sides come loose or fall down or clothing forms

a noose and strangles. Front seat airbags deploy during a crash, killing the small occupant in front. The seat isn't fastened down, or the baby isn't correctly strapped into it, or the baby is too large for it, leading to serious injuries during a crash. Toddlers attempt to climb out, and strangle when they get their necks captured in the V. Napping babies are left unattended. Strangulation occurs when the baby's body slides through leg holes or out gaps, leaving the head behind. Frames fail to lock in the open position, capturing children's fingers and hands in sharp hinges. Babies suffocate in soft surfaces when placed face downward, or when their necks get wrapped up in loose sheets.

PRODUCT

BABY TOYS
SUCTIONED BATH SEATS
WHEELED WALKERS
DIAPER PAILS AND LARGE
    WATERFILLED BUCKETS
SAFETY GATES

FATAL FLAW

Small parts, such as eyes, buttons, or wheels, could work loose. Sharp points and edges might injure. Loose fur or hair can get chewed off. Balloons could pop and catch in the throat. Suction cups on the base of self-standing tub seats don't always hold. Small seats on wheels sometimes move faster than parents anticipate. Toddlers might drop a toy into the water and then reach down to try to retrieve it. Accordion-style gates have X-shaped joints that could work like scissors when they close. Some models have holes in center mesh

panels that a toddler could use for climbing. Stoppers on the side of the gate sometimes fail.

WHAT HAPPENS

Small parts and loose fur are swallowed and get stuck in babies' throats, cutting off the air supply. Sharp points injure during falls. Fur and hair gets caught in the throat. Pieces of latex from popped balloons are inhaled and shut off the baby's air supply. Parents leave the baby unattended. The seat falls over, pressing the baby's face into the water, and the baby drowns within several minutes. Walkers tumble down open staircases, causing severe head trauma. They propel babies into hot stoves, fireplaces, and outdoor swimming pools, where they drown. The baby's heavy head causes him to fall in headfirst and drown. Babies get their hands or fingers crushed when the gate opens. Toddlers use holes in the gate panel to climb over and fall down stairs on the other side. Stoppers on pressure-mounted gates don't hold, causing the gate to fall down stairs with the baby.

Here's some basic guidance for keeping your baby safe:

1. **Keep up with recalls.** Periodically check the Web sites of the Consumer Product Safety Commission and other federal agencies that regulate baby products to see if you own recalled products (see *www.recalls .gov*).

2. **Use straps.** The seat straps in strollers, car seats, high chairs, booster seats, swings, and changing tables are there

for an important reason: They protect babies from falling out or getting strangled. Use them every time you put your baby inside.

3. **Stay nearby.** Stay in the same room if your baby is in a holding device, such as a stroller, high chair, play yard, car seat, or stroller. Feed your baby in your arms instead of using a bottle-propper, and always hold your baby during bathing instead of using a suctioned bath seat that could topple over and drown your baby in only a matter of minutes.

4. **Keep baby away from dangers.** Keep your baby out of range when you're installing, opening, closing, assembling, or doing other things with baby products. You're distracted, and sharp corners, hinges, and edges could cause injuries.

Baby Gear A to Z

Here's our prep course on choosing great baby gear along with our recommendations. We'll be covering not only the basic equipment you'll need before your baby arrives, but also the big-ticket items you're likely to acquire later, such as strollers and high chairs. Everything's in alphabetical order to make it easy to find what you need.

AUTOMATIC BABY SWINGS

If your baby appears to be quickly soothed by rocking and rhythmical motion, then an indoor automatic swing may be just the answer for wooing him into a peaceful, hypnotic state so the rest of the family can eat dinner in peace. These devices come with baby-size seats mounted on a frame that tick-tocks the seat back and forth after you wind it up, or with a switch that turns on a small, battery-operated motor. Keep in mind, though, most swings take up a lot of floor space and are the most useful up to about 6 months of age. After that, there's a danger that your tot may reach out and grab the bars and cause himself to get hurt. A folding travel swing may be a good buy if space is a problem. Or, you may want to consider a rocking baby seat as an alternative. There are basically five styles of automated swings: windup A-frames, battery-operated A-frames, open-front models, multi-use models, and small travel swings. Windup A-frames are equipped with an internal spring that tightens with a hand crank. The spring loosens gradually with each successive swinging motion. They are the least expensive swings you can buy. While some models offer only 15 minutes of rocking time per windup, others will run up to 30 minutes with cranking—a better choice. Battery-operated and plug-in swings have small motors inside to push the swing arm. Battery-only models usually require approximately six C-cell batteries that can run the swing for about 200 hours before the juice runs out. Most versions offer on/off switches and allow a choice of several swing speeds. Some come with built-in computer chip music, which is more likely to drive you nuts than soothe your baby.

While traditional swings have an A-shaped frame to support the swing assembly, some newer designs are configured with an open top, allowing easier access to the seat portion when you're putting baby inside or removing him. Folding travel swings are small, tabletop versions of swings that fold down compactly. They use batteries and may offer sound and music options. Multi-use swings are equipped with both a seat and an interchangeable bassinet (baby bed), either of which lock onto the swing's arms.

Swings

Here's what to look for when you go swing shopping.

- **Seat belts and between-the-legs post.** A sturdy, easy-to-operate seat belt and a permanent post that goes between baby's legs will help to prevent your baby from falling forward into the front bar or slipping out between the seat's legs.

- **Front play tray.** A front play tray can help to hold your baby safely inside, but models with front bars that open and swing out may make it easier to put your baby in the seat. Toys mounted in the tray are nice, but certainly not worth paying extra for.

- **Age and weight limitations.** Be careful to note the age and weight ranges for use of the swing, and do not allow toddlers to swing who exceed the recommended weight limit.

- **Windup running time.** If the swing is a windup model, get the one with the most minutes of swing time.

- **Battery life.** If battery-operated, check how many batteries it requires, what type are needed, and how long the swing is expected to run before the batteries have to be replaced. A plug-in model may be more convenient.

- **The frame.** Measure the amount of floor space the swing requires. If you live in a cramped apartment, choose a miniaturized version, or a rocking baby seat, instead. Newer models have open tops that make installing a baby easier, but the extra price may not be worth the convenience. Check to see if the frame folds for storage.

- **Seat reclining options.** Try out the seat's reclining feature, and check how many positions it offers. A deep recline will be the most comfortable for small babies and for napping.

- **Seat covering.** Choose a seat cover pattern you like, and make sure it's removable and machine washable.

- **Extra features.** Manufacturers add sound, vibrations, lights, deep headrests, suspended moving toys, and even seat height adjustments to induce parents to spend more. Remember: Your baby's swing will likely only be used for a couple of months, so save your money and buy a basic, no-frills model.

SWINGS, *CONTINUED*

- **Windup**. The least expensive option. Babies like the tick-tock sound they make. Models fold easily and are usually very simple, but adequate for the job. They hog a lot of floor space. Winding the swing may be noisy enough to wake up the baby. Sometimes the spring assemblies break from over-winding.

- **Battery-operated and plug-ins.** They're quieter than the windup models, but they cost more; plus, you'll have to pay for the batteries for those models. Seats may be more comfortable and offer recline features that the windups don't. They take up a lot of floor space. Sometimes their small, whirring motors slow down or break. Their batteries and motors make them heavier and more cumbersome to move or store. The computer chip music that adds to the price of the swing can be annoying. Some dogs become aroused by the swing's sounds and movement and may try to attack it.

- **Open-topped, battery-operated.** They're easier to use, and some offer side-to-side rocking in addition to front-to-back motion. Most offer reclining seats. They generally cost more than A-frame models and take up a similar amount of floor space. They don't fold for storage as compactly as A-frames.

- **Folding travel.** They don't take up much space, yet offer rhythmical movement that babies love. They're easy to move from place to place, but they don't offer the full range of motion of larger versions.

- **Multi-use with bassinet.** Gives a young baby an alternative place to snooze without having to sit upright. These systems are huge, and the bassinet section isn't always comfortable for small babies. When rocking, it will knock the baby from one side to the other. There have been recalls when the bassinets have broken loose from the swing's arm.

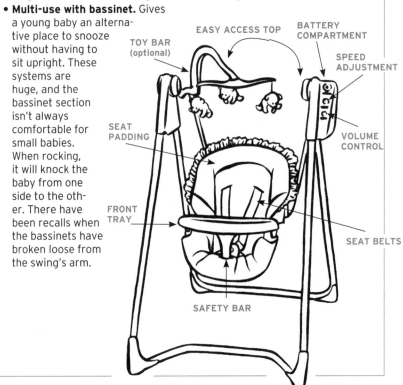

EASY ACCESS TOP

BATTERY COMPARTMENT

TOY BAR (optional)

SPEED ADJUSTMENT

SEAT PADDING

VOLUME CONTROL

FRONT TRAY

SEAT BELTS

SAFETY BAR

BABY BOUNCERS

Baby bouncers are miniature baby seats on a frame that perch a baby where she can watch the action going on around her. Usually the seat portion is made like a padded fabric sling. They may make baby more comfortable after a big nursing by putting her in a semi-upright position, and bouncers give baby a place to watch family members work and play.

Most models jiggle each time a baby moves. Some come with a small, battery-operated motor for soothing vibrations (like a massaging bed). Others have rockers on the bottom, or offer lights and/or music shows to entertain the baby.

Safety is an important issue. Don't ever leave baby alone in the seat, even for a few minutes, and be sure to follow the manufacturer's suggested weight guidelines for use. The safety belt is critical too. It will keep the baby from flipping out of the seat.

A non-skid surface on the seat's base will prevent it from "walking" off table or counter edges. But for maximum safety, seats should be kept on low surfaces to prevent falls. Frames are flimsy and can buckle, so never try to carry your baby from one place to another while she's in the seat. Don't confuse a baby seat with a car seat. The former is lightweight, reclines, and is for use in the house; the latter is a heavy shell with padding to be used only when a baby is strapped into the car, a specially equipped stroller, or in a grocery cart. Don't substitute a car seat for an in-the-house baby seat. It is extremely heavy and can be toppled over by pets or siblings, possibly injuring the baby inside.

Bouncers

A baby seat is a handy place to hold your baby while you work in the kitchen or do housekeeping chores. Those that jiggle offer vibrations, or rocking can substitute for a baby swing and take up a lot less space. Suspended toys or interesting sounds can be momentarily entertaining, but the noise can irritate others.

They're only useful for a small time before the baby can sit up on his own. Baby seats sometimes fall from countertops and tables, resulting in serious head injuries. Don't try to carry your baby in the seat; frames can sometimes bend, toppling the baby out.

- **Stable frame.** Try placing your hand in the center of the seat to test how easily it tips sideways, forward, or backward. Look for a sturdy frame that's larger than the seat, which indicates better stability.
- **Good seat belt.** The bouncer should have a good seat belt to hold baby safely inside.
- **Recline options.** Extra reclining positions will give you some options in finding the most comfortable position for baby.
- **Non-slip base.** Skid-resistant pads on the bottom of the seat are essential

BOUNCERS, *CONTINUED*

and help to keep the baby from walking the seat off a table or countertop when he jiggles.

- **Seat comfort.** Colorful, deeply padded seat covers are a plus, but read the label to make sure they are removable and washable.
- **Toys.** Baby will have fun batting at playful toys suspended from a front toy bar. Just make sure the bar and the toys are well secured and can't work loose.
- **Entertaining extras.** Vibration, music, and rocking are extras that may help to soothe a fussy baby. Buy an extra pack of batteries.

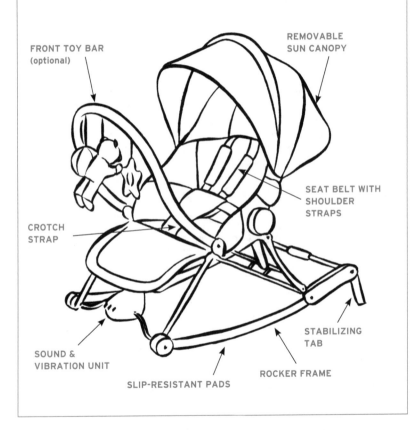

FRONT TOY BAR
(optional)

REMOVABLE
SUN CANOPY

SEAT BELT WITH
SHOULDER
STRAPS

CROTCH
STRAP

SOUND &
VIBRATION UNIT

STABILIZING
TAB

ROCKER FRAME

SLIP-RESISTANT PADS

BATHING AIDS

All new parents are a little scared of giving that first bath to their babies. While your baby's umbilical cord is healing, you shouldn't try to bathe him, and you probably won't need to, anyway. Eventually, the time for bathing will come around, and you're going to have to face the suds challenge.

It's really demanding to try to prepare everything for your baby's bath in advance and then have to deal with a slippery and not-very-happy little one at the same time. (For instructions on how to carry off that first big bath, see page 251.) As for baby bathtubs, they're generally huge, bulky, and a huge pain to manage when they're filled with water that sloshes over the side with the least misstep. Although you may feel more secure using a baby-size bathtub at first, you'll probably soon convert to washing the baby in the kitchen sink lined with a folded bath towel, or taking the baby into the tub with you where you can hold him securely in your lap with someone else helping you lift him in and out. Bath supports are baby-size wire frames shaped like lounge chairs that are lined with a terry or absorbent fabric sling. Once your baby's been bathed, set it out to dry.

Foam bath supports for babies can be useful. They're inexpensive, thick slabs of foam shaped to fit into a baby bathtub that help to hold the baby in place. Once a toddler becomes curious and starts pulling foam pieces off, they should be thrown away. Mildew causes a problem, so wring the foam out and put it in a warm, sunny place to dry after each bath.

Extra Bathing Supplies

Does your baby need special baby soaps for his tender skin? Probably, or at least something very gentle without the harsh chemicals contained in most soap bars. Aveeno and Dove brands are often recommended for baby skin, as are castile soaps labeled specifically for babies. Other than special soap and shampoo, your baby doesn't need a lot of cosmetics—powders, oils, lotions, and ointments that are supposed to be for baby's cleanliness and skin care. They're a waste of money, and some products, particularly those containing perfumes or strong chemicals, may irritate a baby's tender skin. Use a tearless baby shampoo for your baby's scalp instead of soap that leaves a residue. (See "Bathing Basics" on page 251.) Baby powders containing talcum have been connected in some cases with a rare form of baby pneumonia. If the baby spills the powder onto his face and inhales the dust fine particles irritate the lungs and make the baby seriously ill.

If you do use powder, try a talc-free version, such as one made from kaolin clay powder, and gently dust it onto your palms first before applying it to your baby's diaper area.

Knit baby towels aren't very absorbent. Keep your baby dry with your family's regular terry towels laundered in a non-irritating, fragrance-free liquid detergent.

BIRTH ANNOUNCEMENTS

There are literally hundreds of choices for announcements to let the world know that your baby has finally arrived. Most card stores have clever preprinted cards with a place for you to fill in the blanks with your baby's name, date of birth, and weight. Enclose a snapshot if you wish. Office supply stores offer formal announcement cards, similar to wedding announcements, but be prepared to wait a week or so for delivery.

You can find numerous sites on the Internet that sell customized announcements.

BOTTLES AND NIPPLES

Standard baby bottles usually come in 4-ounce and 8-ounce sizes. They can be made of glass or molded transparent plastic. Most newborns get along well with the 4-ounce size for the first few months.

Clear bottles with easy-to-read measurements are the easiest to use. Whimsical bottle shapes, such as those shaped like bears, doughnuts, or baseballs, make it hard to wash out all the milk residue.

Most bottles come with an adjustable, screw-on collar to hold the nipple in place. How tightly the collar is screwed on affects how much air the nipple lets in. A loosened collar will speed up milk flow, a tightened collar will make baby have to work harder to get the milk out.

Baby Bathtub

- **Sturdy sides.** The tub should be made from thick, rigid material with smooth rims so it won't scratch or spill water when you lift it.
- **Small is better.** Miniature body-shaped tubs are easier to manage with newborns than large, one-size-fits-all models. Get one that will fit into your kitchen sink, or simply line the sink with a folded bath towel. (Toddlers usually prefer using the regular bathtub.)
- **Safety features.** A gentle seat angle with support between the legs and slip-resistant surfacing will help hold the baby in place.
- **Tight plug.** A leak-resistant plug on the base makes emptying easier.
- **Folding feature.** Tubs that fold in half for storage take up less room when not in use. Just make sure there are no seams that could pinch a baby or gaps that could leak.
- **Avoid bath seats.** Baby bath seats with suction cups on the base have been implicated in more than 200 baby deaths. The suction cups don't hold, and babies drown. Don't buy or use one.

Sterilizing bottles and nipples is no longer considered necessary. Just use warm, soapy water, a bottle brush, and a small nipple brush to help get out the slimy film that forms on the inside of bottles and nipples. Then, drain them or place them in the dishwasher. Small plastic cages are available for holding nipples and other small baby feeding items together for the dishwasher.

Disposable bottle systems include a circular sheath, vinyl inserts shaped like condoms, a nipple, and a retainer ring. The advantage of vinyl throwaway inserts is that you don't have to wash bottles, but their disadvantage is that they are more expensive. You can run out of liners in the middle of the night, and they may carry a fine vinyl residue that might not be healthy for a baby.

Don't plan to warm your baby's formula in a microwave. Microwaving can cause boiling hot spots that will scald your baby's mouth, and disposable bottle liners have been known to rupture, spewing hot milk on babies. (We discuss choosing baby formula on pages 246–247.)

Nipple Styles

Nipples come in rubber and silicone. Silicone is the best material of the two, because it's more sanitary and less likely to rot or absorb milk residue. But sometimes silicone nipples can develop tears.

It is recommended that new bottle nipples be boiled for 2 to 5 minutes to remove any chemicals involved in their manufacture. Replace nipples every few months just to be safe. Nipples come in different sizes: small for preemies, and standard for most babies. Some nipples are designed with big holes or cross cuts in the outlet expressly made for feeding baby thickened cereals. Nipples also differ in how firm or how soft they are. If a nipple's too soft, it will collapse when baby tries to suck

on it; if it's too firm, it could make your baby have to work too hard for a drink. Some nipples come in an hourglass configuration (orthodontic shape) that allegedly evokes a more natural sucking motion from a baby's tongue. These nipples are difficult to clean, which can lead to rotting in the rubber versions. The type of nipple you use is mostly a matter of preference. Try out different styles until you find one that seems to be the most comfortable for your baby.

BREAST PUMPS AND BREASTFEEDING AIDS

A breast pump is a hand-operated or motor-driven device that creates suction. You could compare a breast pump to a vacuum cleaner but with a gentle, rhythmical action that collects mothers' milk into a baby bottle. Most pumps contain a small motor that creates the suction, a breast shield, and a tube or channel to flow the milk into a collection bottle. If you're planning to stay around home, you'll soon discover your baby is the only breast pump you'll need. So, the concept is to master breastfeeding techniques first; then worry about pumping later.

No pump will work well unless a mother has a letdown, that rush of milk that comes a few minutes after nipple stimulation. In time, an experienced mother can learn to create a letdown by gently massaging the breasts while simply imagining the act of nursing. (Breastfeeding is discussed in detail on pages 238–246.)

Breast Pumps

- **Efficiency.** The best pumps are those that are the most effective at getting the job done. A well-designed manual pump can do the job, but is tiresome. Look for suction control and cycling speed control in electric models.
- **Quietness.** If you plan to pump at work, and there's no private place to do it, the quieter the better.
- **Cleaning ease.** You'll be cleaning the pump daily, so look for easy-to-wash components.
- **Electric adapters.** Don't just rely on batteries. Get a pump that offers an adapter for electrical outlets, and consider purchasing an optional adapter for the cigarette lighter outlet in your car.
- **Shield comfort.** If you have large breasts, the standard shields that fit on the breast may not fit comfortably. Try special adapter inserts.
- **Portability.** Unless you're only pumping at home, the pump should come with an easy-to-tote carry case and be lightweight enough so you can carry it to work each day.
- **Trusted manufacturer.** Some companies offer poor-quality pumps just to fill out their baby feeding lines. Buy from a trusted breast pump manufacturer instead.

With practice, most mothers can become proficient at expressing (squeezing out) their milk by hand without a pump. The technique is called manual expression,

and can be learned from various breastfeeding books and online at breastfeeding sites such as *www .breastfeeding.com.* If you know in advance you'll be returning to work, or you expect daily separations from your baby, or if your baby arrives early and could benefit from the disease-fighting powers of human milk, an effective breast pump may help to keep your milk supply going and allow you to collect it and store it in the freezer until it can be fed to your baby. The most effective pumps are those that are able to mimic the gentle, repeated tugging of a baby during nursing. The most sophisticated pumps have knobs that allow you to adjust both the strength of the suction and timing of the length of time between each suction. Comfort and efficiency are the two most important qualities to look for in a breast pump. Whichever style you choose, it should be simple to use, easy to clean, and not too much trouble to handle.

The best source of information about breast pumps and how they're used is a lactation consultant—a specially trained breastfeeding expert. (See the Resources.) There are five basic kinds of breast pumps on the market, some more efficient than others: inexpensive bulbed models, hand-operated versions, small battery-operated versions, midsize pumps, and large, hospital-grade models. Midsize models are the most popular with most breastfeeders.

Bulbed Pumps

These are the old-fashioned models found in pharmacies that resemble a bicycle horn with a rubber ball on one end to produce the vacuum. The rubber ball is fastened to a glass or plastic milk catcher. These are no longer recommended, because their strong suction can cause bruising and damage to breast tissue.

Hand-Operated Pumps

These rely on your hand action using either a fitted cylinder or a squeeze-grip handle to produce a syringe-like tugging action. Most are designed to screw onto a baby bottle for milk collection and storage. Some offer adjustable suction controls and soft shield adapters to fit most breast sizes.

They're usually lightweight, silent, and easy to tuck into a purse or briefcase. Those with pistol-grip

action and adjustable suction strength work well to collect milk once there's a milk letdown.

They require a lot of effort from you, and your hands and arms can get fatigued. They're simply not as efficient as mid- and large-size electric pumps.

Small, Battery-Operated Pumps

These small pumps are usually sold as kits in baby stores and drugstores. They come with a pistol-grip handle, a place for batteries, shields for the breast, a collection bottle, collection tubes, and a carrying case. Some may offer adapters for electrical outlets or for the cigarette lighter outlet in your car.

They're small, fairly quiet, easy to carry around, and less expensive

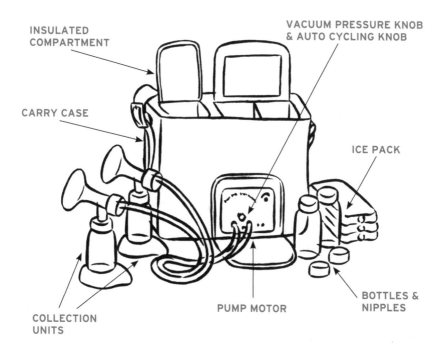

INSULATED COMPARTMENT

VACUUM PRESSURE KNOB & AUTO CYCLING KNOB

CARRY CASE

ICE PACK

COLLECTION UNITS

PUMP MOTOR

BOTTLES & NIPPLES

than larger, more professional versions. They don't work as well as larger pumps, and their small motors have a history of breaking down. They usually have only one milk receptacle instead of two, which makes pumping slower than being able to pump both breasts at once.

Midsize Electric Pumps

These are the work horses of the breast pump world. Some are designed for pumping a single side, while others are able to pump both breasts simultaneously, which saves time. They are normally sold as a kit that includes a small motor encased in a zippered, insulated carry case. Also included are washable tubes that lead from the motor to the breast shields and collection bottles. Units offer adjustable speed and vacuum levels and can run on either batteries or an electrical adapter. Some cases also have a special freezer-pack section for holding bottles of breastmilk until they can be refrigerated or frozen. Breast shields (horns) may have adapters for larger breast sizes. An optional cigarette lighter plug is usually available for pumping in the car and on trips.

- Although not very lightweight, nor very quiet, these units offer excellent efficiency when it comes to collecting milk, and they stimulate the breasts adequately to keep up a mother's milk supply. They're expensive, $100 to $200, but if you're planning to express milk at work every day, the investment will be worth it over the long haul.
- They eat up batteries in a hurry,

so you will probably need an electrical outlet nearby. They're noisy, so people drifting in and out of the ladies' room or health suite at work will know something's going on. Occasionally, mothers have problems with the fit of the breast shields, and cleaning the tubes and components can be time-consuming.

Large, Hospital-Grade Electric Pumps

These are huge, heavy units, about the size of a car battery, that are used in hospitals and cost $500 or more. They can also be rented week by week very economically from most lactation consultants for personal use at home. They do the most efficient job of all breast pumps and are especially useful if you've got a preemie that is dependent on your milk for survival.

- They're highly effective and rapid in gathering milk, and they're useful for emergency situations, such as for providing milk for a hospitalized baby when nursing is interrupted temporarily. (Your breasts need continual suckling to keep producing milk.)
- They're heavy and not very portable, and prohibitively expensive for purchase, but short-term rentals are available from hospitals or lactation consultants. They require an electrical outlet, and make a noticeable churning sound that may feel indiscreet in non-private settings.

CAR SEATS FOR BABIES

Your Baby's Safety Zone

In April 2011, the American Academy of Pediatrics issued a recommendation that all babies age 2 and under should ride facing rearward in the rear seat of vehicles or until they reach the highest weight or height allowed by their car seat's manufacturer. This is because babies have very weak spines and necks and overly large heads in proportion to their bodies, which make them vulnerable to whiplash. During a crash, a baby's head and body will be thrown forward in seconds and then slammed backward. By placing your baby's car seat facing rearward, you are offering firm, solid support to the head and spine to help prevent head, neck, and spine injuries.

Being a backseat passenger gives your baby a buffer zone of airspace between his seat and any impact at the front of the car. More important, front seat air bags, usually located in or just below the glove compartment, deploy with such force they are capable of killing a baby or toddler in a seat, even during a minor fender-bender in a parking lot.

Federal Laws and LATCH

All 50 states and the District of Columbia have laws that require young children to be restrained in a proper safety seat for their size. Even with these laws, most parents (as many as 80 percent) don't install their children's car seats correctly. Part of the problem

Preemies and Car Beds

The American Academy of Pediatrics recommends that all infants born earlier than 37 weeks gestational age be observed in their car seats before leaving the hospital to make sure they don't have potential breathing problems in the semi-reclining position of car seats. If your baby does have a problem, you may need to bolster underneath the seat base to make your baby's position sufficiently reclined, or to purchase a specialized baby car bed.

is getting the seat strapped into the car and in properly fitting the car seat's belts on the child.

In 2001, federal laws were put into effect by the National Highway Traffic Safety Administration to help remedy the issue of correctly installing a car seat. The restraint systems that the law requires are referred to as LATCH, an acronym that stands for Lower Anchor and Tethers for Children. Since the fall of 2002, car manufacturers have had to install special U-shaped bars, called anchors, in the crease of the rear seats of every passenger vehicle in two positions—one for each window seat. Children's car seat manufacturers are also required to provide devices, such as hooks, on the backs of car seats so they can fasten onto these preinstalled anchors.

If you own an older model car, it won't have LATCH, but all children's car seats can also be safely fastened into the car by threading the shoulder and lap belts through special slots in the car seat. Follow the directions supplied by the owner's manual for your car on how to use its particular belting system, and be sure to follow the directions that come with the car seat, usually found in a leaflet fastened on the back of the car seat.

Unfortunately, there are no laws that address the second serious problem: parents not installing their children correctly in the seat.

A Key to Car Seat Terms

- **Buckle.** A metal fastener used to latch all of the straps together in the center of the baby's body, just above the thighs.
- **Three-point harness.** Found on some models of infant-only car seats. There are three straps: the two that restrain each shoulder and buckle together with a between-the-legs strap.
- *Five-point harness*. Found on some models of infant-only car seats and all convertible seats. There are five straps: one strap for each shoulder, one for each side of the waist, and one for between the legs.
- **Harness clip** (or harness tie). A plastic fastener resembling a large hair clip, positioned at the level of a baby's armpits to keep the two shoulder straps together so baby won't be ejected between the straps during a crash.
- **Harness slots.** Slits cut in the rear of the car seat's back and upholstery for adjusting the height of shoulder harnesses to fit babies as they grow. Straps

should be threaded into the frame at or below a baby's shoulder level.

- **Metal locking clip.** A flat, H-shaped metal piece that can be found tucked in back of a baby's car seat. It is used to cinch retracting, one-piece lap-and-shoulder belts in some newer car models. Using the clip may be the only way to firmly hold a car seat in place.
- **Tether.** A black nylon strap that attaches in the rear of convertible seats when they're used in the forward-facing, upright position. It mounts using a hook to bolted hardware into the shelf above the rear seat of the car, or to the hardware on the floorboard of a van or station wagon. The strap stabilizes the seat in the upright position if there's a crash.

What Kind of Car Seat to Buy

There are basically three types of car seats suitable for newborns through the first 6 months of life: rear-facing, infant-only seats; convertible seats; and baby beds for special circumstances.

Infant-Only Seat

Rear-facing, infant-only seats are shaped like small tubs with a slanted, padded seat inside, and a folding, U-shaped carry handle. They're made to protect babies who weigh 4 pounds up to 32 pounds, depending upon the particular model. (Most accommodate babies only weighing up to 20 or 22 pounds.) Some models use a three-point harness system, while others have five-point harnesses. A harness clip latches the shoulder straps together at armpit level.

Most harnesses can adjust to several heights using slots in the seat back. Many of these seats come with a separate base that fastens down in the car either with LATCH hooks or by using the car's shoulder and lap belts so the seat can simply be lifted out leaving the base behind. Federal regulations require that infant seats be equally as safe with or without their bases.

Pros: They're the most lightweight, most portable, and least expensive car seat option for babies under a year of age. Models with five-point harnesses are thought to be safer than those with only three straps. The seat is angled well for the needs of babies born after 37 weeks' pregnancy and it is relatively easy to put the baby inside. The base of the seat has latches on the bottom that lock it into grocery carts or specially equipped stroller frames. You may be able to purchase an additional base for a second car. Some handles are more comfortable than others: The best ones have thick padding or a rotating handle grip to allow the seat to swivel into a comfortable position for carrying.

Cons: This style of seat has been in a number of recalls, particularly when the baby seat portion hasn't attached securely onto the seat's base because of hardware failure. Heavy and awkward when there's a baby inside, they're comfortable only for carrying short distances. Sometimes the sharp pitch of a car's backseat can make the car seat's angle too sharp, causing the baby to flop forward, although most seat bases have a presser foot underneath to adapt for that. A rolled-up towel under the foot of

the seat will work too. Most seats offer a small guide that shows if the angle is correct. You may have to invest in another, better-fitting seat if your baby becomes too tall or too heavy before he reaches his second birthday.

Convertible Seats

Larger than infant-only seats, these restraints have an upright back and resemble an upholstered chair without legs. These seats are designed to recline and face rearward for babies weighing 22 pounds; then, they convert to face forward in an upright position for restraining toddlers until they weigh 40 pounds or are approximately 4 years of age. Most models use a five-point harness system and offer a series of slots for adjusting shoulder belt heights as baby grows. (Not an easy process.) A harness clip holds the shoulder straps together at baby's armpit level. All seats in this category come equipped with a top tether strap that is only to be used in the upright, forward-facing position to fasten the seat to the car's frame as directed.

Pros: You are basically getting two seats for the price of one. Since most of these models can accommodate babies weighing more than 20 pounds, a larger-than-average baby can still face rearward through age 2. The frames are all one piece, minimizing the dangers of infant-only seats snapping off their stands during a crash.

Cons: The seats are not very portable, and they take up a lot of space when they're slanted in the rear-facing position. That

Infant-Only Car Seats

Here's what to look for when you shop for a rear-facing, infant-only car seat:

- **Five-point harnesses.** Models with a five-point harness system (a strap for shoulders, waist, and between the legs) offer more security than models with three-point systems (only shoulders and crotch).
- **Higher weight range.** Seats that safely carry larger babies are a better value. Look for a model that can restrain a 22-pound baby, or even heavier. That way, if your baby is larger than average, you won't have to change seat models before his first birthday.
- **Carry handle.** A curved carry handle with dense foam cushioning will make toting the car seat on your arm more comfortable.
- **Canopy.** A generous, adjustable sunshade will help to keep your baby protected from glare and bright sunlight.
- **Base.** Most seats come with a separate base to lock the seat in place using your car's LATCH anchors (see below), or by threading adult seat belts through the base. Get a base that has an adjustable presser foot so the seat angle can be adjusted according to the slope of your backseat.
- **Directions.** Follow the directions that come with the seat and the installation directions found inside your auto owner's manual.
- **Avoid used seats.** Don't buy a used infant seat unless you're sure it hasn't been on a recall list and that it's never been in a crash.

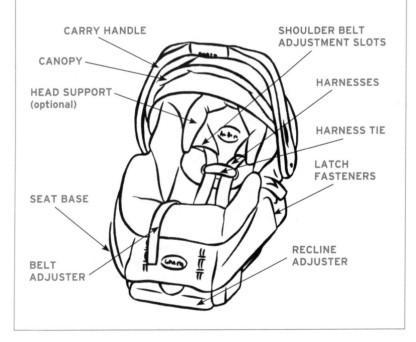

could present a problem if you don't have a lot of space in the rear compartment of your car. The distance between the crotch strap and the back of the seat may mean a tiny baby will not get good strap contact. Models with a front shield, rather than a five-point harness system, are thought to be less safe than those relying on the direct body contact of five-point harnesses.

Stroller/Car Seat Combos

Some manufacturers combine their strollers and infant-only car seats together and sell them as a single package. They have matching colors and upholstery. Sometimes buying the stroller/car seat combination costs less than purchasing each item separately. Typically, the carton holding the travel system will contain the stroller, the car seat, the car seat's base, and an adapter bar or railing that fastens into the stroller frame so the car seat can be clicked onto the stroller.

Usually, the car seat is positioned so it faces toward the rear of the stroller, where the parent is pushing. Some dual strollers can hold two infant car seats for twins. If you want wheels for your baby's car seat, but don't want to invest in a stroller to support it, consider buying an inexpensive rolling stroller frame made specifically for infant seats, such as Baby Trend's Snap-N-Go series (*www.babytrend.com*).

Pros: A convenient marriage between two pieces of baby equipment that allows you to use a simple snap-out-of-the-car-and-into-the- stroller maneuver. Your

baby in his car seat gets to face you in the stroller. You'll probably save money on this two-for-one deal.

Cons: Rear facing, infant-only seats have some limitations. You'll use the rear-facing seat for only 1 to 2 years, depending upon the weight and height limits set by the manufacturer, but the stroller for 3 to 4 years, and purchasing the system commits you to the stroller that comes in the package. Most strollers now come with universal adapters that fit all name-brand infant car seats, and the stroller model you're forced to buy with the seat may not be the most compact, lightweight, or maneuverable option you could find. Consider purchasing your baby's car seat and stroller separately on their own merits—for example, the car seat because it has a five-point harness system and holds heavier babies, and the stroller because it is lightweight and the best size and wheels for your lifestyle. (Long walks: big wheels; city maneuvering, shopping, and travel: small wheels.)

The Test for Good Car Seat Installation

Whether you buy a rear-facing, infant-only seat, or a convertible infant-toddler seat, the safety of the seat will depend upon its being tightly fastened down in the rear-facing position in your vehicle's backseat using either the LATCH anchors in the car or the car's seat belts if there are no anchors. The ultimate test of a good installation is that the seat won't budge. If you fail to fasten the seat in correctly, it will wobble to the left, right, or rear when you press down on it. Try

Convertible Car Seats

- **Compatibility.** Check out the dimensions of your car's backseat. If you're driving a compact or a sub-compact, you may not be able to fit some of the larger models into your backseat in the semi-reclined position.
- **Crotch strap.** If you're using a convertible with your newborn, make sure the seat's between-the-legs strap is positioned closely enough to the back of seat so it will provide direct contact with your baby. (Some manufacturers offer two positions for the strap.)
- **Shoulder slots.** Look for four or more shoulder harness slots in the back that allow you to adjust the height of the straps as your child grows. (The straps should be positioned at or below your baby's shoulders.)
- **Recline feature.** Examine how the seat reclines. It should offer several recline positions depending upon the needs of your baby and the slant of your vehicle's backseat.
- **LATCH fasteners.** The hardware and straps to fasten your seat to the LATCH anchors that come with your car should be easy to fasten and unfasten.
- **Tether strap.** The tether strap coming from the upper back of the seat is designed for use only when the seat is in the upright, forward-facing position for toddlers weighing more than 20 pounds.
- **Directions.** Follow both the directions that come with the seat, and those that are printed inside your auto owner's manual.
- **Avoid used seats.** Don't buy a used convertible seat unless you're sure it hasn't been on a recall list and that it's never been in a crash.

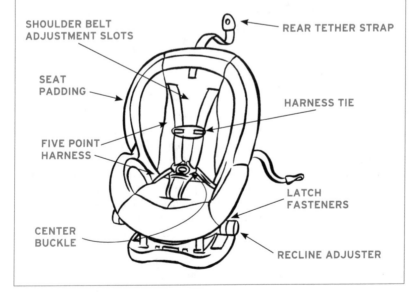

SHOULDER BELT ADJUSTMENT SLOTS

REAR TETHER STRAP

SEAT PADDING

HARNESS TIE

FIVE POINT HARNESS

LATCH FASTENERS

CENTER BUCKLE

RECLINE ADJUSTER

grasping the seat near the armrests on either side, and see if you can pull the seat away from the car's seat or make it move from side to side. It should not slide more than about an inch.

Then, without your baby inside, firmly push the top edge of the seat above where your baby's head would be in the direction of the floor of the car. Although the vehicle seat cushion may give, the safety seat should stay firmly in place, and the back of the car seat should stay at approximately the same angle (reclined about halfway back). (It's okay if you can push the top of the seat toward the rear of the car.)

The seat should be so firmly implanted in the auto's seat that it won't budge. You should get someone else to help you so the seat is implanted as tightly as possible. Press the seat deeply into the car's upholstery with your knee while your assistant helps to tighten the straps that hold the seat in place.

If you have an older model car with a retracting, one-piece shoulder and lap belt, you will need to use the H-shaped metal locking clip that comes attached to the back of the car seat. It acts as a cinch to hold both parts of the belt together. First, knee the seat so it imbeds deeply into the upholstery. Have your helper stretch the seat belt out as far as it will extend. Then, use the metal piece that fastens into the car's seat buckle to thread the seat belt loop through the holes in the back of the car seat for that purpose. Fasten the seat belt buckle, then pull tightly on the shoulder portion of the belt until there's no give. Use the locking

clip to fasten the lap section to the shoulder section just above the buckle. When it comes to installing your baby into the seat, your baby's weight and height should fall into the stated ranges for the seat; shoulder straps should be taut and allow no more than two fingers of space between the straps and your baby's body; these straps should be at, or a little below, your baby's shoulders; the crotch strap should have contact with your baby's body; the harness tie (see above) should be at armpit level; and the seat should be angled so that your baby lies back, rather than hunches forward (refer to the angle indicator on the side of the seat).

Products to Make Traveling Easier

- **Travel mirror.** If you're worried about not being able to see your baby in the backseat, you may be able to find a mirror that suctions onto your rear window so you can glance at your baby through your rearview mirror. Just make sure it doesn't interfere with your ability to safely negotiate lane changes, and don't get distracted while driving in traffic.
- **Travel toys.** Soft toys and teethers are safe for baby's play during travel, and some can be purchased on a flexible, padded bar. Avoid hard toys that could do their own harm during a crash.
- **Extra supplies.** Keep extra diapers, a box of wipes, several changes of baby clothing, paper towels, a changing pad, an extra blanket, and a bath towel in a bag in the backseat in case your baby vomits or makes a mess. Also use the bath towel to protect the

seat from getting too hot or too cold when you're out shopping. If you're not nursing, you should store several bottles of unopened, pre-bottled liquid baby formula.

- **Soothing sounds.** Save a CD of children's songs or lullabies from around the world to soothe the savage beast during meltdowns.

CHANGING TABLES

Changing tables are special stands made just for diaper changing. There are five basic kinds of changing tables: a dedicated changing table with a pad and storage compartments underneath; a folding, wooden top that comes fastened onto a wooden chest of drawers; thick, vinyl-covered foam changing pads that screw onto chests; changing table adapters for cribs and play yards; and thin, lightweight changing pads that come in diaper bags or can be purchased separately.

Dedicated changing tables are somewhat expensive, rectangular-shaped tables that position a baby on top of a cushioned pad. They come with a waist belt to hold baby on the table, and guard rails on two or all sides to help protect babies from falls.

They are usually constructed of wood or rattan and have storage shelves or drawers underneath. Some manufacturers have created fold-out diapering tops that come attached to wooden nursery chests and have changing pads and waist belts. The units can be removed by taking out the screws once the baby no longer needs changing.

Vinyl-covered thick foam

hanging pads are available from baby specialty stores. These thick pads are made to screw onto the tops of preexisting chests. They are indented in the center, and usually come with a small vinyl safety belt. Some baby specialty stores sell rimmed plastic changing table shelves that are designed to fit over the bars of a standard-size crib.

They come with a pad in the center and a safety belt for baby's waist. Some portable play yards also come with a removable changing table unit that has a pad and a small safety belt.

The most inexpensive option of all is a simple folding (or rolled up) changing pad, like those that come in diaper bags that can be used on the floor or on a bed, or stuffed in a backpack or purse. They don't offer safety straps, so you'll have to use them on a surface where your baby can't roll off.

What Changing Option to Buy

Here is a comparison of your options for places to change your baby's diapers.

CHANGING TABLE

Pros: They raise the baby to a comfortable height for changing. You can place them wherever it's convenient, or have one for each floor in your home. They come with a waist belt to hold baby in place. Railings on the sides will help to prevent a baby's rolling over and falling out.

Cons: Babies are injured when they squirm and roll overboard, falling headfirst to the floor below. Using a retraining belt is important, but it can get in the way of diapering. Open shelves

Changing Tables

Here's what to look for when you shop for a changing table:

- **Comfortable height.** Get one that is high enough so you don't have to bend over to change your baby, yet not so high that you can't control your baby at all times.
- **Good waist belt.** Look for a sturdy belt with an easy-to-use buckle that snaps together.
- **Guard railings on all sides.** The taller the railings, the better protection for your baby should you neglect to belt him.
- **Shake test.** Give the table a good rattling to test how sturdy the joints are.
- **Storage.** Until your toddler reaches the exploring stage, open storage shelves can come in handy.
- **Extra safety precautions.** Always belt the baby down, and never leave the baby alone on the table, such as to fetch diapers or to answer the telephone.

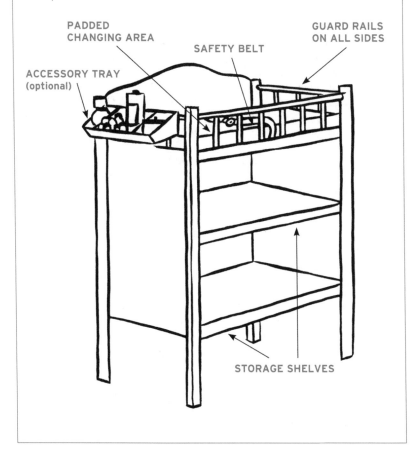

PADDED
CHANGING AREA

GUARD RAILS
ON ALL SIDES

SAFETY BELT

ACCESSORY TRAY
(optional)

STORAGE SHELVES

underneath may be an invitation to toddlers to pull things out onto the floor.

NURSERY CHEST TOPPERS

Pros: The chest can coordinate with your other baby furniture, and it will adapt for use during childhood.

Cons: There have been stability problems with the foldout changer frames that can cause the chest to topple forward. Most chest models don't have a protective railing in the front to prevent a baby from falling.

CHANGING PAD

Pros: They present an inexpensive option for adapting any chest for a diaper changing station. They're lightweight, and easy to fold for carrying in a diaper bag, backpack, or briefcase.

Cons: They're only safe if they are screwed down on the chest. Seat belts are often flimsy and difficult to thread. Even though they often have an indented channel in the center to hold the baby, none offer the safety of side rails that a standard diaper-changing table has to prevent accidents.

PLAY YARD DIAPERING ADAPTERS

Pros: Diaper changing platforms fit on top of the railings of standard-size cribs. Some play yards come with a small diaper-changing accessory that fits over the top bars of the yard. Both are less expensive than buying a separate changing table, and both offer cushioned pads and seat belt options.

Cons: The crib shelf may be too high to be comfortable, and an unrestrained baby can easily roll out, which could lead to injury. The attachment will have to be removed each time you put the baby to bed. Portable play yard changers are very small and low, so they will only be useful for a short while, and could lead to a backache. Rollouts are a dangerous possibility for an unrestrained baby.

CLOTHES

Babies have very tender skin, and most hate getting dressed and undressed. Their biggest complaint is when parents pull clothes over their heads—it makes them think they're suffocating, and most will fuss every time. Other than that, your baby will be generally oblivious to what you make her wear.

When it comes to buying baby clothes, you basically get what you pay for. Inexpensive baby clothes tend to be thin and their finishing may be so poor that there are loose strings and scratchy seams, and they will fade and come apart after a couple of washings. On the other extreme, designer brands in upscale department stores and from the Internet will be dense and buttery soft. The only problem is that your baby is going to grow like wildfire, practically doubling weight in the first 4 months.

Investments in tiny luxury just won't pay off, especially if the duds have to be dry-cleaned (though you may be able to minimize your loss by reselling at a consignment shop).

Rather than dressing your baby to the hilt, think simple comfort instead. The best baby duds are super-absorbent and soft. Avoid shirts or clothes with scratchy seams, especially around the arm and leg holes.

Also avoid appliqués that are rough on the inside and can cause skin irritation. Watch out for garments with sharp metal-backed snaps. They can scratch, and if they aren't enameled, the raw metal surface may cause a skin rash. Avoid unshielded metal zippers that could scratch or capture a baby's fragile skin. Plastic zippers are better. Constantly monitor all garments for loose threads that could wrap around a baby's fingers or toes and cut off circulation.

There is no uniform industry standard for sizing baby clothes, and there are wide differences among brands. Most prepackaged baby garments have a weight chart on the back to help you choose the right size for your baby, but it's always better to err on the large side.

Don't hesitate to open packages to look at the size or to compare the quality of garments from different manufacturers. Although it's nice to have several shirts in a baby's actual newborn size, you'll quickly learn to buy shirts, Onesies (shirts that snap at the crotch), and nightgowns in 6- and 12-month sizes so they'll last longer. Sleeves can always be rolled up. Shirts should either open from the front or have generous, wide necks or neck flaps to make pulling them on and off a quick and easy task.

Everyday baby shirts usually come in either all-cotton or cotton/ polyester blends. The blends are less likely to wrinkle, and they're often cheaper, but pure cotton knits are more absorbent and less likely to stain.

Cotton garments tend to shrink and become denser and more absorbent with laundering. Most manufacturers have compensated for that by making the cut of their prewashed garments larger. If you go the all-cotton route, buy items that are at least one, or even two, sizes larger than your baby's current weight just to get more wear out of them.

Babies soil clothes several times per day. So how many shirts, Onesies, or gowns you buy depends mostly on how easy and convenient it is for you to do laundry. If you live in an apartment with all the washers and dryers in the basement, then stock up on lots of baby shirts so you can wait longer than a day before being forced to take that long trek down to the laundry room.

Baby nightgowns can be handy in the early days, especially those gowns with small flaps to cover the baby's fists. This feature will keep the baby from scratching his face with his fingernails until you gain confidence in fingernail filing or cutting. Softly elasticized bottoms on gowns will help to keep them down over the baby's legs while he sleeps.

Since babies outgrow clothes so quickly, consider loading up on baby shirts and garments at thrift stores and tag sales. Almost all baby hand-me-downs are likely to have formula stains down the front that can usually be removed by a soaking in bleach, using oxy-based cleaners, or spotting with stain removers.

Minimum Clothing to Have on Hand

TYPE OF GARMENT	DESCRIPTION	NUMBER	COMMENT
BABY T-SHIRTS	All-cotton baby T-shirts that snap on the side, or slip over the head with wide necks.	6	Your baby will outgrow them quickly. Buy two in the newborn size just to have something that fits perfectly, but buy the rest in the 6-month size or larger. Get short sleeves for warm weather and long sleeves for winter, or a combination of the two, and use the short-sleeve versions for undershirts. Check for soft inside seams, and inspect for loose strings after every laundering.
ONESIES	All-cotton knit shirts with wide neck openings that snap at the crotch. Choose 3- or 6-month sizes.	4	Choose long sleeves for winter, short sleeves for summer.
NIGHTGOWNS	Full length, all-cotton, or cotton/poly blends with an open or gently elasticized bottom.	4	These keep babies' legs covered in the night. Fold-over cuffs for the hands can keep baby's fingernails from scratching his cheeks.
FOOTED SLEEPERS	Stretchy, baby-style pajama suits with long sleeves and covered feet.	3	Buy the 6-month size, and roll up the sleeves if they're too long. Avoid metal snaps if the skin side is not enameled. Inspect the inner seams after every washing to make sure there aren't any loose strings that could wrap around tiny toes.

MINIMUM CLOTHING TO HAVE ON HAND *CONTINUED*

SLEEP SACK (BABY BUNTING)	A baby sleeping bag made from fleece or quilting for cold weather.	1	Use it instead of a blanket and a cover sheet in the crib in cold weather. Look for the 6-month size with a shielded zipper down the front, or flat snaps that give access to the diaper area. Avoid versions with scratchy appliqués on the front.
SOCKS	Cotton knit with soft cuffs.	4	They stay on better than booties and help to keep a baby's feet warm. Tie the socks together in a knot, or stuff them in a zippered lingerie bag for washing so they won't get lost in the machine.
BABY SWEATERS	Choose tightly knit cardigans that zip or snap up the front. Use for winter warmth or in buildings with air conditioning.	2	Get the 6-month size, and roll up the sleeves. Should be washable and without extra lace, appliqués that could scratch or that use a loose knit that could capture tiny fingers.
HAT	A small, knitted toboggan if it's winter. For summer, a brimmed hat with a neckband to hold it on and a flap to cover the back of the neck for protection.	2	Most babies hate wearing hats, but they can help to keep a baby from losing heat in the cold, and shield the baby from sunburn in warm weather.
BIBS	Small, washable bibs with easy-open neck closures.	4	Babies constantly drool and spit up, so use them to protect clothing.

Other Clothing to Have on Hand

TYPE OF GARMENT	DESCRIPTION	NUMBER	COMMENT
RECEIVING BLANKETS	Choose the 28-inch or 36-inch size in a soft, absorbent cotton flannel or a waffle weave.	5-6	These handy, washable blankets are great for protecting your shoulder or for swaddling up a fussy baby.
WATERPROOF PADS	Small fabric-backed with waterproof (rubber) pads.	4-5	Use them under the baby in the crib to protect the sheet from wetness, and on your lap or shoulder for spit-up protection.
REUSABLE DIAPERS	Thick, soft, prefolded terry or flannel with outer covers that use Velcro side closures.	12 diapers, 4-5 outer covers	Handy when you run out of disposables in the night. Also handy for cleaning spit up.
CHEAP WASHCLOTHS	Buy several large packs.	1 to 2 dozen	Use them to wipe baby's messes. If they get stained and won't wash clean, just toss them.
BABY SNOWSUIT (FOR COLD CLIMATES)	The suit should have insulation, a hood, legs, and a zipper to the ankles for diapering.	1 (winter)	If your baby is born in late summer or early fall, go for the 12-month size to take your baby through the entire winter. For a midwinter baby, buy the 6-month size. For a late-winter baby, a sleep sac (see above) may work, but only if there are slots inside the garment to adapt to the shoulder and between-the-legs straps of the car seat.

Hidden Fire and Heat Hazards

When it comes to sleepwear, the U.S. Consumer Product Safety Commission (CPSC) has issued several warnings: One is against using loose-fitting, all-cotton garments as pajamas because they ignite rapidly if exposed to a flame. As a result of burns to toddlers, the commission has required that children's loose clothing labeled as sleepwear be flame resistant. Form-fitting clothing is considered safe.

Unlike toddlers, newborns are not likely to wander near flames, but if you or someone in your household smokes, you use a wood stove or kerosene heaters, or you have open-flamed stovetop units, flame retardancy in your baby's clothing is important.

Smoke detectors are critical lifesavers. Make sure all of them are operational before you bring your baby home. Install a carbon monoxide detector as well. Ask your local fire department about putting a special sign on your baby's window indicating a child is there, and make sure your house number is brightly displayed at the bottom of your driveway.

Babies can be seriously burned by hot water coming from the faucet. Lower your water heater's thermostat to no hotter than 104°F, and if your sinks and bathtubs have a hot and cold knob, make it a practice to always turn the hot water off first.

The Sleep Sack Option Instead of Blankets

The CPSC also warns against using loose top sheets and blankets to cover your baby at night. That's because babies can strangle when they've become entangled in them. One suggestion is to place baby with his feet nearly touching the end of the crib, and then to carefully fold sheet and blanket so that they are only to the level of your baby's armpits.

One clothing option for safe sleeping is to use no top coverings at all, but to place your baby, face up, in a sleep sack, a one-piece bag that encloses baby's legs. Sacks can be found in large retail baby product stores. A small, strapless knit cap can help your baby to conserve body heat if you turn down the thermostat at night, or if it's drafty in his bedroom.

After the first few weeks, your baby will adapt to home temperatures that are comfortable for you. Babies' feet are always colder than the rest of their bodies, but some parents have found that keeping small socks on a baby's feet helps him to feel safer and more comfortable.

It's important to not overdress your baby if he is ill and has a fever. The concept of sweating out an illness is dangerous and even can be fatal for a sick baby. A baby's internal thermostat is primitive, and he doesn't sweat like children and adults in order to cool down. Some babies have died from heatstroke when they had fevers and were purposely overheated by their clothing.

CRIBS AND OTHER SLEEPING OPTIONS

During the first 2 years of life, your baby will be spending more time sleeping than being awake. And most babies spend the majority of their sleeping careers in full-size cribs. In the early days after you bring your baby home, though, you'll probably want to keep your baby near you so you can monitor him and make sure he's all right. The problem is that a full-size crib is huge, too large to roll though a doorway, and difficult to assemble and disassemble. So you'll probably want to leave it in your baby's room.

Full-Size Cribs

It goes without explaining that full-size cribs are the rectangular baby beds with bars on the side that can be found in virtually every baby store. You can buy a crib, or you can buy a whole bedroom suite for baby that includes an armoire and a chest with a diaper-changing platform on top. Note that crib mattresses (discussed on page 308) are sold as a separate item. The quality and prices of cribs range from less than $100 for a model with rough finishing up to $1,000 or more for an heirloom-quality crib that is actually a piece of furniture—huge, finely finished, and fit for a prince (or princess)—but no less subject to safety recalls and hazards. But remember: Cribs are the biggest baby killers in the baby product world. Malfunctioning older cribs that parents continue to use even though bars are missing, the drop sides fail to hold, or mattress supports have broken cause most baby deaths.

All cribs are subject to federal regulations regarding interior dimensions, bar spacing, and safety

of components: (1) The interior dimensions of the crib must be uniform so that there are no gaps between the mattress and sides that could capture a baby's head. (2) Bars must be spaced no more than 2⅜ inches apart so babies can't slide out between them, body first, and get strangled. (3) The regulations also address basic crib safety, such as how high the bars must be even in the lowest position.

Cribs also have a voluntary certification standard overseen by the American Society of Testing and Materials (ASTM) and the Juvenile Products Manufacturers Association (JPMA). To be certified, crib brands must undergo extra testing for sturdiness. Certified cribs will usually have a sticker somewhere on the frame with the words JMPA and CERTIFIED on it. Being certified isn't an absolute guarantee of safety. For example, some certified cribs have undergone federal recalls because of loose bars. A big price tag isn't necessarily a sign of how safe or durable a crib is. Extremely expensive cribs may have a solid feel of quality to them, but could be recalled because of a serious flaw.

Cribs come in a variety of colors and finishes. There are pastel painted versions in light greens or creamy whites as well as models with furniture stains, such as cherry and pale blond, and natural-looking finishes. Lighter wood finishes are less likely to show scratches than darker cherry and mahogany stains, and often the darker stains are used to cover up visible flaws in less expensive wood cuts.

The best strategy for buying a crib is to shop middle-priced models, choose a smooth finish that goes with your home décor, and examine the quality of crib components, such as well-glued slats and sturdy hardware. If the service is available, consider paying the store to deliver and set up the crib. It's a two-person job that can last an hour. Make sure you set it up in the room where it is to stay, since cribs are too large to be moved out of rooms without being disassembled.

Pros: The biggest advantage of buying a crib, rather than using other baby beds, is that they are governed by stringent federal regulations. That means that they are constantly watched for flaws and recalled when they fail to pass the tests and requirements. In addition, they are also covered by JPMA certification standards, which means that those manufacturers who choose to can have their cribs tested and certified for additional safety compliance.

Cons: Full-size cribs are so large they can't fit through doorways. Newborns and young babies don't need all that room. Poorly functioning older cribs and new models with poor craftsmanship can be hazardous.

Crib Mattresses

Once you've chosen your baby's crib, you may be surprised to discover that even though mattresses are displayed inside cribs in stores, cribs don't come with them. And salespeople are trained to immediately walk you to their mattress displays while you're in the flush of your crib decision

Safety Warning: Cribs Can Kill!

Nearly fifty babies a year die in malfunctioning or old cribs, heirloom cradles, and bassinets. Rickety beds with weakened screw holes and broken hardware fall apart, entrapping heads and causing strangulation. Loosened or widely spaced bars allow a baby's body to squeeze through, leaving the head behind to strangle. Crib components and drop side hardware can fail.

Babies can be poisoned by lead-containing varnish or paint when they gnaw on wooden sides. Poorly fitting or mushy mattresses can lead to suffocation. Protruding carved areas on end boards can strangle a baby if clothing gets captured or small heads become trapped.

to encourage you to buy the most expensive version in the store.

Your baby will be sleeping on a crib mattress for approximately 2 years—and maybe a couple of years longer if you buy a pint-sized toddler bed the same dimensions as a crib. Firmness is more critical than internal structure or padding. Granted, getting a quality mattress is important, but there's no need to pay extra bucks because a sales pitch claims your baby needs extra back support. He doesn't. Babies' bodies are quite flexible. It's the grownups who carry them around who need the help.

Federal regulations enforced by

Cribs

- **Certified.** A JPMA-certified sticker means the crib brand passes a voluntary safety test overseen by manufacturers.
- **Fixed sides.** Cribs with sides that can be lowered (drop sides) are most likely to experience hardware problems since they contain more moving parts and have more non-rigid connections than those with firmly attached sides. Drop side corners can come loose from the tracks that are on each end of the crib ends, or other components can break, allowing the side to fall or come off.
- **Frame integrity.** Make sure the frame doesn't rattle when shaken. The bars (slats) should be well fastened and should not twist or move.
- **Finish.** All surfaces must be smooth and splinter-free.
- **Well-glued slats.** Slats, or bars, should be firmly attached. Glue residue spilled out onto the wood is a sign of poor craftsmanship.
- **Teething rails.** Most models have a small plastic railing to line the tops of the railings on the sides. Make sure it doesn't have sharp edges and can't be pulled loose.
- **Mattress supports.** The metal support that goes under the mattress should be sturdy with no sharp points that could puncture the underside of the mattress. Make sure it fastens to the crib with strong, thick hardware.
- **Locking wheels.** If the crib has wheels, they should be lockable to prevent a baby's motion from moving the crib.
- **Underside storage drawer.** Storage drawers that slide or roll out from under the crib can be useful, but check their quality before paying extra for them.

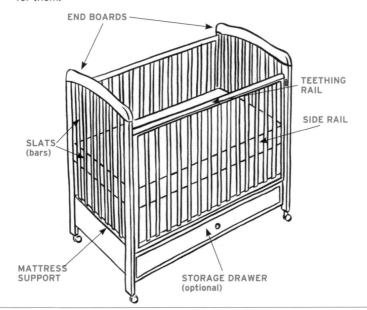

END BOARDS

TEETHING RAIL

SIDE RAIL

SLATS (bars)

MATTRESS SUPPORT

STORAGE DRAWER (optional)

the U.S. Consumer Product Safety Commission mandate that all crib mattresses be the same length and width so that they will fit flush against the sides of cribs. In turn, full-size cribs must also have identical interior dimensions.

There are basically two generic types of mattresses for babies: innerspring and foam. The coverings on crib mattresses, called ticking, come in a variety of colors and materials, such as quilted, moisture-resistant fabric, laminated vinyl, or a combination of fabric and vinyl.

Ticking should be thick and resist moisture and stains. The best coverings are triple-laminated, meaning they offer three thick layers of material heat-welted together. How the mattress ticking is sewn can be important. The binding around the edges of the mattress should be durable and double-stitched to prevent ripping and tearing. And it will help to keep seams from splitting when a toddler jumps around on the mattress. Higher-quality mattresses have fabric bindings all around the seams, rather than vinyl, and the seams are tightly double-stitched so they won't come loose.

Air vents—small, metal-lined holes along the side of the mattress or pocket-style openings at both ends—allow the insides of the mattress to breathe. Inexpensive mattresses may have small metal vents fastened onto thin vinyl on the sides that could be easily plucked off and swallowed by curious tots. Sometimes manufacturers will claim that a mattress has antibacterial qualities. That means that an antibacterial chemical has been added to the vinyl used in the laminate to help destroy bacteria on the surface of the mattress. Unfortunately, a baby's continual wetting is more than any surface material can handle.

Some mattresses claim they are non-allergenic or hypoallergenic. That simply means they're made of foam instead of cotton and other fibers that attract dust mites and can cause allergic reactions.

Manufacturers will also use the selling ploy of a lifetime warranty to get parents to pay more for their baby's mattress. But you'd better comb through the fine print, since the actual warranty may come with lots of loopholes in favor of the manufacturer, such as special conditions and a payback scale that depends upon the age of the mattress.

We suggest using a quality, washable pad to protect the mattress, turning the mattress over frequently, and following the manufacturer's directions for cleaning (usually wiping the surface down with a mild soap solution and then cleaning off the soap residue using a cloth dampened with clear water).

Innerspring Mattresses

Innerspring crib mattresses resemble miniature adult mattresses. Underneath the ticking are thick layers of padding, a series of metal coils, and thick metal support wires to hold up the edges of the mattress. As for adults, better innerspring mattresses for babies generally have more coils than less-expensive versions, and the coils are made from higher-quality metal, such as steel.

As the name implies, innerspring mattresses have springs inside, and the quality and price of the mattress often depends upon the number of coils, such as "180 tough steel springs and steel-reinforced edges."

Pros: The main advantage of an innerspring mattress is that it offers variable support to different parts of your baby's body as he grows and gains weight.

Cons: Their biggest drawback is that they're substantially heavier and less flexible than mattresses made from foam. That makes sheet changing, which you'll be doing once, possibly twice per day, more of a hassle than with a foam mattress. Plus, most tots like to use innerspring mattresses like trampolines, which could lead to falls and injuries.

Foam Mattresses

Foam mattresses come in a variety of prices and grades. The higher the quality of foam, the heavier it weighs and the denser it is. Denser versions are less squishy when you squeeze them. Poor-quality mattresses will be lightweight, have a single layer of vinyl for a covering and vinyl bindings.

There are two quick tests for the denseness of a foam mattress. One is to take it down from the shelf (or out of the display crib), and to lean on the mattress with the top edge braced under your arms. A less dense mattress will bow into a curve under your weight.

The second test is to press your palms together with the mattress in between. A dense mattress will stay put without compressing inward, a less dense mattress will change shape under the pressure of your hands.

Usually, foam mattresses are constructed from a single foam slab, but sometimes higher-quality versions will offer more than one density—a firm surface where baby sleeps, and a tough, non-springy edge to reinforce the outer rim of the mattress.

Pros: Quality foam mattresses can be really firm, almost like a brick—an advantage when it comes to preventing a pocket of exhaled air. They're lightweight too and have clear-cut corners that help keep fitted sheets on.

Cons: Inexpensive foam mattresses can compress and sag in the area where your baby lies. Some have only a single layer of vinyl that's poorly bound on the sides, which can lead to tears and stretching. (Stick with a name-brand manufacturer that uses thick, reinforced upholstery.)

Alternative Sleeping Options for Babies

There are a number of smaller-than-crib options for keeping your baby in your bedroom during the first months after birth.

Bassinets. Bassinets are compact baby beds on wheels. Most frames are made either out of tubular plastic or from woven rattan with wooden legs. Most have wheels or casters that make them easy to roll.

Their charm is in their appealing ruffles in baby-style fabrics such as lacy white or pastel prints. Canopies are a cute extra, but models without such a topper are simpler to use and may cost less.

Pros: While a standard-size

Look For: Bassinet

- **Good mattress.** A well-fitted, quality mattress is a must. It should be extra firm and extend completely to the edges and corners of the bassinet's interior.
- **Rigid sides.** Solid sides in the baby's sleep area are safer than soft fabric sides that could allow a small neck or head to get trapped in pockets caused by loose fabric sides.
- **Washable fabrics.** Fabrics and liners should be completely washable. (Read the instructions.)
- **Leg locks.** Folding legs should lock firmly in the open position to prevent accidental collapse.
- **Locking casters.** Wheels are handy. Lockable, multi-direction casters are the best buy. They'll keep siblings from pushing the bassinet around.
- **Rocking feature.** Some bassinets have a rocking option, which could be comforting for a fitful baby. Look for locks to keep the bassinet motionless for sleep; otherwise, your baby may end up pressed into one side when his weight shifts.
- **Size limits.** Follow the manufacturer's weight and age instructions for the best time to graduate your baby to a full-size crib (usually when he is able to roll over or pull up).
- **Face up for sleep.** For safety's sake, always place baby on his back for sleep, and keep out suffocating soft pillows, quilts, or stuffed toys. (See sudden infant death warnings on page 233.)

crib can't fit through a doorway, bassinets come with wheels and can easily be rolled from one room to another. So, bassinets are one option for keeping your baby close during that first crucial month when you are more likely to worry about your newborn's well-being.

Cons: Soft mattresses can smother and components including legs and hardware may malfunction, causing the bassinet to collapse.

As with full-size cribs, a baby should always be placed on his back for face-up sleep. And soft quilts, pillows, or stuffed toys should be kept out of the bassinet to protect against baby suffocation or the potential for sudden infant death syndrome (SIDS).

Cradles. Cradles are the traditional bed for newborns. They come in two basic styles: those with rockers on the base, and those that rock by being suspended on a footed frame by a hook or rocking mechanism at the top.

Unfortunately, small babies have little body control, and they may be rolled back and forth with the rocking motion, or become trapped. Heirloom cradles with widely spaced bars (more than 2⅜ inches apart) and those with soft, poorly fitting mattresses can be life threatening. Young babies can slide through the bars leaving their heads behind, causing strangulation, and they can also get wedged between the cradle side and the mattress, causing suffocation.

Pros: They have a romantic, all-baby feel to them. They offer rocking that should be soothing to a baby.

Cons: Unfortunately, most cradles simply roll a baby's body back and forth from one side to the other, and babies can get trapped against the side that's lowest.

Portable Cribs. An alternative product option is a small-scale crib with wheels. These are actually a safer choice since many models from major manufacturers have passed special safety and durability tests to earn a JPMA (Juvenile Products Manufacturers) certification sticker.

Pros: These are simply miniature cribs, small enough to roll through doorways. Most have adjusting legs so that they can later be used as a playpen. They tend to be safer than other bedding alternatives because of the strict regulations they have to follow. Legs may lower to allow the portable crib to sit on the floor like a playpen for use later.

Cons: Most use nonstandard-size sheets. They may offer only one mattress height. Some models have soft, instead of rock-hard, mattresses. Babies should only sleep on extra-firm versions.

Bedside Sleepers. These are low, small, three-sided cribs with mattress pads designed so that newborns can sleep directly beside their parents. They're made to attach to the side of an adult bed using long straps that go across the adult's bedsprings to strap the sleeper firmly against the side of the bed. The concept of this design is to give parents easy access to their babies without the risk of SIDS, or the potential roll-over hazard of an adult bed. The downside is that many models of co-sleepers have been recalled

themselves due to entrapment hazards. Your pediatrician's office and/or *www.cpsc.gov* places are good places to go for the latest information on the safety of co-sleepers.

Pros: The beds are handy and allow the baby to be quickly moved back and forth for nursing and feeding with parents not having to get up.

Cons: The beds take up a lot of space on the side of an adult bed, and make it difficult for the adult to get in and out of bed herself. Babies tend to fall asleep at the breast, and arousing them by removing them from the warmth of the parent's body to put them onto the cold sleeper surface is likely to awaken them in the same way that lifting them and placing them in a crib or bassinet will.

DIAPER BAGS

Going out in the world with your baby will require toting a humongous load of baby gear too. The list of what to pack includes spare diapers, a change or two of clothes, baby bottles, toddler snacks, diaper wipes, and a distracting toy or two. Diaper bags come in a huge variety of sizes and designs. Outer finishes range from colorful, baby-friendly quilted fabrics to serious, down-to-business black and navy bags at home in the office. Most bags offer a wide range of pockets and extras, including removable diaper changing pads, moisture-proof storage pouches, insulated bottle holders, and even loops to hold car keys or snap-on toys.

Diaper Bags

- **Sturdy upholstery.** A heavy-duty outer covering will resist moisture, dirt, and wear. Dense, moisture-resistant nylon weaves and thick canvas last better than thin cotton quilting or lightweight fabrics.
- **Handle comfort.** Carry handles need to be short enough so the bag won't drag if you're carrying it with one hand. Check underarm carrying comfort too.
- **Less is better.** Light and simple are best. Too many pockets and sections weigh the bag down and make it harder to find lost items.
- **See-through pouches.** The best inside pouches and dividers are clear vinyl or mesh so you can spot what you're seeking.
- **Zippered closure.** Zippering the bag closed will help prevent spills and keep small hands out of mischief.
- **Reinforcements.** The best bags have reinforced stitching or heavy-duty braids where handles and straps join the body of the bag.
- **Great alternatives.** Backpack bags with padded straps and a center carry handle are an advantage: they allow multiple carrying options, including hands-free porting for babes-in-arms. If nothing else works for you, try morphing your favorite large purse or a backpack into a diaper bag by inserting inexpensive waterproof pouches and a lightweight changing pad.

DIAPERS

Your baby will use up nearly sixty diapers a week in the early months. That rate will gradually slow down, and a mature toddler verging on potty training will use only a few per day.

During your baby's entire diapering career, you'll be changing diapers between five thousand and eight thousand times. Can you imagine? It makes sense to decide on the type of diapering system you're going to use before your baby arrives. Things to weigh: how much a particular diapering option will cost over 2 years, and how demanding the system will be on your time and energy.

Here are your basic options: reusable fabric diapers, disposables, and—in some larger cities—diaper services to launder fabric diapers for you and deliver them to your door.

Each system has its advantages and disadvantages. You don't have to be dedicated to just one solution. You can use a combination of systems, e.g., a diaper service for starters, reusable cloth diapers for most of the time, and disposables for going out. Whichever system(s) you choose, you'll need ample diapering supplies on hand before you bring your little wetter home.

When it comes to diaper pails: You'll need a soaking pail with a locking lid for fabric diapers (or you can simply throw them directly into the washing machine until you have enough to run). If you're using disposables, you can buy a milk jug–shaped pail that takes rolled-up diapers and wraps them in a vinyl sleeve to help keep odor down, or you can simply use a lidded can and throw-away plastic liners.

Fabric Reusables

Laundering your own diapers is the most economical option, and you'll probably save more than $1,000 during your baby's entire diapering career. But when you compare diapering costs, also try to factor in the wear and tear on your washing machine from laundering fabric diapers every few days, plus your utility and detergent costs, and the value of your time and labor—all of that can translate into hundreds of dollars a year. Some parents feel that fabric diapers, like woven cotton underwear, are more natural and comfortable. Another group prefers reusables out of concern for the environment, such as the depletion of forests and the impact of disposables on community waste management systems.

Whatever system you settle upon, your decision should be based on your judgment about what's best for both you and your baby. Gear yourself up for a regular, day-to-day laundering schedule to keep on top of the dirty diaper pile that baby will generate. For the most efficient diaper cleaning, it's best to use unscented liquid detergents that won't leave a residue behind. Don't use a fabric softener; its perfumes can be irritating to baby's nose and skin, and it also tends to clog the vent screen of dryers, which slows down the drying process. A sturdy washer and a dryer are essential.

Since cotton is more absorbent than other materials, it's the material of choice for reusable diapers. In decades past, parents could choose from only one or two fabric weaves: mostly bird's-eye, which resembles old-fashioned white dishtowels, or loosely woven, more porous gauze.

Standard, old-fashioned diapers are usually packaged by the dozen and come in one of three basic models: unfolded, folded, and shaped. Unfolded diapers are simply a single, large square of fabric. The packaging usually gives instructions on how to fold them to fit your baby so that absorbency is concentrated in the middle of the diaper where it's most needed. (Usually they're folded in a triangle: one point for each side of the baby and a point to fit between the legs. The three points are brought together at baby's middle and pinned.)

Pre-folded diapers are rectangular-shaped and have extra fabric folds sewn into the center for absorbency. Fitted diapers can be shaped like an hourglass or the profile of an airplane. They're hourglass shaped to leave less bulkiness and chafing between the legs, but you have to stock them according to your baby's size.

Avoid plastic pants with sewn-in diaper interiors. They don't launder well, take forever in the dryer, and harbor bacteria that can lead to diaper rash.

Combination diaper-and-cover systems that are far more sophisticated than prepackaged cotton diapers are the best (and most expensive) reusable option. Often imported, these systems consist of lightweight, breathable, but moisture-resistant outer coverings that use Velcro-type closures, and a thick inner core that is smaller, but thicker than a regular diaper and comes closest to mimicking the absorbency of disposables.

Nowadays diaper systems come in a variety of fabrics from bamboo (highly absorbent and soft), burley-knit terry, fleece, hemp, microfiber, and combinations, such as bamboo/cotton/viscose and poly micro. You can save money by sewing your own diapers. That allows you to customize the diapers and choose from a wide variety of patterns and fabrics available online (see *www.verybaby.com*). You can also purchase samples of different products to find the system that will work the best for you. When you search diaper e-tailers on the Internet, try combining the words "diapers" and "cotton" using your favorite search engine, then shop around.

It makes sense to order single samples of two or three diapering systems to check out their quality and absorbency before you invest heavily in a single brand. The company will advise you how many diapers you will need to get started, and most company Web sites offer good diaper laundering advice too.

Pros: After your initial investment in a fabric diaper system, you can expect to save hundreds of dollars in the years that follow. Some parents consider fabric diapers kinder to baby skin, and also to the environment; plus, you'll never run out as long as your washing machine and dryer keep chugging along. Old-fashioned pre-folded versions have other practical uses, too: stuffing in your bra to catch letdowns and soaking up spit-ups on your shoulder, and they'll still be around to use again with your next baby.

Cons: They're more labor-intensive to launder and require a hefty up-front investment for getting started. Except for the very expensive versions, most diaper fabrics don't absorb wetness as readily as disposables, nor do they have an outside dampness barrier to protect your clothing and furniture. So, you'll need to buy a supply of waterproof outer pants too—preferably made of breathable materials that won't turn your baby's bottom into a hothouse for bacteria. If not well laundered, they are associated with more diaper rash.

Diaper Services

Diaper services flourished in decades past, but they've almost all gone out of business due to the competition from disposables. You may still have the option of using a diaper service if you live in a major U.S. city. (See: *www.realdiaperindustry.org* for a member directory of diaper service companies.)

Here's how a diaper service works: You choose the style of diapers you want to use. These diapers, and only these, are allotted to your baby—so the fear of contamination from another baby isn't founded. Once or twice a week, a truck pulls up and takes away the soiled diapers you've stored in a mesh bag inside a pail furnished by the service. In their place, you're left neatly wrapped stacks of clean, white diapers laundered at extremely hot temperatures that can't be matched by home machines. Most services let you sign up for as long or short a time as you wish.

Pros: If there is a diaper service in your community, you can pay a monthly fee to be supplied with weekly stacks of soft, ready-to-use fabric diapers. They free you from laundering chores, and it may help prevent diaper rash, too. Plus, diaper services are cheaper than disposables.

Cons: The service costs more than doing your own laundering. The likelihood of finding a service in your area may be slim. You may not be able to use the sophisticated diaper systems with heavyweight flannel or terry inserts that are the most absorbent. Occasionally, you may run out of diapers before your next pickup.

Disposables

Disposables are convenient and usually effective in wicking moisture away from your baby's skin, a help in preventing skin irritation. Expect to buy about 5,000 of them in all, for an investment of between $1,200 and $1,500. A good disposable should be snug and not too tight. It should be non-irritating with no redness, rashes, or chafing. And, it should prevent leaks from leg holes or around the waistband. Disposables continue to improve every year, mostly because of the steep competition between Kimberly-Clark (Huggies) and Procter & Gamble (Pampers)—the

two giants that manufacture disposables. Over time, these diapers have become more absorbent, fit babies better, and are easier to fasten than ever before. And prices are always changing. Most parents settle down to a preferred disposable brand after trying a few different versions. They may like a particular type of diaper because it seems to fit better, because it appears to be more absorbent, because they like the way it fastens on the sides, or simply because it's cheaper.

Disposables come in five or six sizes. Some start at a preemie size and go up, others offer the newborn size as the first size. As your baby grows, the diapers get larger too, and that means getting fewer diapers in each package you buy, even though the package prices remain roughly the same.

There are a couple of ways to save some money on disposables. You can purposely get on the company's mailing list to get coupons in the mail. You can sometimes do that by calling their toll-free telephone numbers, signing up on one of their sponsored Web sites, by using a baby registry (see page 77), or subscribing to free baby magazines. You can also save a lot by buying your baby's diapers by the case from large discount chains, such as Sam's Club, and watching for special sales. Generic diaper brands offered by discount stores can sometimes be a real bargain, especially in bulk quantities. But the quality of these brands sometimes can be inconsistent.

It makes sense to purchase several different brands and take them home to actually test them on your baby. You're looking for fit, comfort, leak resistance, and economy. While one brand may work well on small babies, another may do just fine for toddlers, so remain open to different options.

Pros: They're the most convenient of all options and tend to fit babies better than one-size-fits-all diapers. Their absorbency truly does keep dampness away from a baby's bottom, and that may mean fewer diaper rash breakouts. Newer diapers are especially designed to prevent leaks around the legs and waist.

Cons: They're your most expensive option, costing more than twice as much as reusables. If you're sensitive to perfume, you'll probably also be sensitive to the strong, undeniable chemical smell of some disposable brands. Some parents nix disposables out of concern for the depletion of forests and environmental issues. Piles of disposables can stink while they wait for garbage day, and, yes, parents do run out of them in the middle of the night.

HIGH CHAIRS

High chairs have come a long way from the old wooden models of bygone eras. Now they offer reclining features and almost infinite height adjustments. (But they cost more too.)

Since your baby won't have the strength to sit up on his own until he reaches 4 to 6 months of age, you may want a chair that has a recline option so you can use the seat as a baby holder in the kitchen, or you can simply postpone buying a high chair until it's time for baby to start experimenting with eating—at about 6 months.

There are cheap, bare-bones models with flimsy trays, but they usually can't be trusted to hold up to everyday wear and tear. At the other end of the spectrum are trendy imported chairs priced well over $200.

Since your baby will be using a high chair multiple times per day for several years, it might be worth the extra investment to get a quality piece of equipment that can hold up to the day-by-day wear and tear that toddlers dish out.

Scale is important. Some manufacturers have gone overboard with their high chair designs and have made trays and seats so huge that they completely overshadow the small baby seated inside, not to mention eating up a lot of kitchen floor space.

The chair doesn't need a huge tray, just one that has a lip on all sides to catch liquid spills. The tray should also slide effortlessly on and off with one hand and the barest push of a button or squeeze of a latch.

Most chairs now offer adjustable heights so seats can be raised for spoon feeding, lowered to slide up to the dining room table, or even lowered flush with the floor to make a toddler chair.

Quality models have seats that effortlessly adjust to numerous positions. Poorly designed models make adjustments difficult and

High Chair

- **JPMA approved.** Look for a "JPMA (Juvenile Products Manufacturers Association) certified" sticker on the frame. That means the model lives up to tough safety standards.
- **Seat belt.** The sturdy seat belt should fasten around the waist and between the legs and feature a toddler-proof buckle.
- **Easy-to-use tray.** The tray should be removable with one hand and have a deep, spill-catching rim. It should lock in different positions with an audible click.
- **Crotch post.** A between-the-legs post will help to protect your baby from sliding under the tray (submarining) and getting his head captured, which can be deadly.
- **Seat adjustments.** Multiple seat heights will let the chair fit under a table rim or lower down to the floor for use by a toddler. Reclining positions allow the chair to be used as a baby seat before baby can sit up by himself.
- **Stability.** A wide footprint means the chair will be less likely to tip over when a toddler pulls on the chair or tries to get in on his own. Wheel locks help too.
- **Washable upholstery.** Select a chair with upholstery that's easy to remove and throw in the washing machine.

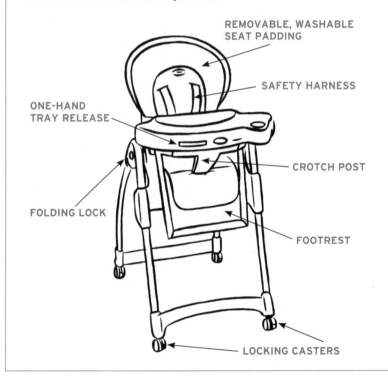

REMOVABLE, WASHABLE SEAT PADDING

SAFETY HARNESS

ONE-HAND TRAY RELEASE

CROTCH POST

FOLDING LOCK

FOOTREST

LOCKING CASTERS

awkward. They take up a lot of floor space.

Pros: High chairs raise your baby up to your level for feeding, and they give him a bird's-eye view of the kitchen while you're fixing his meal. Some models have adjustable heights so you can lower the chair and remove the tray for pulling your baby up to the table during family meals. Trays with deep rims can help to catch spills. One-handed tray removal can come in handy.

Cons: High chairs can take up a lot of kitchen space. High chairs aren't reliable babysitters, so always stay close. Babies stand up and fall out, or try to slip out under the seat when they're not safely belted in.

MONITORS

There are different options for listening in on your baby during pregnancy and also after he arrives. While you're pregnant, you may enjoy tuning into your baby's sounds using a battery-operated amplifier that you place on your belly. If you place it correctly, you may be able to pick up the rapid beating of your baby's heart (120 to 160 beats a minute) and the whooshing sound of blood moving through your baby's umbilical cord.

Some companies now rent sophisticated, handheld Doppler devices for more precise amplification. A "Pregaphone" is a simple handheld device you place on your belly to amplify your voice while you talk to your baby in the womb. Okay, so it's silly, but hey, who knows?

Nursery, or baby, monitors are 2-piece electronic devices that allow you to keep tabs on your baby while he's sleeping and you're in another room. They're like walkie-talkies, but most without the talkie part.

There are two parts to the monitor. The part that goes in the baby's room is called the transmitter, and it sends out the noise signals. The part that parents carry around with them, usually battery-operated and with a small antenna, is called the receiver. It acts like a radio to amplify your baby's noises through a small speaker.

Most monitors have volume controls so you can listen to baby's every rustle, or you can choose to be signaled only for outright fussiness. Some have light bars that let you see as well as hear your baby's noises, while others borrow from cell phone technology and vibrate to baby's sounds.

You may need to try out more than one monitor model to find one with the sensitivity and power that suits your particular environment. Your monitor may lose power if you stray too far. Sometimes barriers, such as brick walls, can block monitor signals. Or batteries can weaken, causing transmissions to fade. Fortunately, most models have a low-battery indicator light.

Parents living in apartments sometimes report that their monitor picks up the sound of another baby, not their own. And some monitors can interfere with cell phone reception, or they transmit annoying sounds

Monitor

- **Clear reception.** Buy a monitor with a different channel mix, such as channels A through D, instead of only A and B, and one that uses 900 MHz, which is less crowded than the traditional 400 MHz channels and can pick up signals better.
- **Rechargeability.** Monitors gobble up batteries. Rechargeable receivers can save up to $50 a year in battery costs. Also, make sure both the transmitter (baby's unit) and the receiver (yours) have plug-in electric outlet adapters and a low-battery indicator.
- **Portability.** An easy-to-use belt clip and flexible antenna improve portability. But note: A too-small receiver gets lost quickly. (Search under the couch pillows.)
- **Sound lights.** Indicators that light up to signal the intensity of baby's sound are useful for judging when it's time to head for the nursery, even when you're vacuuming.
- **Walkie-talkie feature.** Monitors that allow you speak soothing sounds from another room or carry on a conversation with your partner are useful.
- **Useful extras.** A light display that lets you see baby's sounds as well as hear them; a warning light or alarm that signals when you're out of range; a nightlight feature for baby's room.

from police cars or other passing vehicles.

Static and interference from cell phones and even crying from a baby in another apartment with a monitor on a similar channel can be annoying.

Less expensive monitors sometimes use the crowded 400 MHz channels, but now most quality monitors use 900 MHz for less interference and a wider sound range. Some monitor brands appear to have better clarity than others. Check parents' ratings of monitors on Web sites that offer unbiased product feedback from parents.

You may be able to buy a monitor set that includes an extra receiver so both you and your partner can listen in, or you can keep one permanently stationed in the kitchen or your bedroom.

And, at the high end of the monitor price range are monitors that allow you to talk to the baby remotely from your receiver, or turn on a nightlight, play traditional lullabies or night sounds, or offer a wider variety of transmission channels from which to choose.

Pros: A monitor can give you more peace of mind that your baby isn't crying when you're out of earshot.

Cons: Nothing can replace staying close and checking your baby every so often. A monitor can't tell you if your baby has stopped breathing. A monitor may make you more jumpy about normal baby sounds and momentary fussiness that get amplified by the receiver. Static and interference are often problems. Unless your monitor is rechargeable, it can eat up a lot of batteries.

PLAY YARDS

Portable play yards are
rectangular like a crib, but
instead of being constructed from
wood, their frames are made out
of tubular metal and covered in
moisture-resistant fabric with
see-through mesh sides. Instead
of having legs, they sit close to
the ground on casters, or they
may have two legs on one end
and two wheels on the other.
They're lightweight and fold
compactly for storage. Parents
use them for travel, or to restrain
a baby indoors or outdoors in the
shade.

Unlike cribs, play yards are
narrow enough to roll through
doorways. The hinged sidebars and
folding floorboards are padded
for baby's safety and comfort. For
safety's sake, it's important to
study the manufacturer's directions
about how to fold and open the
yard before your baby uses it for
the first time.

Most models squeeze shut like
the ribs of a travel umbrella when
you release the sidebars using a
button and twist and pull up on
handle of the flat hub located in the
center of the yard under the floor's
padding.

Opening the play yard is a
challenge—the hinged sidebars
must stand nearly upright before
the yard will open completely so
its sidebars can be firmly locked
into place. While some play yards
feature open mesh on all four
sides, others have fabric panels on
both ends with a storage pocket
sewn on the outside. The fabric
on the sides and floorboard can

be damp mopped with a mild soap
and water solution.

Some models offer an optional
bassinet feature that fastens to
the frame's sidebars, and most
companies also offer models with
a small diaper-changing station
that fits over one end of the yard's
frame.

Safety Issues

Over a million portable play yards
manufactured in the past decade
have undergone federal recalls
or corrective actions when the
sidebars of some models failed
to completely lock in the open
position.

A V shape was formed when
the sides were left limp instead
of being locked firmly into place,
causing babies to strangle when
their necks got caught in the gap
and they couldn't right themselves.
The recalls have provided repair
kits or other remedies for older
models—but for maximum safety,
we recommend purchasing a new
model if you're not sure about the
safety status of an older version.
Don't use a portable play yard as
a substitute for a crib. Its loose
mesh sides and puffy quilting can
be dangerous for unsupervised
sleeping. Babies can get entangled
in loose sheets and bedding too,
so don't add a sheet or pillowcase
as a cover for the floor or bassinet
section.

Remember, all babies should be
placed face up and not belly down
to lessen the danger of suffocation.
(See sudden infant death syndrome
discussion on page 231.) Older-
model play yards may come with
a ribbed dome that fits into small
holders on the top corners of

Anatomy of a Portable Play Yard

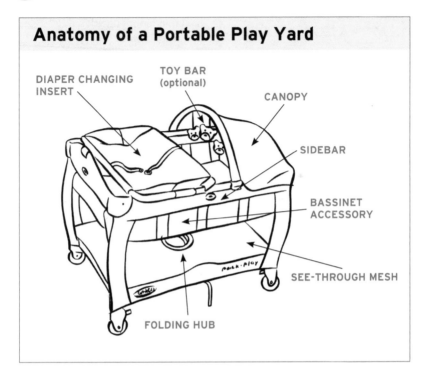

DIAPER CHANGING INSERT

TOY BAR (optional)

CANOPY

SIDEBAR

BASSINET ACCESSORY

SEE-THROUGH MESH

FOLDING HUB

the yard. The dome comes with warning signs not to use it in direct sunlight because of the danger of serious heat buildup inside. Most manufacturers have discontinued making the domes because of the danger of babies getting heatstroke or entrapped between the dome and the play yard railing.

Pros: Portable play yards are lightweight, have wheels, and fold compactly for storing or carrying in the trunk of the car. Their dimensions allow them to be rolled from room to room. The mesh sides let babies peer out. The bassinet feature allows small babies to snooze, but only with close supervision. Some models come with a carry case that makes porting easy.

Cons: Opening and folding play yards is a hassle, and if the sidebars don't click into place, as with some older models, a toddler's life could be endangered. Mattress pads tend to be soft and cushy, and their moisture-resistance makes them less porous and breathable, which could affect a baby's air supply in the facedown position. Pad covers aren't removable for laundering, and placing sheets or other bedding on top of them can entangle the baby.

ROCKERS AND GLIDERS

Babies and parents both gravitate toward gentle rocking motions for soothing, nursing, and resting together. Surprisingly, if you've got a fussy baby on your hands, the rougher the rocking motion, the better (as long as there's good neck and head support).

You can use a rocker or glider as the center of your "baby nest," which is most convenient when it's near your baby's crib. You'll use the chair hundreds of times for those l-o-n-g, middle-of-the-night feeding sessions while you both snooze.

Put a table beside the chair for your CD player, a book to read, tissues, some fabric diapers for milksops, and a big, trucker-size container of water with a straw for fueling up. Consider stocking your chair with a couple of large, soft pillows and a small blanket to cover both you and baby.

If you're not using a recliner, you may want to purchase a separate footstool so you can prop your knees up to help hold the baby. A semi-circular nursing pillow (Boppy) can serve to give your arms a rest if you're nursing. You have three choices for your official baby chair: an old-fashioned rocker made of wood or wicker, a rocker recliner, or a glider. Wooden rockers are usually (but not always) the least expensive option. Sometimes you can find old but sturdy versions in antiques stores. Make sure their scale fits your dimensions: the armrests should be the right height for your elbows, and your feet should rest comfortably on the floor without pitching you forward. You should be able to add your own cushions for seat and back comfort. Rocker-recliners come in a variety of sizes and upholstery finishes. Needless to say, babies make messes, so it makes sense to choose a

moisture-resistant upholstery finish, such as pleather, that you can wipe clean with a damp cloth.

Make sure the chair fits to your body. Check out the armrests and the ease of reclining. Don't spend a lot of money on a recliner equipped with massage and vibration features; you probably won't use them enough to justify the expense.

Gliders are usually made from wood or metal frames. They offer deeply padded cushioning and a smooth, back-and-forth swaying motion that comes from the chair being suspended underneath the seat portion. Most come with matching ottomans that also rock. Hopefully, cushion covers can be unzipped and can survive numerous machine washings.

Which style of rocker you choose depends upon its fit to your body, how comfortable it is, and your budget. All versions have one flaw: The rockers or the hardware underneath the chair for the reclining or gliding features can be positively hazardous to small exploring fingers or feet. Be careful when using these chairs around toddlers and children, and don't let children play on them.

SAFETY GATES

Safety gates enclose doors and openings to restrain your tot so he won't wander where you don't want him to go—down staircases, where pets sleep, or into your kitchen when you're cooking or loading the dishwasher or the oven door is hot.

Gates are usually made of wood, metal, or plastic, or combinations of these materials. There are three types of safety gates: those that attach to the side of the wall using screws (hardware-mounted gates), those that cling to the wall using rubber gaskets (pressure-mounted gates), and those that are circular fences that can be used to corral kids inside them.

Some models close and open like an accordion, while others swing open and shut like a gate. The centers of gates can be molded plastic mesh, nylon fabric, or clear poly. Some models also allow the gate's opening direction to go only one way so they won't swing out over stairs. Although a safety gate can't completely stop your determined toddler from vaulting down the steps or getting into other mischief when he sets his mind to it, it can give you a few extra minutes to figure out what's going on. Hardware-mounted gates are considered the safest—in fact, they're the only type of gate you should use at the top of staircases or to shut off dangerous areas. Pressure-mounted gates can be used in less risky settings since they can sometimes work loose from the wall—especially if your toddler rolls into one in a walker, or if children are roughhousing. Old-fashioned accordion gates with wooden slats shaped like Xs at the top are positively dangerous and shouldn't be used. They could capture a child's neck or crush small fingers. Most new-version gates are designed to minimize harm and to help prevent toddlers from crawling over them.

Here are qualities of a good gate: the latches are easy for you to use but hard for your tot to operate, there are no finger-pinching places, and the placement of slats or pattern of plastic mesh won't allow your tot to get a foothold for climbing. Specialty gates are available to help you shield wide and unusual openings in your home, such as dining room entries or open stairs with iron railings on the side. Taller-than-normal gates are also available for containing super-active kids and large pets. For safety's sake, remember that safety gates aren't foolproof. You'll still want to keep constant watch over your active toddler.

One important caution: Thousands of parents and siblings of babies receive bruises and arm fractures when they attempt to step over the gate and crash on the other side, rather than open the gate. Always open and close it each time and caution others in the house to do the same.

Pros: Safety gates can help to keep your toddler off the stairs and help to keep him out of the kitchen or other places that may be unsafe.

Cons: Sometimes gates give parents a false sense of security about their babies. Parents routinely forget to lock gates, use gates that don't hold well, or trip and fall down the stairs themselves when they try to step over the gate instead of going to the trouble to open it and walk through. Gates with X joints can strangle and kill, and those with sharp parts, such as molded mesh holes, can actually injure babies' hands and feet.

Gates

- **Use hardware mounting.** Gates that screw into the wall are the safest by far. Gates that use thick rubber stoppers to hold the gate in place can be pushed over by a determined toddler, possibly causing falls.
- **Metal is sturdier.** It also makes gates more expensive and heavier. But if you've got a dangerous stairwell to protect, they're the best solution.
- **Measure first.** Look on the packaging for the gate. It will specify the gate's maximum width.
- **Choose the tallest version.** The taller the gate, the more protection you'll get from a climbing toddler or a nosy pet.
- **Easy-to-open hardware.** Try out the hardware that opens the gate. It should be easy to operate and not break fingernails in the process.
- **No floor interference.** Avoid gates that place a bar across the floor. They could cause you to trip.
- **No toe holds.** Avoid gates with sharp holes in the center panel that a tot could hurt his fingers on or try to use for climbing.

SOFT CARRIERS AND SLINGS

Mothers and fathers have fastened babies onto their bodies throughout human history. Doing so frees parents' arms to do other things and gives babies the rhythmical rocking movements that soothe them by reminding them of life in the womb.

There are basically three types of baby carriers that parents wear on their bodies: soft carriers made of fabric, slings that go over one shoulder and are also constructed of fabric, and hard-framed carriers for older tots that support a baby who rides on a parent's back. Since backpacks are an option to be postponed until your baby gets older, we will only cover soft carriers and slings.

Soft carriers usually consist of an inner seat pocket for the baby and an outer fabric covering that also offers a fold-down firm headrest for newborns, padded shoulder straps for the parent, and waist straps to help support the baby's weight. Slings resemble small hammocks with pleats that are designed to hold a young baby in a reclining or semi-reclining position.

Some parents prefer slings because they feel it gives baby rounded back support instead of making the baby sit bolt upright as soft carriers do, but there have been some major safety issues with them.

If you use a sling, make certain that you can see your baby's whole face at all times and that your baby's chin is not being compressed into her neck.

Soft Carriers

Pros: They're made of comfortable fabric, which is easy to wear. They put your baby's head at your chin, and you can provide natural warmth and comfort with your hand on baby's back.

Cons: Some models are a complex mesh of straps that makes putting on the baby a challenge. They can be hot in the summer. Poor hardware or too-large leg holes have led to baby injuries in the past.

Slings

Pros: They allow babies to lie in a more natural, semi-reclined position. The sling can be quickly adjusted to provide coverage for discreet nursing.

Cons: They're difficult to adjust, and you may need coaching from another user on finding the right position and length for your and baby's comfort. There are no straps to hold the baby in, which could be a problem if you lean over to pick something up. Rather than being evenly distributed, all of baby's weight is carried on one shoulder and across your back, which may cause body alignment problems.

Soft Carriers

- **Washable.** One spit-up can ruin a whole day! Fabric should be sturdy, soft, and able to withstand lots of machine washing.
- **Simple to use.** Avoid models with a jumble of straps to figure out.
- **Padded shoulder straps.** Parents' shoulder straps should be adjustable, densely padded, and spaced so they don't rub the neck or slip off the shoulders.
- **Head support.** A cushioned head support will be needed for the first few months. Fold it down or snap it off after that.
- **Adjusting seat.** Baby's seat should adjust to different heights using sturdy snaps that won't rub his belly. (Extra safety loops or a backup pouch will help to prevent accidental falls.)
- **Front or rear facing.** Some models allow facing outward as well as toward the chest, or riding on the back too—handy options for porting toddlers.
- **Nursing position.** Read the directions on how to nurse your baby while he sits in the carrier.
- **Great options.** Other extras: snap-on, flannel burper bibs; elasticized pockets for carrying small items; adjustments for discreet nursing; reflector strips for evening strolls; breathable mesh or special porous fabric for air circulation.

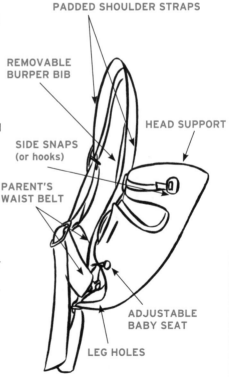

PADDED SHOULDER STRAPS

REMOVABLE BURPER BIB

HEAD SUPPORT

SIDE SNAPS (or hooks)

PARENT'S WAIST BELT

ADJUSTABLE BABY SEAT

LEG HOLES

STROLLERS

It takes careful searching to locate the best possible stroller for you and your baby-to-be, and other than a crib, it is probably the most expensive piece of baby equipment you'll buy. It is also the most complex baby product, and it can be the biggest investment other than a crib and mattress.

Strollers come in a huge variety of sizes and weights. Most manufacturers offer a basic model, followed by step-up options that drive the price up, making it hard to decide what you really need and what are useless extras. You'll have to pay more for those loaded with fancy extras than those offering only basic comfort.

Here's our breakdown of the different types of stroller models out there. (Mind-boggling, isn't it?)

- **Lightweight and inexpensive.** Commonly called umbrella strollers, these are usually flimsy, with single wheels on each axle, hammock-like seats with no padding, an almost useless canopy, and no reclining options. They're usually priced under $40 or $50. Some parents buy one or two in their babies' riding careers just to take on trips or to run fast errands.

- **Mid-priced and mid-weight workhorses.** These are the mainstream vehicles for pushing baby around. They come with dual wheels on the front and comfort features such as reclining seats, thick upholstery, wrap-around canopies, and deep storage compartments. Some offer removable front trays. They're priced in the $40 to $150 and $140 and up ranges.

- **Lightweight and costly imports.** These are the sports cars of the stroller world. They're stuffed with gizmos and feature trendy fabrics, luxury padding, and loads of extras, such as padded headrests, cup holders, and sleek folding mechanisms. They're priced between $150 and $400.

- **Heavy travel systems.** These are bulky models with large wheels, mostly designed to support their own snap-out car seats, $180 and up.

- **Carriage-stroller combinations.** Huge, fully reclining carriage/stroller combinations—basically baby beds on wheels, $300 and up.

- **Jogging and sports strollers.** These are even larger, three-wheeled strollers with air-inflated, bicycle-style tires for use by sports and fitness enthusiasts, $300 and up, depending on wheel size.

Price Doesn't Make Perfect

Most parents make the mistake of believing that when a stroller costs a lot, it will automatically deliver more quality, durability, and safety than less expensive models. That strategy might work with cars, but it doesn't work for baby wheels. Parents sometimes use strollers as status symbols. Instead of bragging about their Mercedes, BMW, or fancy SUV, they brag about their baby's Maclaren, Peg Perego, or Aprica—all imports with price tags starting around $200 and rising to $400 or more. Never mind the show-offs! The $400 Maclaren is a bummer to open

Strollers

Plan to take a variety of stroller models on a test drive before you settle on the one you want to buy.

- **Folding.** Test how readily the stroller folds up and reopens for locking into the upright position. Expect to feel awkward. In fact, you may need a sales clerk to help you locate elusive release latches. Lightweight strollers are the easiest to open and fold single-handedly and are great for racing to airport gates. They're too lightweight, small, and jiggly, though, for negotiating sidewalks and steep curbs on long, leisurely walks.

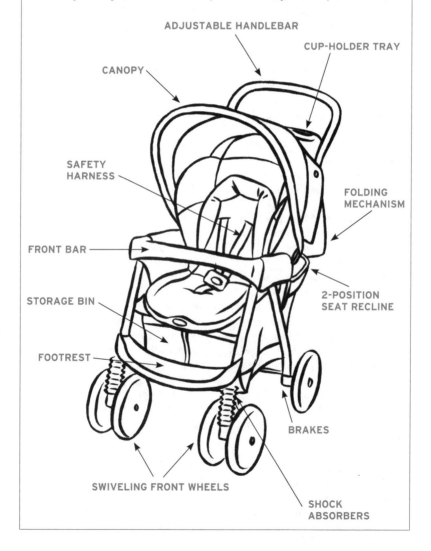

ADJUSTABLE HANDLEBAR

CUP-HOLDER TRAY

CANOPY

SAFETY HARNESS

FOLDING MECHANISM

FRONT BAR

2-POSITION SEAT RECLINE

STORAGE BIN

FOOTREST

SWIVELING FRONT WHEELS

BRAKES

SHOCK ABSORBERS

STROLLERS, *CONTINUED*

- **Steering.** Try pushing the stroller with one hand. The model should roll straight ahead without veering to one side. Most mid-priced models have swivel wheels with dual tires on the front or a single front wheel that lock into a straight-ahead position by a foot pedal on the wheel assembly. A toddler's weight affects stroller steering. A stroller may push straight when you're testing it in the store without your baby, but veer when your baby grows into a weighty toddler. Bring along a friend with a toddler test passenger to help narrow down your choices.
- **Seat recline.** Check out how easy it is to recline the back of the seat and the number of positions offered. The more reclining options, the better, but sides of the stroller should be well-padded to protect the baby's head and arms from slipping through when the seat is in its fullest recline position. Only large, combination carriage/stroller models recline fully into a protected bed. A semi-recline will do.
- **Seat belt.** The seat belt should have straps that come together to click into a center buckle at the baby's waist. Your baby will also require a strap between the legs to prevent slide-outs. The safest models also offer shoulder straps to hold a restless toddler in place. Superior five-point harness systems offer an adjustable strap for each side of a baby's waist, a between-the-legs strap, and adjustable shoulder straps.
- **Canopy or sunshade.** A deep, folding sunshade will help to protect your baby from wind, rain, and glare. Some models offer a small, vinyl window in the back of the canopy that keeps the baby in sight.
- **Storage bin.** A roomy storage bin underneath the stroller seat comes in handy for toting your purse, a diaper bag, or other items. If the bin sags too far down when it's filled with packages, it may scrape the ground when you try to go over curbs.
- **Weight considerations.** An aluminum frame, although a little more expensive than steel, will be sturdier and lighter.

and fold. The Peg Perego is jiggly to a fault. And although Apricas are admittedly plush, you can get the same amenities, feature-by-feature, but perhaps with a little more poundage, from a less expensive Combi, or commonplace Graco or Evenflo models. In truth, all strollers are vulnerable to wheel and frame alignment problems and safety issues.

Stroller dangers include metal joints and hardware that can crush small hands and fingers during folding as well as leg holes and gaps that can cause strangulation if a baby is left alone to nap but isn't belted. Sometimes, stroller latches aren't strong enough to prevent the frame from accidentally folding while in use, tossing the baby out, or capturing and injuring his hands on the sides of the frame during the collapse.

What Size Do You Need?

The weight and size of your stroller are important to consider. You'll come to hate the huge, bulky model that eats up your trunk space, leaving no room for suitcases or groceries.

You'll also despise a giant model that weighs so much you feel like you're breaking your back every time you have to fold it and lift it in and out of the back of your car—an act you'll repeat about a thousand times before your baby can walk.

Super-lightweight models are great for negotiating tight store aisles, but their tiny wheels don't work well for leisurely walking on uneven sidewalks. Your baby will get jolted with every seam in the pavement and practically vault out the front when you try to roll down over curbs.

Some parents ultimately settle for two strollers: a compact, easy-to-maneuver version for shopping, and a larger, sturdier model for taking baby on afternoon walks. Postpone buying a jogging stroller until your baby is mature enough to have good head and body support (about 6 months of age). By that time, you'll know whether you have the time and energy to resume your pre-pregnancy exercise program.

Purchase a competitively priced, sturdy, midweight (10 to 17 pounds) stroller from a mainstream manufacturer. Look for an aluminum frame and a model that isn't burdened with a lot of accessories. Later, consider adding a less-expensive, lightweight umbrella-style stroller (read: throwaway) with good brakes and at least one reclining position for running quick errands and negotiating airports. (Be sure to pack the stroller in a box for flying, since the frame is likely to get bent if you check it like baggage.)

Optional Stroller Items

Here's our list of handy but costly stroller add-ons:

- **Full recline.** A seat that fully reclines is available only on huge carriage/stroller combinations. Your baby can sleep just fine in a semi-reclined position.
- **Car seat support.** Should you buy a heavier-than-normal stroller just so you can tote baby around in an infant car seat? Only if the supporting stroller is lightweight.
- **Reversible handlebars.** Some strollers offer a frame that allows the handlebar to reverse from back to front of the seat so baby can face toward you or outward. Others have seats that lift off the frame to reverse, and companies are experimenting with stroller seats that can be shifted to allow facing either direction. Most of these features add extra pounds, and, after the first few months, most babies prefer facing the world, rather than their parents.
- **Front play tray or bar.** Many strollers come with trays or padded bars fastened onto the front of the stroller. Some come with attached toys. Although babies like to grip onto these front pieces, mostly they get in the way when it comes to strapping baby in and taking him out. If you buy a stroller with a tray or front bar, make sure it can be removed so your independent toddler can get in and out by himself.
- **Cup holders.** Some strollers come equipped with parent and baby cup holders. This may not be a necessity for your baby.
- **Giant wheels.** Huge sport wheels are great for going over

rough terrain, but they add extra weight to the stroller and eat up valuable trunk space when the stroller is folded. If you plan to do a lot of country walking, buy a model with medium-size wheels. If you're a city dweller, go for the most compact and lightweight model you can find in the mid-price range.

• **Snap-on boot.** The most expensive strollers offer a snap-on boot for covering baby's legs during cold weather. The hitch is that you're likely to pay fifty dollars or more for the luxury of it. Consider using a blanket, or buying a well-padded baby sack.

TOYS AND PLAY EQUIPMENT

Do babies really need toys? Parents, grandparents, and other gift givers seem to think so. They spend millions of dollars every year to provide their babies with the latest fads in Toyland. In truth, parents are baby's most cherished toys. That said, babies like to slowly track colorful rattles and toys. They like to grasp onto rattles and teethers. They're drawn to sharp contrasts, bright patterns, and bold colors. The best toys are those that respond to some action taken by a baby.

Mobiles

A mobile suspends and rotates toys to music over a baby's head as she lies in the crib. It fastens onto the crib's side bar with a clamp and has a long arm that reaches out into the center of the crib where small stuffed toys or painted images slowly rotate above the baby's head. The best mobiles use very bright, intriguing toys that are faced downward toward the baby.

A mobile should only be used during the first 5 months of a baby's life or until a baby begins to roll over or tries to sit up. Then, it should be removed from the crib and put away, since a mobile's toys and strings aren't considered safe playthings after that.

Simple mobiles use wind-up music boxes with a small rotator bar to provide both the sounds and the motions. The most sophisticated versions are battery operated; present a huge array of motions and graphics; play classical music, lullabies, or children singing; and may even offer a remote-control option so you can start it going without baby even knowing you're there.

Pros: Mobiles play pleasant music and offer clever, rotating toys for babies who are too young to sit up.

Cons: Most babies don't spend much time on their backs staring up at mobiles. When they're awake, they want to be held, diapered, and fed. Mobiles are dangerous for babies who can sit up and pull them over, so they're only useful for a few months, and they may get in the way of lifting your baby out of the crib.

Rattles and Teethers

These are the basic items that most babies will play with once they get a little eye-hand coordination, but they really aren't all that interesting to babies until about 5 months of age, although a newborn will track a brightly colored rattle with his eyes if you move it slowly enough. Shop for mainstream brands from known and trusted toy manufacturers, and avoid inexpensive imports found in drugstores or airports that are flimsy and could easily break. The best rattles make a lot of noise for not a lot of work and are the right scale for a baby's small fists.

Teethers resemble small necklaces or cushioned bracelets that a tot holds in his hand to gnaw on when he gets to the drooling stage. Again, buy from a reputable toy manufacturer, and be careful that there are no small parts that could come loose and be swallowed by the baby.

Pros: Babies are intrigued by the sound and motion of rattles. Once they gain some hand skill, they can hold onto it themselves.

Cons: Babies like to throw rattles on the floor from high chairs and changing tables. Sometimes their bulbs come loose, or they break, exposing sharp shards of plastic and small objects that can be swallowed.

TIP

If an item can pass through the center of a toilet paper roll, it's too small and your baby might choke on it.

Soft Toys

Your baby is likely to gather a huge menagerie of stuffed toys from well-meaning gift givers. Be cautious about inexpensive stuffed

---

Safety Warning: Toy Boxes

Don't be tempted to use a wooden box with a hinged lid for storing your baby's toys. There have been numerous baby deaths attributed to toy box lids. The baby lifts the lid, peers down into the box, and the lid slams shut on his neck, entrapping him and leading to suffocation. The best way to store toys is to display them on a low shelf that's been bolted to the wall with an L-shaped bracket so it can't be pulled over by the baby. Rather than put everything out, store toys on closet shelves in boxes so they're out of sight, and then rotate your display from time to time to keep your baby intrigued.

---

toys like the type you win at the fair. They may have loose eyes or hair that could choke a baby.

Large stuffed animals should be kept out of a baby's crib because they pose a suffocation hazard, and toddlers will use them as props for climbing out. Probably the best solution is to use your baby's animal menagerie as part of your nursery décor. Sit them on a colorful shelf fastened far away from baby's reach, or suspend them in a mesh hammock, also well out of reach.

Another genre of soft toys is excellent for baby play. They're the worms, flower faces, and baby-size fabric balls that offer a variety of textures, colors, and crinkling sounds to intrigue small explorers. The best versions offer bright colors, whimsical patterns, and a variety of unexpected sounds or textures.

Pros: They're cute and appealing just like babies are.

Cons: They're not safe in baby cribs because they can lead to suffocation. Sometimes babies can pull off their ribbons, eyes, or fur, and ingest them.

Electronic Toys

Increasingly, baby toys are being outfitted with small batteries, sound chips, and flashing lights. Although they are initially fascinating to a baby, most tots enjoy toys that respond to their squeezing or gnawing, rather than those that simply put on a show. (And don't forget the joy of wooden spoons, plastic cups and containers, and pots and pans as freebies that are perhaps more fun because they are things you use, too.)

Pros: They offer momentarily exciting stimulation, sometimes fascinating and unexpected to babies.

Con: Some babies are annoyed or frightened by unexpected sounds and lights. These toys eat up batteries too.

Play Gyms

These are small play areas designed especially for babies lying on their backs. Arches hold suspended toys, mirrors, and other playthings that babies can bat with their hands and feet. Most gyms fold down compactly into a carrier when you're on the go. Specialized foot toys encourage leg movements, such as presser bars that make noise when a baby's foot taps on

them and booties with noisemakers imbedded inside that sound with every kick.

Pros: Babies seem to enjoy the sense of mastery they get from making sounds and motions happen, and it's silly and fun to watch them.

Cons: They're sometimes quite pricey, and babies are only interested in them for a short time before they begin to roll over, sit up, and crawl.

WALKERS AND EXERCISERS

Walkers and exercisers are designed to entertain babies who can sit up on their own (around 6 months of age), but who can't walk yet (1½ years of age). Both walkers and exercisers are made from molded plastic frames and feature a seat suspended in the center. Some walkers have adjustable, X-shaped metal joints on the side. The difference between walkers and exercisers is that walkers have wheels on the bottom that let a baby propel himself around by pushing on the floor with his toes.

Exercisers have a solid base for a baby's feet and are designed to stay in one place, but offer a baby a jiggling or rocking motion when he moves with his legs and body.

Most walkers and exercisers have toys installed on the tray that can help to keep baby entertained. And some models have battery-operated noisemakers and electronic sound and light enhancements.

A safety certification program from the Juvenile Products Manufacturers Association (JPMA)

Exercisers

- **Adjustable seat height.** Offers at least three seat heights so the walker can grow with your baby.
- **Comfy seat padding.** Thick padding, good head support, and smooth seams around the leg holes will keep baby comfortable.
- **Smooth seat rotation.** The seat should rotate effortlessly using hidden ball bearings.
- **Toy joys.** The toys should be short enough so they won't block your baby's view, be the right scale for small toddler hands, and offer numerous actions and sounds to keep a baby interested.
- **Springy motions.** Look for spring action that will reward your baby's movements.
- **Lockable rocking.** There should be small flip-down latches that let you lock the rocking so you can feed baby and stop him from propelling the exerciser across slick floors.

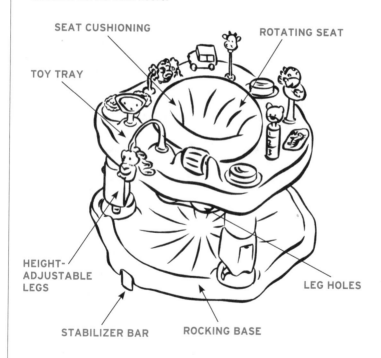

SEAT CUSHIONING

ROTATING SEAT

TOY TRAY

HEIGHT-ADJUSTABLE LEGS

LEG HOLES

STABILIZER BAR

ROCKING BASE

and the American Society of Testing and Materials (ASTM) now provides an extra margin of walker safety for those units with the certified sticker.

Walkers that get certified must either have a wide-enough base that they won't fit through doorways or have a stopper foot or other device underneath the walker frame to help halt the walker before it topples down stairs.

So, it's important to buy a new JPMA-certified walker rather than relying on an older, less safe walker for keeping your baby safe—especially if you've got stairs in your house. But, keep in mind that walkers with stoppers and skid-resistant bands on the bottom that are supposed to prevent them from rolling down stairs can go down anyway if your child rolls sideways or backward into the stairwell.

Install hardware-mounted gates at the tops of all stairway openings, including the basement, and keep them locked. Or better yet, don't buy a walker at all. Stationary exercisers, sometimes called Exersaucers after Evenflo's original models, are a much safer alternative than a walker. They stay in one place, but offer jiggling and rocking actions. They've got lots of play toys all around their trays that a baby can manipulate as he rotates his seat around using his hands and feet.

Pros: Babies like sitting in them temporarily. The toys are in easy reach of small arms.

Cons: Babies sometimes slip through the leg holes or climb out. In addition, toys can be pulled off, exposing sharp edges, and the seats might give way.

The Big Picture

For most mothers, there's a gap between the birth of their baby and the time when the deeper, more meaningful rewards of parenthood start to set in.

Unless you've had a baby before, it's hard to imagine what life might be like with a baby. Even if you are an experienced parent who has been through pregnancy, birth, and baby care before, no two babies are ever alike. That means having to adapt to a whole new set of baby rules each time.

We promise that at some point, your body won't hurt any more, you'll get 8 hours of sleep—give or take a few—and your baby will gradually transform from being a need machine into a human being you can relate to, and not just any human being, but the most interesting, entertaining person you can ever hope to know.

It will take about 2 years before your child can begin to communicate with you in words you can understand and about that amount of time to get out of changing poopy diapers. And those 2 years can seem like a long time when taken day by day. Rest assured, though, that in time, and after you've recovered from pregnancy and the demands of a newborn, you'll start to discover the joy, rewards, and fulfillment of parenting. You can expect worthwhile, intensely valuable moments will come, one small moment at a time.

Someday, having a child in your life will feel as natural to you as having fingers. Life before baby will be as hard to recall as trying to picture your parents' lives before you were born. You won't wish your old life back for anything in the world, at least most of the time.

Bonding is a lifelong experience, not made in a single day, month, or year. It doesn't matter if you feel how you're "supposed" to feel, or if you do what you're "supposed" to do in the way experts say you should. What truly matters is that you and your baby not only survive, but thrive.

The joys will outweigh the pain, and all of the attention and affection you've poured into your baby will reap positive results. Even though pregnancy has caused your body to undergo subtle (and not so subtle) changes, your mind and heart will be stronger for the experience.

You may hear people say that "there's no such thing as a perfect mother." But that's not true. You are your baby's perfect mother. Whatever your choices are, you are your baby's only, best mother, and no one can do your job better. Your love for your baby may take the form of tenderness or affection so huge that you fear it may overwhelm you, or sometimes your love may feel more like duty.

It doesn't matter if you're single or married, sad or serene. Your love for your child will not be any less if you go back to work the day after delivery or stay at home until he or she leaves the nest.

What does matter is that you do your best to do what's right for your child. Your love is perfect and whole because you are your baby's only mother, the best and only mother your baby will ever have.

Resources

Trying to find pregnancy information on the Internet can be hit or miss—it's not always easy to tell quality information from stuff that's poorly sourced, commercial, or flat-out untrue. Also, a lot of pregnancy and parenting sites sell parents' names, addresses, and due date information to mailing-list brokers who sell them to marketers, eager to heap you with junk mail selling diapers, formula, baby life insurance policies, cord-blood banking services, and so on. Occasionally, though, you may get mailed stuff you actually want, like a free baby magazine subscription, coupons, or product samples.

More reliable are sites from national not-for-profit organizations. The March of Dimes, the American Academy of Pediatrics, La Leche League, and Childbirth Connection are valuable sites to bookmark. They all carry well-researched articles of interest to parents on their Web sites. Google, the *New York Times*, and other major newspapers also offer news posting services that allow you to have topics of interest e-mailed periodically to you.

HOW TO SEARCH FOR MEDICAL INFORMATION

Finding quality medical research about pregnancy, birth, and babies online can be tough—the language of research studies can be dense and technical, and it can be hard to tell which studies are weak, or even misleading. It's great that we have all of this information about safety at our fingertips now, but it also presents the problem of trying to figure out just how much to worry about what.

Still, if you want to know the answer to a specific medical question, medical literature is the place to go. PubMed is the most popular Web site for searching abstracts of medical literature. Its main address is *www.ncbi.nlm .nih.gov/PubMed*. Using PubMed is free (or rather, already paid for by your tax dollars). You can search for specific terms, such as "twins," "labor," "pregnancy," or "breastfeeding," or you can conduct a more formal search based on key terms used by the site, which is called a MeSH (medical subject heading) search.

When you uncover an abstract of an article that appears to address your concerns, you'll find a "Related Articles" option to the right of the article title in PubMed that will uncover even more studies.

DON'T FORGET BOOKS AND MAGAZINES!

We're not just saying that because we wrote this one. A well-researched book on pregnancy and childbirth can help you synthesize information and bring everything into perspective the way a collection of Web articles can't. But like Web sites, books can also have biased, incorrect, or outdated information: beware of books from fly-by-night publishers that are biased toward a particular point of view.

National magazines, such as *FitPregnancy*, are also valuable resources. Unlike books or Web sites, major market magazines employ fact-checkers who make sure that everything you read is timely and accurate (or at least they still do as of 2012). You can also get news by following "pregnancy" as a keyword on your Google news page or with national newspapers, but again, be wary of news stories about small, single studies (though do pay attention to recommendations from major organizations like the American Association of Pediatrics).

Cochrane Reviews (*www2 .cochrane.org/reviews*) from the UK are thought to offer the "gold standard" of evidence in medicine, including obstetrics. Most reviews combine the findings of numerous, well-conducted studies based on thousands of patients in order to reach conclusions about the best medical practices on any given topic. You can search abstracts on cesarean sections, induction, amniocentesis, and many other procedures used during pregnancy.

HELPFUL WEB SITES FOR EXPECTANT AND NEW PARENTS

Note that Web sites come and go. These listings and reviews were up-to-date at the time this manuscript was completed (2012), but changes are to be expected. If we've missed any of your favorite sites, or you're with an organization and would like to have your address listed here, please write us in care of our publisher or on our Great Expectations Pregnancy Facebook page and we will try to include your address in our next edition.

Alternative Pain Relief Options for Birth

NAME	DESCRIPTION	WEB ADDRESS
Acupuncture .com, home of traditional Chinese medicine	All about the use of Chinese herbs and the use of acupuncture for relief of discomforts during pregnancy and labor.	www.acupuncture.com

| HypnoBirthing | Find doulas that practice and the Mongan Method, which aims to teach "women and their birthing companions to trust birth and release all fear and limiting thoughts." | www.hypnobirthing.com |
| Pain Relief Options During Childbirth | Information and animations on pain-relief options for birth from anesthesiologist and Harvard medical school professor Bhavani-Shankar Kodali. | www.painfreebirthing.com |

Baby Loss, Stillbirth, and Miscarriage

NAME	DESCRIPTION	WEB ADDRESS
AGAST	An all-volunteer organization dedicated to helping grandparents through the trauma, stress and grief after the loss of a grandchild.	www.agast.org
Center for Loss in Multiple Birth (CLIMB)	An international site of resources for people who have experienced the death of one or more, both, or all of their twins or higher multiples at any time from conception (including selective reduction) through birth, infancy, and childhood.	www.climb-support.org
Helping After Neonatal Death (HAND)	A resource network of parents, professionals, and supportive volunteers that offers information online and a variety of services throughout Northern California and the Central Valley.	www.handonline.org

The Hygeia Foundation, Inc., and Institute for Perinatal Loss and Bereavement	Online journal for pregnancy and neonatal loss support and information.	www.hygeia.org
MISS Foundation	A volunteer-based nonprofit organization committed to providing crisis support and long term aid to families after the death of a child from any cause. Site has forums and support for children, parents and grandparents.	www.missfoundation.org
The National Stillbirth Society	A nonprofit with the goal is to "educate, agitate and legislate" for greater stillbirth awareness, funding, and the passage of legislation nationwide to recognize births by requiring states issue a "Certificate of Birth Resulting in Stillbirth."	www.stillnomore.org
A Place to Remember	Books, resources, and bulletin boards for parents and grandparents facing stillbirth or neonatal death.	www.aplacetoremember.com
Share Pregnancy and Infant Loss Support Inc.	A nonprofit to support individuals touched by pregnancy loss, via stillbirth or in the first few months of life. Offers resources and online support groups and mails out free informational packets.	www.nationalshare.org

Baby Products and Product Safety

NAME	DESCRIPTION	WEB ADDRESS
The Car Seat Lady	Supplies detailed information on seat installation and safety.	www.carseatdata.org
Consumer Reports	Provides free articles on baby products and subscription-only access to baby product ratings.	www.consumerreports.org
Diapers.com	Disposable diaper delivery as well as maternity clothes and baby products.	www.diapers.com
Dr. Toy	The site for Dr. Stevanne Auerbach, a child development expert who oversees an annual national rating for the best toys for babies and children.	www.drtoy.com
MyRegistry	Allows users to build a registry with items from any Web site on the Internet.	www.myregistry.com
One Step Ahead	A catalog of carefully chosen baby products with an emphasis on uniqueness and quality.	www.onestepahead.com
Rattle & Roll Baby Boutique	An online source for "simply irresistible kids' stuff," including furniture, prints and murals, and personalized items.	www.rattleroll.com
SafetyBeltSafe USA	A great resource for studying car seat safety: take a look at their technical section.	www.carseat.org
Seat Check	A free children's car seat inspection locator service.	www.seatcheck.org
Toy Industry Association	The professional organization of toy manufacturers America (TIA) Offers toy safety tips.	www.toy-tia.org

Urban Baby Runway	A single-mom-owned boutique specializing in carefully chosen edgy baby fashions from other small businesses.	www.urbanbabyrunway.com

Birth Defects

NAME	DESCRIPTION	WEB ADDRESS
March of Dimes	A nonprofit organization with information about birth defects, testing, suggestions for having a healthy pregnancy, newborn feeding tips, and vaccinations. Accepts questions by e-mail.	www.modimes.org
National Society of Genetic Counselors	The Web site of genetic counselors' professional organization lets you search for a counselor by area of expertise and by zip code.	www.nsgc.org

Birth Information

NAME	DESCRIPTION	WEB ADDRESS
American Association of Birth Centers (AABC)	A nonprofit organization founded by Childbirth Connection that establishes standards of care and promotes best practices for birth centers. Site visitors can also locate birth centers in a particular state.	www.birthcenters.org
The American Congress of Obstetricians and Gynecologists (ACOG)	Their patient page has downloadable pamphlets on a variety of topics.	www.acog.org
Association of Women's Health, Obstetric and Neonatal Nurses (AWHONN)	An organization of nurses that works to promote the health of mothers and newborns. The AWHONN Web site has position papers on best practices; health4mom.org is an informational site for parents-to-be and new mothers.	www.awhonn.org www.health4mom.org

Birth Balance	Information, birth stories, and resources for parents and labor assistants about water birth.	www.birthbalance.com
Birthing from Within	Resources, products, and events for expectant parents, families, and birth companions.	www.birthingfromwithin.com
Born Free!	Born Free! Site for Laura Shanley, an advocate for the unassisted childbirth movement. Site includes articles on natural birth and birth stories.	www.unassistedchildbirth.com
The Bradley Method	Find Bradley Method childbirth classes and student resources.	www.bradleybirth.com
Brigham and Women's Hospital	The nation's oldest women's hospital in Boston has helpful medical information on labor, analgesia, and c-sections.	www.brighamandwomens.com
Centering Healthcare Institute	An organization that supports prenatal care groups with journaling, group discussions, and educational and self-care activities in conjunction with prenatal medical care.	www.centeringhealthcare.org
Childbirth.org	Pregnancy information, including week-by-week calendar, an interactive birth plan and testing information, and forums hosted by about.com.	www.childbirth.org
Childbirth Connection	Formerly known as the Maternity Center Association, Childbirth Connection is a nonprofit that uses research, education, and advocacy to improve maternity care for women and their families.	www.childbirthconnection.org
Childbirth Solutions	Advice and articles on birth options.	www.childbirthsolutions.org

Doulas of North America	The oldest and largest doula organization. Sets standards of practice and certifies birth doulas. The site features a directory of birth and postpartum doulas.	www.dona.org
Gentle Birth	Lots of articles on birthing, comfort measures, fathers' roles. Offers a helpful online brochure, "Planning Your Childbirth," describing commonly used analgesics and anesthetics.	www.gentlebirth.org
Home First	The Web site of a large home-birthing practice in Chicago that also offers several home birthing stories from parents and reviewed links to other sites of interest to families electing home birth.	www.homefirst.com
International Birth & Wellness Project	Group that offers a Childbirth Educator Training and Certification Program. The site lets visitors locate birth doulas and childbirth educators.	www.alace.org
International Cesarean Awareness Network	A nonprofit that works to prevent unnecessary cesareans through education, provides support for cesarean recovery, and promotes vaginal birth after cesarean (VBAC). Site has information on c-sections and recovery, and connections to local support groups.	www.ican-online.org

Lamaze International	A nonprofit organization that promotes childbirth education. Online you can find childbirth classes, watch birth videos and ask questions of birth expert Henci Goer.	www.lamaze.org
Leapfrog Group	A nonprofit organization that compares hospitals on national standards of safety and quality; consumers can compare hospital safety based on overall patient safety or the safety of certain procedures, including normal and high-risk deliveries.	www.leapfroggroup.org
Midwives Alliance of North America	A professional organization for midwives; parents can locate a midwife, find an accredited birth center and learn about the laws regarding direct-entry midwives and homebirths in their state.	www.mana.org www.mothersnaturally.org
Natural Childbirth	An Internet resource for people interested in natural childbirth education and midwifery	www.naturalchildbirth.org
Science & Sensibility	A blog on pregnancy and postpartum research from Lamaze International.	www.scienceandsensibility.org
Society for Obstetric Anesthesia and Perinatology	Organization's site has information on types of pain relief for labor.	www.soap.org
Waterbirth International	Provides water birth education, training, programs, consultations, and referrals for parents and practitioners; lets you compare makes and models of inflatable homebirth pools and order pools and accessories.	www.waterbirth.org

Breastfeeding

NAME	DESCRIPTION	WEB ADDRESS
International Lactation Consultant Association	The professional organization of lactation consultants; the site offers referrals to consultants and information on evidence-based breastfeeding practices.	www.ilca.org
Kelly Mom	Web site from an international board-certified lactation consultant that provides evidence-based information on breastfeeding, sleep, and parenting.	www.kellymom.com
La Leche League	An international organization providing education, information, support, and encouragement to women who breastfeed or are planning to. Holds monthly living-room meetings in many communities. Provides a hotline to answer questions and a Web site with publications and FAQs.	www.lalecheleague.org
Nursing Mothers Counsel	A California-based non-affiliated, nonprofit organization with the goal of helping mothers and their babies enjoy a relaxed and happy feeding relationship. Offers 24-hour help lines staffed by volunteers.	www.nursingmothers.org

Circumcision

NAME	DESCRIPTION	WEB ADDRESS
Circumcision Information and Resource Page	Internet resource with information about all aspects of circumcision.	www.cirp.org
National Organization of Circumcision Information Resource Centers (NOCIRC)	An educational nonprofit organization "committed to securing the birthright of male, female, and intersex children and babies to keep their sex organs intact."	www.nocirc.org

Child Care

NAME	DESCRIPTION	WEB ADDRESS
ChildCareAware	A hub of information for parents and child care providers, with a toll-free hotline to help you find care in your area.	www.childcareaware.org
National Network for Child Care	A site from the U.S. Department of Agriculture that lets you search child care resources by state.	www.nncc.org
National Resource Center for Health and Safety in Child Care and Early Education	A center funded by the Maternal and Child Health Bureau, U.S. Department of Health and Human Services, Health Resources and Services Administration to promote health and safety in out-of-home child care settings. Site has resources including day care licensing requirements, checklists for determining quality care, and tips on dental care and preventing obesity.	www.nrckids.org

Child Health

NAME	DESCRIPTION	WEB ADDRESS
American Academy of Pediatrics	A variety of information on child health, including circumcision, immunizations, and car seats.	www.aap.org
Kids Health	Created by the medical experts at the Alfred I. Du Pont Hospital for Children and the Nemours Foundation, with in-depth information on pregnancy and newborns.	www.kidshealth.org
Mayo Clinic	Public information on pregnancy, childbirth, and baby care.	www.mayohealth.org

Safe Kids USA	A nationwide network of organizations working to prevent unintentional childhood injury, the leading cause of death and disability for children ages 1 to 14. Information on childproofing, car seats, and other injury prevention; provides child safety seats, helmets, and smoke alarms to families who need them.	www.safekids.org
Zero to Three	A national nonprofit organization that informs, trains, and supports professionals, policymakers, and parents in their efforts to improve the lives of infants and toddlers. Site has information on development, mental health, nutrition, sleep, and play.	www.zerotothree.org

Fatherhood

NAME	DESCRIPTION	WEB ADDRESS
At-Home Dad	News, statistics, and links to stay-at-home dads' blogs	www.angelfire.com/zine2/ athomedad/index.blog
The National Center for Fathering	A nonprofit educational organization "whose mission is to champion the role of responsible fatherhood by inspiring and equipping men to be more engaged in the lives of children." Site includes articles and information on topics such as "how to bond with baby."	www.fathers.com

Maternity and Breastfeeding Wear

NAME	DESCRIPTION	WEB ADDRESS
Expressiva Nursingwear	Nursing tops, dresses, bras, swimsuits, and nightgowns. Also carries plus sizes.	www.expressiva.com
Gap Maternity	The popular retailer also sells maternity clothes and nursing wear online and in certain retail locations.	www.gap.com/maternity
Hot Mama Ink	Maternity wear with tattoo-inspired artwork.	www.hotmamaink.com
Motherhood Maternity	Maternity wear and pregnancy accessories, including work clothes, formal wear, outerwear, swimsuits, and nursing clothes.	www.motherhood.com
Motherwear	Maternity clothes, nursing tops, bras, dresses, swimsuits, and plus sizes.	www.motherwear.com

Parenting Styles and Situations

NAME	DESCRIPTION	WEB ADDRESS
John Rosemond's Traditional Parenting	Site of a psychologist, parenting columnist, author, and speaker who advocates biblically based parenting advice	www.rosemond.com
JustMommies	Pregnancy and parenting news, information, and forums	www.justmommies.com
Looking Glass	A site that offers clinical and supportive services, training, and research for families in which a child, parent, or grandparent has a disability or medical issue.	www.lookingglass.org
NICU Parent Support Site	A site with a blog, newsletter, and free e-book download for parents of babies in a NICU.	http://www .nicuparentsupport.org/
Parents with Disabilities Online	Links to organizations, products, periodicals, personal stories, and other resources for disabled parents.	www.disabledparents.net

| Peaceful Parenting | A site supporting **attachment** parenting, breastfeeding, and genital integrity. | www.drmomma.org |

Pregnancy, Miscellaneous

NAME	DESCRIPTION	WEB ADDRESS
Baby Shower.com	Site with lots of ideas for baby shower games, cakes, party themes, invitations, baby shower favors, and gifts.	www.baby-shower.com
BabyZone	Information and message boards for parents covering preconception to toddlerhood.	www.babyzone.com
Childbirth Connection	A national not-for-profit organization dedicated to improving the quality of maternity care.	www.childbirthconnection.org
HealthGrades	An independent ratings organization that rates doctors and hospitals.	www.healthgrades.com
InfantRisk	A site from the Infant Risk Center at Texas Tech University Health Sciences Center, the definitive source for information on the safety of medications during pregnancy and lactation. The center also sponsors help lines for depression, nausea and vomiting, and substance abuse.	www.infantrisk.com
iVillage	News, information, message boards, and pregnancy expecting clubs.	www.ivillage.com www.forums.ivillage.com
MotherRisk	Sponsored by the Canadian Health Network, offers information on how to protect yourself and your baby from health risks, including research updates and discussions of occupational hazards, smoking, and substance abuse.	www.motherisk.org

Motherstuff	Links to pregnancy and birth information, including sample birth plans, methods, complications, home births, and more.	www.motherstuff.com
The Organization of Teratology Information Specialists (OTIS)	Provides evidence-based clinical information to patients and healthcare professionals about exposures during pregnancy and lactation. Posts fact sheets on a number of different hazards and links to medical providers who provide free counseling for prospective parents and medical providers.	www.otispregnancy.org
Prenatal Music	Site by a doula and music therapist with information on music therapy for pregnancy and the birthing experience.	www.prenatalmusic.com
Transition to Parenthood	Research-based information on pregnancy, birth, newborn care, and breastfeeding for parents and birth professionals.	www.transitiontoparenthood.com

Pregnancy, Special Circumstances

NAME	DESCRIPTION	WEB ADDRESS
Plus-Size Pregnancy	A Web site with information and support for "women of size."	www.plus-size-pregnancy.org

Pregnancy Dictionary

A

ABORTIFACIENT
A drug or device that ends a pregnancy within the first several weeks after conception.

ABORTION
Giving birth to an embryo or fetus in the first 20 weeks of pregnancy. Abortion may be spontaneous, called a miscarriage, or induced, when a pregnancy is terminated on purpose. After 20 weeks of pregnancy, it is called a live birth or a stillbirth. Spontaneous abortion in the first half of pregnancy is synonymous with miscarriage.

ABRUPTION (Placental Abruption, Abruptio Placentae)
Any sudden breaking away. During pregnancy, the term is usually used to refer to the premature separation of the placenta from the uterus prior to the delivery of the baby. When this happens, a woman's body may deliver the baby early. Bleeding is the number one symptom, and there can also be severe, premature contractions.

ACNM (The American College of Nurse-Midwives)
The American professional organization of midwives (midwifery) that maintains the certification process for midwives.

ACOG (The American College of Obstetricians and Gynecologists)
The professional organization of obstetricians and gynecologists who specialize in the care of women's reproductive needs. (See Resources on page 343.)

ACTIVE LABOR (See DILATION and EFFACEMENT)
The phase of labor when the cervix (mouth of the uterus) is in the process of expanding and thinning—usually between 4 and 10 centimeters (sometimes expressed as fingers). Contractions are usually 2 to 5 minutes apart. Typically, the cervix dilates about 1 centimeter (one finger), or more, per hour.

ACTIVE MANAGEMENT OF LABOR
An approach to managing the labors of a first-time pregnant mother that calls for continuous nursing support; continuous monitoring (electronic fetal monitoring), routinely breaking the mother's waters upon admission to the hospital (amniotomy) when the mouth of the uterus (cervix) is at least 3 centimeters dilated, and artificially speeding up labor using drugs to make contractions stronger when labor fails to progress within set time limits.

ACUPUNCTURE
The ancient Chinese medical practice of inserting and pulsating thin needles in selected locations on the body that is thought to help balance the body's energy flows and soothe pain. It can be used to help a mother through labor.

AFEBRILE
Not having a fever. A sign that you, or your baby, are not suspected of having an infection.

AFTERBIRTH
The placenta and membranes expelled by the uterus after the baby is born. The "birth" of the placenta is called the third stage of labor. (The first stage is when contractions position the baby to move down into the birth canal for delivery; the second stage is the pushing stage after complete dilation of the cervix that results in the baby being born; the fourth stage is the recovery after giving birth.)

AFTERPAINS (See INVOLUTION)
Cramping caused by the contraction of the uterus while it is returning to normal size.

AIDS (Acquired Immunodeficiency Syndrome) (See HIV)
A virus transmitted from one person to another through the exchange of bodily fluids—primarily through blood, blood products, semen, and vaginal fluid. In women, AIDS is often caught through intravenous drug use or sexual exposure through an infected partner. There is no evidence that pregnancy accelerates AIDS, but women in advanced stages of AIDS may be more likely to give birth prematurely or to have a low-birthweight baby or a baby that dies before or after birth. Most babies born to mothers with AIDS do not become infected, but some do. Mothers who take medicines to fight the disease rarely transmit it to their babies.

ALBUMINURIA
Excess protein detected from testing urine (urinalysis).

Sometimes, but not always, it can be one of the symptoms of preeclampsia. It also shows up temporarily as a side effect of vigorous exercise.

ALPHA-FETOPROTEIN TEST (AFP, a-Fetoprotein test, triple test, triple screen, MSAFP-plus, AFP-plus)
A blood test administered between the fifteenth and twentieth week of pregnancy to screen mothers for increased risk of having a baby with Down syndrome, neural tube defects (NTD), and abdominal wall defects. The test registers levels of alpha feto protein (AFP), human chorionic gonadotropin (hCG), and estriol (uE3). Some tests also register the presence of inhibin, a chemical produced by the ovaries and placenta. A low AFP reading is associated with Down syndrome. The test is used to decide whether a mother should undergo a more invasive test, such as amniocentesis. Most women who test positive for these disorders give birth to a baby without the disorder.

ALVEOLI
Grape-like clusters of glandular tissue in a woman's breast where milk is made. The cells of the alveoli secrete the milk that is then expelled into the tiny tubes (ductules) that deliver the milk to the nipple for the baby.

AMA
Stands for the American Medical Association, the largest professional organization for physicians in the United States. (Also sometimes used by providers for advanced maternal age, as a mother's age at 35 or older at the expected time of delivery.)

AMBULATION (See THROMBOPHLEBITIS)
Getting up and walking after surgery or giving birth. Nurses are likely to urge mothers to get out of bed and walk as soon as possible in order to help prevent blood clots from forming.

AMENORRHEA
Absence of menstruation.

AMNIOCENTESIS
The testing of the fluid inside the amniotic sac that surrounds the baby. A long, thin needle is used to obtain the fluid, and the results help to detect fetal abnormalities by examining the baby's skin cells sloughed off by the baby that float in the "waters."

AMNIOINFUSION
Injection of solutions into the amniotic fluid in an attempt to cushion the umbilical cord and prevent it from being squeezed during labor.

AMNION (amniotic sac, bag of waters) (See AMNIOTIC FLUID)
One of the membranes that make up the sac, which contains the amniotic fluid in which the baby floats during pregnancy.

AMNIONITIS (CHORIOAMNIONITIS)
An infection of the amniotic sac and amniotic fluid that sometimes happens, usually after the membranes (bag of waters) break.

AMNIOTIC FLUID
A clear, slightly salty fluid with flecks of white skin cells floating in it that fills the sac that surrounds a baby during pregnancy. It protects the baby from being injured from

outside, and maintains an even temperature. Approximately one-third of the fluid is replaced every hour. At term, it is primarily composed of the baby's urine and fluid made in the baby's lungs.

AMNIOTIC FLUID EMBOLISM
An extremely rare event, when amniotic fluid escapes into the wall of the uterus or where the placenta is implanted and into the mother's bloodstream usually during labor, causing the mother to go into shock.

AMNIOTIC SAC (See AMNION)

AMNIOTOMY
The intentional rupture of the amniotic sac using an instrument that resembles a long crochet hook. Doing so may speed up labor but may increase the chance of amnionitis. Having an amniotomy commits a mother to giving birth.

ANALGESIA
A medical intervention that reduces the sensation of pain.

ANALGESIC
A drug that helps to relieve or reduce the sensation of pain.

ANEMBRIOTIC GESTATION (blighted ovum) (See MISCARRIAGE)
An implanted egg that dies during the early months of pregnancy, which leads to miscarriage weeks later.

ANEMIA
Any condition of the blood in which the number or shape of red blood cells is altered. It is discovered by a blood test. When the red blood cell content is low, it is more difficult for the body to supply sufficient oxygen to the tissues of the body. Anemia is

a common condition during pregnancy.

ANENCEPHALY
Defective development of a baby's brain combined with the absence of the bones normally surrounding the brain.

ANESTHESIA
A general term for all techniques used to alleviate pain. During childbirth, you may undergo general anesthesia (being put completely to sleep, such as during an emergency c-section), local anesthesia (you remain conscious, but a small area of your body becomes numb), or analgesia (reduction of your pain that allows you to remain conscious and relaxed with discomfort minimized).

ANESTHETIC
An agent or drug that is able to produce partial or complete loss of feeling (anesthesia).

ANESTHETIC BLOCK
Numbing of a part of the body. In obstetrics, this usually refers to an epidural or spinal anesthetic that is used for cesarean deliveries.

ANOMALY
An abnormality, a deviation from the normal.

ANOXIA
A lack of oxygen.

ANTENATAL (prenatal)
Before birth.

ANTENATAL GLUCOCORTICOID THERAPY
Drugs administered to a mother in danger of giving birth prematurely to prepare her baby's immature lungs for breathing.

ANTEPARTAL
Happening before delivery.

ANTERIOR POSITION (anterior presentation) (See POSTERIOR PRESENTATION)
During the descent through the birth canal, the baby's face is turned toward the spine of the mother. This is the most common position for emerging babies.

ANTIBIOTIC
A medication that kills or stops the growth of bacteria.

ANTICIPATORY GRIEF (See GRIEF, STAGES OF)
When a person experiences numbness, shock, and fear that causes them to emotionally pull away from the dying person. Parents may distance themselves from their premature or sick newborn out of fear of impending loss and death. They may, for example, postpone naming their baby while they wait to see if it survives.

ANTICIPATORY GUIDANCE
Guidance given in advance of a difficult event. During pregnancy, it is counseling offered to expectant parents in advance to help them in coping with the needs of their newborn, or for how to cope with a baby diagnosed with a physical disorder.

ANTIPHOSPHOLIPID SYNDROME (APS)
Up to 5 percent of all pregnancy failures are thought to result from this little-known immune disorder that is associated with the formation of blood clots in the body. The body attacks certain fatty molecules (phospholipids) that make up part of a cell membrane, and the result is

inflammation and blood clots. Pregnant women with APS are more likely to develop blood clots and preeclampsia and to have repeated miscarriages. When APS causes blood clots in the placenta, it can result in fetal growth problems, fetal distress, preterm birth, or pregnancy loss. There is no known cure, but low doses of aspirin and daily injections of a blood-thinning drug, heparin, may be recommended.

APA
Refers to antiphospholipid antibodies, the antibodies that cause antiphospholipid syndrome (APS).

APGAR SCORE (APGAR rating)
Ratings taken of a baby's condition at 1 and 5 minutes following birth that assigns 0, 1, or 2 points for each of the following factors: tone, pulse, grimace, color, and respiration. The maximum total score is 10 points, but most babies get around an 8 or 9. An extremely low score indicates a baby that needs immediate medical attention.

APNEA (See POSITIONAL APNEA)
A temporary pause or complete cessation of breathing that frequently occurs in premature and low-birthweight babies.

APNEA MONITOR
A motion detector that sets off an alarm when a baby ceases to breathe for a period of time. Portable monitors are available for home use but are suggested only for premature and low-birthweight babies with an apnea problem.

APPROPRIATE FOR GESTATIONAL AGE (AGA)
When a baby's weight falls within normal range based on the actual age of the baby, rather than the date the baby was born.

AREOLA (plural: AREOLAE)
The dark ring of skin that surrounds the nipple of a breast. To milk the breast correctly, a nursing baby needs to latch onto much of the areola as well as the nipple.

ARRHYTHMIA
Irregular, abnormal, or missed heartbeat.

ARTERY
Blood vessel that carries blood away from the heart.

ARTIFICIAL RUPTURE OF THE MEMBRANES (AROM)
(See RUPTURE OF MEMBRANES and AMNIOTOMY)

ASPHYXIA, PERINATAL
The lack of oxygen in a fetus or baby that can lead to the excess buildup of carbon dioxide waste, which can lead to death if not corrected.

ASPIRATION
Using suction to draw air or a substance in, out, up, or through the breathing passages. During the birth process, a baby may aspirate meconium, which can block and irritate the airways, potentially causing damage to the baby's lungs. As soon as their faces emerge during birth, the mouth and nose are usually aspirated using a bulb-like suction device to help prevent aspiration of meconium-stained fluids. Aspiration also refers to the extremely rare event of a woman aspirating the acidic contents of the stomach while under general anesthesia, which can potentially

harm the lungs. Healthcare providers may administer an antacid to a woman prior to a cesarean delivery to neutralize the acids.

ATONY, UTERINE (ATONIC UTERUS)
When a uterus relaxes and fails to contract during birth, or when it fails to tighten after birth, which potentially leads to excessive bleeding.

ATROPHY
When a part of the body (an arm or leg, cells, organs, or tissues) shrinks and withers from lack of nourishment or use.

ATTACHMENT (bonding, love)
The strong bonds of affection that form between a parent and a baby. Sometimes feelings of attachment are felt immediately; other times, the feeling takes time to develop.

AUGMENTATION OF LABOR
An intervention to make labor contractions stronger after they have already started.

AUSCULTATION
Listening to the sounds made by various organs of the body, including the heart, to determine their condition.

AUTOLOGOUS TRANSFUSION
A transfusion of a person's own blood previously donated by her in anticipation of surgery.

B

BABINSKI REFLEX
An automatic response in newborns that causes a baby to curl his big toe and spread out his other toes when his foot is stroked from the heel upward and across the ball of the foot.

BABY BLUES (postpartum blues) (See POSTPARTUM DEPRESSION)
A feeling of sadness and letdown that affects 40 to 70 percent of all new mothers. It usually starts a few days after birth, and usually goes away within 2 weeks.

BACK LABOR
When most of the pain of labor is felt in a mother's lower back. A baby's facing toward a mother's front instead of toward her back (occiput posterior) may contribute to it as can back problems prior to labor.

BACTERIA
Small microscopic organisms that can cause infection in the body.

BACTERIAL VAGINOSIS (BV)
A common infection of the genital tract that causes vaginal itching and an abnormal fishy-smelling discharge and that may be associated with an increased risk of preterm labor, premature rupture of membranes, preterm birth, and infection of the amniotic sac. (See discussion on page 154.)

BACTERIURIA
The presence of bacteria (germs) in the urine. Usually a sign of infection.

BAGGING
Placing a mask over a newborn's nose and mouth and rhythmically squeezing oxygen from an attached bag to help the baby breathe.

BAG OF WATERS (See AMNION)

BALANCED DIET
Properly nourishing yourself by eating the right amount of nutrients in correct proportions.

BETA HUMAN CHORIONIC GONADOTROPIN (SS-HCG) (See HUMAN CHORIONIC GONADOTROPIN)

BETAMETHASONE
A drug given by injection to the mother that helps develop the baby's lungs. Administered when doctors anticipate that the baby may be born prematurely.

BETA-THALASSEMIA
An anemic condition found mainly in persons from Mediterranean countries such as Greece, Italy, or the Middle East that can be passed along genetically to a baby.

BILILIGHTS
Special fluorescent lights placed above a baby's bed to treat jaundice. Usually, the baby's eyes are covered to protect them from glare.

BILIRUBIN (See JAUNDICE and KERNICTERUS)
A yellowish-red coloring pigment produced by the body as red blood cells break down. An excess of bilirubin in the bloodstream leads to temporary jaundice (yellowing of the skin and whites of the eyes) in a newborn. Excessive levels may harm the developing baby's brain.

BIOFEEDBACK
The use of sensitive, computer-driven instruments to measure and display the patterns of physical processes such as brain activity, blood pressure, muscle tension, heart rate, and other bodily functions. The feedback from the devices is used to enable individuals to master skills in controlling and managing their body's reactions. Once mastery is achieved, the instruments are no longer needed. Biofeedback training is used to give pregnant women skills in coping with the stress and pain of labor.

BIOPHYSICAL PROFILE (BPP)
A test to assess the health of an unborn baby. The profile measures a series of things: breathing rate, movement rate, muscle tone, the baby's heart rate, and the volume of amniotic fluid in the amniotic sac where the baby floats. It combines the use of a non-stress test together with ultrasound. Not enough amniotic fluid in the uterus is called oligohydramnios.

BIOPSY
The removal of a small piece of tissue from the body to examine it more closely with a microscope.

BIRTH ASSISTANT (labor assistant) (See DOULA and MONITRICE)
Someone who is trained in basic childbirth support skills who attends to a birthing mother's health and comfort needs before, during, and after labor.

BIRTH CANAL
The passage the baby goes through from the uterus (womb) until delivery. It includes the vaginal canal and the bones of the pelvis that the baby passes through.

BIRTH CENTER
A medical facility that serves as an alternative to giving birth at home or in a traditional hospital setting. Birth centers can be in houses, in medical

buildings, or in separate rooms inside hospitals. Out-of-hospital birth centers often use midwives. Birth centers try to simulate a home-birth experience while providing additional medical resources.

BIRTH DEFECT

A mental or physical problem in a baby caused by an error in how a part of the baby developed. A birth defect may or may not be inherited (passed through a parent's genes or chromosomes). According to the American College of Obstetricians and Gynecologists, approximately 3 percent of babies born in the United States are born with a major birth defect.

BIRTHING BALL (PT BALL)

A large, sturdy, inflated ball that can be used during labor as a comfort measure. A mother can bounce, rock, sit, or lie on top of it.

BIRTHING ROOM (See BIRTH CENTER)

Rather than moving a mother into a delivery room that resembles an operating theater when birth nears, many hospitals now offer special, homelike rooms where labor and delivery can take place.

BIRTH PLAN (birth wishes, birth goals)

A plan created by an expectant mother that expresses her desires for how she would like her labor to be managed.

BIRTH TEAM

The people a mother chooses to support her during labor and birth.

BISHOP'S SCORE

A rating system used by healthcare providers to assess how prepared the cervix is for labor. Physicians use it to decide when an induction of labor is most likely to be successful.

BLADDER (See CATHETER)

The membrane, or sac, inside the body that stores fluid. Sometimes the bladder, which holds urine, can become infected, causing pain. You may be asked to have a full bladder when you go for a sonogram to allow for clearer pictures of the uterus. During some epidurals and a cesarean section, a catheter is inserted in the bladder to protect it by keeping it drained.

BLASTOCYST

What a fertilized ovum (egg) is called once it enters a mother's uterus.

BLIGHTED OVUM (See ANEMBRYONIC GESTATION)

An egg that fails to form into a baby.

BLOOD GLUCOSE (blood sugar, plasma glucose, serum glucose) (See GLUCOSE TOLERANCE TEST)

The amount of glucose (blood sugar) present in the blood. It can be measured by a drop of blood collected from a fingertip or earlobe and placed on a glucometer, a device for measuring glucose levels. Levels are expressed as a number with 100 considered normal and higher numbers, such as 150 and above, indicating the body's inability to handle glucose.

BLOOD PATCH

The treatment of a severe spinal headache that sometimes is the result of the sac surrounding the spinal cord getting punctured during an epidural. Sterile blood from the mother is injected into the epidural space to form a clot that prevents further leakage of spinal fluid.

BLOOD PRESSURE (See PREECLAMPSIA)
A measurement for the force that the blood exerts against the walls of arteries that enables the blood to flow. Blood pressure is expressed as two numbers. The top number, systolic pressure, is the pressure exerted when the heart contracts. The bottom number, diastolic pressure, is the pressure exerted between heartbeats when the heart is relaxed. It is normal for a pregnant woman's blood pressure to decrease during the second trimester.

BLOODY SHOW (See SHOW)

BM
Abbreviation for bowel movement.

BODY MASS INDEX (BMI)
The relationship of a person's height to weight, which is used to determine if a person is underweight, normal, overweight, or obese. The formula is calculated by dividing a person's weight in pounds by height in inches, dividing this figure a second time by height in inches, and then multiplying the figure by 703. Overweight is defined as a BMI of 25 to 29.9, while obesity is defined as a BMI of 30 or above. These calculations do not apply to weight during pregnancy.

BONDING
The feeling of attachment or love between a parent and a baby. Sometimes the feeling emerges soon after birth, but, just as with grown-up relationships, bonding with a baby may be gradual and take more time to grow.

BRACHIAL PLEXUS PALSY
Dysfunction of the nerves that affects the function of a baby's arm. May be caused by an injury to the shoulder during labor and delivery.

BRADLEY METHOD (husband-coached childbirth)
A childbirth method that encourages natural breathing, husband support, and breastfeeding. (See discussion on page 188.)

BRADYCARDIA (sometimes called a brady spell) (See FETAL HEART RATE)
Excessively slow heartbeat. A newborn's heartbeat is considered too slow when it is measured as fewer than one hundred heartbeats per minute.

BRAXTON-HICKS CONTRACTIONS (false labor) (See CONTRACTIONS)
Contractions of the uterus that occur throughout pregnancy and serve to prepare the uterus for ejecting the baby. During the last weeks of pregnancy, they become more noticeable, but, unlike the contractions of labor, they usually aren't painful or predictable and don't get stronger or closer together over time.

BREAKING OF WATERS (SEE RUPTURE OF MEMBRANES)

BREECH PRESENTATION (breech birth)
When a baby's buttocks, knees, or feet appear first during birth, instead of the head. The position is rare during labor, occurring in fewer than 5 percent of births. Labor with a breech baby is more

challenging and tends to take longer. Most doctors prefer to deliver breech babies by cesarean, as recent studies suggest that it may be a safer for the baby. Before proceeding with a cesarean, many doctors will first attempt to turn the baby into a headfirst position by external cephalic version (ECV), in which the doctor pushes on the mother's abdomen. Frank breech means the baby's hips are flexed and the legs are extended upward toward the baby's face. Complete breech means the baby's legs and arms are folded, Indian-style.

BRETHINE (See TERBUTALINE SULFATE)

BROWN FAT
A special tissue found in newborn babies that helps to fuel the body's energy and produce body heat.

BROW PRESENTATION
When a baby's head is bent backward during birth, rather than the typical flexed, chin-on-chest position. Presentation is determined by examining the baby's skull using the provider's fingers during a vaginal examination. If the baby's head fails to change to a chin-down position during labor, then an intervention, such as a cesarean section, may be necessary.

BSN
Bachelor of Science in Nursing.

C

CAFÉ-AU-LAIT SPOTS
Light or coffee-colored birthmarks sometimes found on a newborn's arms, legs, or body.

CANDIDA (*Candida albicans*, Monilia) (See YEAST INFECTION and THRUSH)
A yeast-like fungus that usually grows in the intestinal tract of the body, but can infect other parts of the body causing a variety of symptoms.

CANNULA
A small tube. For example, a small cannula may be inserted into the vein when getting an IV, or into the cervix as part of measuring contraction strength.

CAPPA
Stands for the Childbirth and Postpartum Professionals Association, a professional organization that certifies labor doulas, postpartum doulas, childbirth educators, and lactation educators.

CAPUT SUCCEDANEUM
A lump or swelling under a newborn's scalp present at birth that is caused by pressure exerted on the baby's head during the birth process. It can be caused by vacuum extraction. The location of the swelling will depend upon the position of the baby's head during birth. It usually disappears within 24 to 36 hours.

CARDINAL MOVEMENTS
The series of passive movements, such as flexing and rotating, that a baby's body makes in order to be born.

CARDIOMYOPATHY, PERIPARTUM
Rare, pregnancy-related heart failure in women not related to a previous heart condition that occurs during the last month of pregnancy

or during the first 5 months after birth. The cause is unknown, but one-quarter to one-half of women who develop this problem die due to congestive heart failure, irregular heartbeat (arrhythmia), or a blood clot that affects the heart (thromboembolism). Between 1991 and 1997, there were 245 pregnancy-related deaths due to cardiomyopathy, or 7.7 percent of all maternal deaths, or a mortality ratio of 0.88 per 100,000 live births. The risk of dying from this condition increases as women age, and African-American mothers are 6.4 times more likely to die from it than Caucasian mothers.

CARDIOTOCOGRAPH
A machine to measure a baby's heart rate and a mother's contractions. It provides a printout of the information it records.

CARDIOVASCULAR
Pertaining to the heart and blood vessels.

CARPAL TUNNEL SYNDROME (See DEQUERVAIN'S TENDONITIS)
Numbness and/or a pins and needles sensation in the hands and fingers caused by fluid collecting around the wrist joints, which press on the nerves that thread through the narrow channels in the wrist bones leading to the hand. It is thought to affect approximately one out of three pregnant women and disappears within a few weeks following birth.

CASE MANAGER
A person, a nurse or social worker, who is assigned to help parents whose babies have been identified as having specific conditions and who may benefit from counseling and help.

CATARACT
When the lens of the eye is coated with a milky tissue that affects vision.

CATHETER (being catheterized, being cathed)
A small, hollow tube used to flow fluids into, or out of, the body. A catheter is used to help protect the bladder from being bruised or injured. During some epidurals or a c-section, a catheter may be inserted into a mother's urethra, the passage that flows urine out of the body. It will be threaded into the passage until it reaches the bladder. The other end of the catheter empties urine into a plastic bag.

CAUL
A thin, filmy membrane (amnion) that sometimes covers the head of a newborn baby.

CDC
Centers for Disease Control and Prevention

CEPHALIC PRESENTATION
When a baby is proceeding through birth in a head-downward position.

CEPHALOHEMATOMA (cephalhemotoma)
Bleeding under the thick membrane that covers a baby's skull. It can be caused by prolonged pressure of his head against the cervix or a mother's perineum or pubic bones, or from the pressure of vacuum extraction. It can also be caused by the blades of forceps, attempting to rotate a baby's head, or rapid compression and relaxation on the

head with precipitous birth or an extremely rapid labor that lasts less than 3 hours. Swelling and redness may not appear until a few hours after birth, and it may grow larger, and can take 6 to 12 weeks to disappear.

CEPHALOPELVIC DISPROPORTION (CPD)
When a baby's head is too large to fit through the mother's pelvis.

CERCLAGE
A stitch placed in the mouth of the womb (cervix) to hold it closed in order to help an "incompetent" (weak) cervix to keep a baby inside until birth.

CEREBRAL PALSY
A condition that affects a child's ability to move, which is thought to be caused by brain injury. It may result in seizures or mental retardation. Its causes are not completely understood, although infection, injury, or lack of oxygen while the brain is developing may play a part.

CERTIFICATION (CERTIFIED)
When a person or agency has received approval from a professional organization by meeting specific standards. Baby products can also be certified if they have met specific standards set by the juvenile products industry.

CERTIFIED NURSE-MIDWIFE (CNM)
A nurse who has completed either a certification program or a master's degree program and has met the certification requirements of the Certification Council (ACC) of the American College of Nurse-Midwives. Certified midwives are able to independently provide pregnancy, childbirth, after birth, and women's reproductive health services.

CERTIFIED REGISTERED NURSE ANESTHETIST (CRNA)
CRNAs are advanced practice nurses with specialized graduate-level education in anesthesiology. During birth, a CRNA may work with your obstetrician or with your anesthesiologist (physician anesthetist) to administer pain management medications to you.

CERVICAL CAP
A flexible contraceptive device designed to tightly fit over the cervix to prevent sperm from entering the uterus and fertilizing the egg.

CERVICAL INCOMPETENCE
When the neck and mouth of the uterus begin to open too soon without contractions before a pregnancy is ready to end. The condition can cause preterm delivery during the second and third trimesters of pregnancy.

CERVICAL OS
The opening in the mouth of the uterus at the tip end of the cervix.

CERVICAL RIPENING (cervix ripening) (See INDUCTION)
The process by which the cervix softens and thins in preparation for labor. It occurs naturally at the end of pregnancy, or it can be accomplished artificially. The cervix may be widened with a balloon-tipped Foley catheter, or softened using medications such as misoprostol or prostaglandin (PGE-2).

CERVICOGRAM (partogram)
A way of charting, on an hourly basis, the progress of labor. It is

done by using a graph that represents the dilation of the cervix in centimeters and the descent of the baby (station) as measured (in plus or minus centimeters) by the position of the baby's presenting part in relation to the ischial spines over time.

CERVIDIL

A medication used to "ripen" or soften the cervix (mouth of the womb) before labor is induced. Sometimes it can be used to induce labor.

CERVIX

The necklike lower part of a mother's pear-shaped uterus that shortens and thins (effaces) and opens (dilates) during labor to allow a baby to be pushed out of the uterus. The cervix is about 1 to 2 inches, or 2.5 to 4 centimeters long. The center of the cervix is called the cervical canal, which the baby passes through during birth.

CERVIX, RIPE

During the process of birth, the cervix, the mouth of the womb will move from the back of the mother, near her spine, to the front of her abdomen, and it will begin to soften. If a cervix is not ready for artificially starting labor (induction), it will be firm and springy to the touch like the tip of a nose. When the cervix is considered ripe, it will have the texture of lips, soft and mushy, and will spread open more easily to allow the baby out than one that is firm and thick. If the cervix isn't ripe, an induction of labor is more likely to result in a cesarean delivery.

CESAREAN SECTION (c-section, cesarean birth, cesarean delivery, C/S, also spelled Caesarean) (See VBAC)

Surgically removing a baby from a mother's uterus through an incision (cut) made in her abdominal wall and through the uterus. There are several varieties of c-sections, differing mainly on the location of the incision. The mother is usually given an anesthetic that numbs her lower body, such as an epidural or combined spinal epidural (CSG), and is draped with a curtain between her chest and the surgery. The baby is removed, followed by the placenta.

CHADWICK'S SIGN

Dark blue or purplish discoloration of the cervix (mouth of the womb), or vagina that is one early sign of pregnancy.

CHICKEN POX (varicella, varicella zoster virus [VZV])

A highly contagious virus transmitted by droplets of mucus and the ooze from the itchy skin sores of the disease. Pregnant women who work with children are at risk. In about 2 percent of cases, it can have serious consequences for a fetus during the first 20 weeks of pregnancy. If a person has previously had chicken pox, she will be immune to further outbreaks. Immunity can be detected by a blood test. If a pregnant mother is not immune and is exposed to the virus, she may be treated with zoster immune globulin (ZIG) to protect her baby from congenital varicella syndrome that includes eye, bone, and brain problems, and sometimes early death. Non-pregnant women who have never had chicken pox should be vaccinated against this disease before they become pregnant (the vaccine cannot be given during pregnancy). (See discussion on page 132.)

CHILD HEALTH NURSING
Also called pediatric nursing, it is the field of nursing that focuses on the care of children and their families from birth onward.

CHLAMYDIA (PRONOUNCED CLAH-MID-I-AH) (See OPTHALMIA NEONATORUM)
The most common sexually transmitted bacterial disease in the United States, it has been labeled "The Silent Epidemic." Women ages 15 to 24 represent 70 percent of all cases. Most victims experience no symptoms. Antibiotics can quickly cure the infection, but left untreated, it can lead to pelvic inflammatory disease (PID), ectopic pregnancy, or chronic pelvic pain. Infected women who deliver a baby may pass the infection on to the baby in the form of severe eye infection or pneumonia. All babies are given antibiotics in their eyes within an hour after birth to protect them against this infection.

CHLOASMA (chloasma gravidarum, the mask of pregnancy)
Increased skin coloring (pigmentation), brownish-yellow patches that some women develop on their faces during pregnancy. It occurs in the area under each eye and resembles the shape of a butterfly.

CHORIOAMNIONITIS (See AMNIONITIS)
Infection of the amniotic sac and the fluid inside.

CHORIOCARCINOMA (See GESTATIONAL TROPHOBLASTIC DISEASE [GTD])
An extremely rare, highly malignant cancer that grows in the uterus during pregnancy or at the site of an ectopic pregnancy.

CHORION (See AMNION)
The outermost fetal membrane that makes up one layer of the amniotic sac.

CHORIONIC VILLUS SAMPLING
A medical technique that removes a small amount of tissue from a mother's placenta in order to test for chromosomal, metabolic, or DNA abnormalities. The test is generally performed between the tenth and twelfth week of pregnancy. Chorionic villus sampling carries a 2 to 3 percent chance risk of miscarriage, and its risks may be higher than for amniocentesis, which is usually done later in pregnancy. (See discussion on page 35.)

CHROMOSOME
A large molecule found in the center (nucleus) of a cell, which carries the genes that determine which parents' characteristics a baby will inherit. Every cell contains forty-six chromosomes except for sperm and egg cells, which each carry twenty-three.

CHRONIC HYPERTENSION (See PREGNANCY-INDUCED HYPERTENSION)
A form of high blood pressure. A mother can have it before she gets

pregnant; it can show up before the twentieth week of pregnancy and stays longer than forty-two days after her baby is born.

CIRCUMCISION (See FORESKIN, FRENULUM, and GLANS)
The surgical removal of the foreskin covering the end of a newborn male's penis. (See discussion on pages 216–219.)

CLAVICLE, FRACTURED
When a baby's collarbone gets broken during the process of delivery. It requires no treatment and usually heals on its own.

CLEANSING BREATH
A deep, voluntary breath through the nose expelled through the mouth that is used in some comfort management strategies during labor. It is used at the beginning and end of contractions to help restore normal breathing and to help manage stress.

CLEFT LIP (CL)
A malformation found in newborns (approximately one out of eight hundred live births), a groove (cleft) in a baby's upper lip. It can be corrected with surgery.

CLEFT PALATE (CP)
Cleft palate (CP), which is less common than cleft lip (one out of two thousand babies), is a deeper groove that can extend all the way through the lip and into the nose and bony structure at the roof of the mouth. It can be inherited or the result of exposure to harmful drugs or environmental toxins in the womb. It is usually repaired right away by surgery because it can affect a baby's feeding and sucking.

CLINICAL NURSE SPECIALIST (CNS)
A nurse who has completed a master's degree in a specialty, such as neonatal medicine, who can provide expert care to patients, participate in educating and conducting research with other healthcare professionals, and serve as a special consultant to parents and healthcare providers.

CLUBFOOT (See TALIPES)

CM
Stands for certified midwife.

CMV (See CYTOMEGALOVIRUS)

CNM (Certified Nurse-Midwife) (See CERTIFIED NURSE-MIDWIFE)
Signifies a certified nurse-midwife.

COAGULATION
The function of the blood to form clots and scabs.

COCAINE (See NEONATAL ABSTINENCE SYNDROME)
A so-called recreational drug that acts to decrease blood flow to the placenta, causing a temporary but dramatic drop in oxygen available to the baby. Cocaine can cause the placenta to tear away from the wall of the uterus, causing a life-threatening loss of blood (hemorrhage). Some studies now suggest that babies whose mothers have used cocaine during pregnancy can experience withdrawal after birth, and some may have permanent nervous system (neurological) problems.

COLIC (COLICKY BABY)
Prolonged and frequent crying by a baby with no known cause. It usually appears a few weeks after

birth and subsides within the first 3 months of life.

COLOSTRUM
A thin white or yellowish fluid produced by the breasts of a pregnant mother in the latter months of pregnancy and soon after birth that transfers concentrated protein and specific immunities to the baby. A mother's breasts may secrete tiny amounts of colostrum as early as the sixteenth week of pregnancy.

COMA (in a coma, becoming comatose)
When a person goes into a deep sleeplike state and cannot be awakened. Can be caused by a severe form of preeclampsia.

COMPLETE ABORTION
When all the products of conception (baby and tissues) are expelled from the uterus.

CONCEIVE (getting pregnant)
When a sperm fertilizes an egg.

CONCEPTION (fertilization)
When the sperm succeeds in penetrating the egg.

CONDOM (rubber)
A sheath of rubber that fits over an erect penis to catch semen when a man ejaculates during sex to prevent pregnancy. It is the most effective contraceptive for preventing the transmission of sexually transmitted diseases.

CONDUCTION HEAT LOSS (See CONVECTION HEAT LOSS)
When a baby loses body heat through contact with a cold surface.

CONDYLOMA
A wart near the vagina or rectum.

CONGENITAL CATARACT
Cloudiness of the lens of the eye of a baby that is present at birth.

CONGENITAL DISORDER
A condition present from birth.

CONJOINED TWINS (Siamese twins)
Twins with joined bodies. Some may share vital organs, which makes surgical separation risky.

CONSTIPATION
Sluggish bowels. Bowel movements may be irregular and are hard, dry, and difficult to push out.

CONTAGIOUS (communicable)
When a disease can be passed from one person to another.

CONTINENCE (See STRESS INCONTINENCE)
Being able to control bladder or bowel function.

CONTRACEPTION
Methods used to prevent a woman from getting pregnant during sex. Could mean the use of a condom (rubber), a specially fitted diaphragm, a contraceptive sponge, or refraining from sex during the times when a woman is fertile and able to conceive. Other methods include contraceptive pills, patches, vaginal rings, intrauterine devices (IUDs), and sterilization.

CONTRACTION (labor pains) (See BRAXTON-HICKS CONTRACTIONS)
Tightening of the abdomen and uterus to expel the baby for birth. They can be strong and regular (happening every 3 to 5 minutes), or they can be weak and irregular. Contractions are considered "real" when they work to dilate (stretch)

and efface (open) the cervix, or they are sometimes called "false" when they don't cause cervical changes.

CONTRACTION STRESS TEST (CST)
A test used during pregnancy to assess how a baby is doing inside the mother's uterus. It measures a fetus's heart rate in relation to the contraction activity of the uterus. It is rarely used now because of its high rate of "false positives" (suggesting problems when there are none).

CONVECTION HEAT LOSS (See CONDUCTION HEAT LOSS)
When a newborn loses heat from drafts and cold air. Newborns are quickly wrapped in a blanket or towel to help keep them warm.

CONVULSION (SEIZURE)
A series of spasm-like contractions of the body's muscles. Sometimes babies have convulsions as the result of a rapid rise in temperature from a fever, or a mother may have a convulsion if she has eclampsia.

CORD (See UMBILICAL CORD)

CORD BLOOD BANK
A commercial or public facility that oversees the collection and storage of blood from newborn's umbilical cords for harvesting stem cells for future medical use. Commercial facilities charge fees for the collection, processing, and storage of the blood.

CORD COMPRESSION
When a baby's umbilical cord gets squeezed, usually during birth, so that blood flow is slowed or stopped.

CORDEE (chordee)
An abnormal curvature of the penis most often caused by a congenital abnormality.

CORDIOCENTESIS
A way of getting samples of fetal blood and giving babies blood transfusions in the womb. It can be used for diagnosing hereditary blood disorders such as hemophilia and infections such as rubella, and to assess the levels of oxygen and baby metabolism in intrauterine growth retardation, or fetal anemia in red cell isoimmunization. It is an outpatient technique using local anesthesia.

CORD PROLAPSE (See PROLAPSED CORD)

CORE TEMPERATURE
The temperature deep inside a mother's or baby's body. The normal body temperature as measured by mouth is 98.6°F (37°C). A higher temperature (fever) may indicate the presence of infection in the mother or baby. Sometimes an epidural can also raise a mother's temperature without an infection being present.

CORONA RADIATA
A protective layer of cells surrounding an egg after ovulation that must be penetrated by a sperm to fertilize the egg (ovum).

CORPUS LUTEUM
A structure in the ovary, which develops after an egg has been released, that produces progesterone.

CORTISOL
Called the stress hormone, cortisol is produced by the adrenal glands in

the body. Typically, a woman's cortisol level is significantly higher than normal during pregnancy, more than double her non-pregnant levels. This rise in cortisol is thought to be related to the actions of other hormones, including progesterone. If a mother is under extreme stress, her cortisol can cross the placenta to her baby, but its effects are not completely understood. The baby's own cortisol is critical for the maturation of his lungs, liver, and other organs.

COUVADE SYNDROME
When fathers exhibit the same symptoms as their pregnant partners, including weight gain or loss, digestive disturbances, fatigue, headache, and backaches. (See discussion on page 52.)

CPD (See CEPHALOPELVIC DISPROPORTION)

CPM (Certified Professional Midwife)
A designation achieved after passing national NARM (North American Registry of Midwives) examination for midwives.

CPSC (Consumer Product Safety Commission)
The government regulatory agency that oversees all baby products, except the crashworthiness of children's car seats, which is the responsibility of the National Highway Traffic Safety Administration (NHTSA).

CRADLE CAP
(seborrheic dermatitis)
A skin condition in newborns that causes scaly, yellow patches. It usually appears on the scalp, but sometimes it affects the eyelids,

eyebrows, or the genital area. It is common in newborns under 3 months of age. Your healthcare provider may suggest special cleansing routines, or instruct you simply to leave it alone and wait for it to go away by itself.

CRETINISM
When a baby has insufficient thyroid function. It can lead to mental retardation and other mental and physical changes.

CRNA (See CERTIFIED REGISTERED NURSE ANESTHETIST)

CROWNING (the baby has crowned)
When birth is about to happen because the baby's head has descended so far down into the birth canal that it can be viewed, encircled by the stretched skin of the vagina. Birth typically follows within minutes.

CROWN-TO-RUMP LENGTH
The measurement of a baby's size from the top of the head to the buttocks, typically used during ultrasound examinations performed during the first trimester of pregnancy to determine the gestational age of the pregnancy.

C-SECTION (C/S) (See CESAREAN SECTION)

CTX
Shorthand for contractions.

CURETTAGE (See DILATION AND CURETTAGE)
The scraping of the lining of the uterus with an instrument called a curette to remove the products of conception. It is also performed

following a miscarriage, in order to remove a polyp, or to obtain a sample for examination in a laboratory. (See discussion on page 24.)

CYSTIC FIBROSIS
An inherited (genetic) disorder that affects a child's lungs and digestive system. It generally occurs among children who are Caucasian and of Northern European descent.

CYSTITIS
Inflammation of the bladder, the saclike organ that stores urine.

CYTOMEGALOVIRUS (CMV)
A herpes-like virus that can cause damage to an unborn baby and also can be caught by the baby during the birthing process if its mother has the infection. In adults, CMV has silent or very mild symptoms similar to mononucleosis, such as fatigue, aches, and fever. About eight thousand babies a year in the United States develop lasting disabilities from being infected by their mothers during pregnancy and birth, including mental retardation, learning disabilities, and hearing or vision loss.

D

D&C (or DNC) (See DILATION AND CURETTAGE)

D ANTIGEN (See: Rh FACTOR, and RHESUS ANTI-D GAMMA GLOBULIN INJECTION)
A protein on the surface of red blood cells that is missing for mothers who have Rh-negative blood. This condition occurs in about 15 percent of Caucasians of European ancestry, 5 percent of African-Americans, and 1 percent of Asians. If the baby has Rh-positive blood, the D antigen could be interpreted as a foreign intruder by the mother's immune system, causing her body to generate antibodies (fighter cells) that cross the placenta and attack the baby's blood cells, resulting in anemia.

DEATH, EARLY NEONATAL
When a baby dies within 7 days of being born.

DEATH, LATE FETAL
When a baby dies after the twenty-eighth week of pregnancy.

DECIDUA
The outermost layer of the lining of the uterus (womb). This is the layer of the lining of the uterus (endometrium) into which the pregnancy implants.

DEHYDRATION
A condition caused by the body losing more fluid than it is taking in. In adults, it is signaled by a dry mouth and scant urination. Dehydration can be fatal in babies, and its symptoms are extreme sluggishness and failure to wet diapers.

DEMEROL
A narcotic commonly used to reduce the sensation of pain during labor and delivery and following birth. Constipation is one potential side effect.

DEOXYRIBONUCLEIC ACID (DNA)
The chemical structure in the body that contains all of the genetic information cells need to duplicate themselves. DNA is the building block of chromosomes.

DEQUERVAIN'S TENDONITIS

A painful hand condition caused by inflammation of the tendons in the thumb that sometimes happens to new mothers. Its causes are not completely understood, although it is thought to be related to post-birth hormonal changes and the stress of lifting the baby. Treatment options include anti-inflammatory medications, splinting the thumb to take pressure off the tendon, and instructing mothers to hold the baby with rigid rather than flexed wrists.

DEVELOPMENTAL DELAY

When the development of a baby or child is slower than normal.

DIABETES (diabetes mellitus, glucose intolerance) (See GESTATIONAL DIABETES, and GLUCOSE TOLERANCE TEST)

A serious disease that affects the body's ability to absorb glucose from the bloodstream, the body's source of energy. It is caused by the body's not producing enough insulin (a hormone made in the pancreas), or an insensitivity to insulin in the tissues of the body. Diabetes is characterized by high levels of glucose in the blood. Left untreated, this disease can cause dysfunction of various organs in the body, including the heart, kidneys, and blood vessels, and may result in death. During pregnancy, untreated diabetes can cause miscarriage, birth defects, and overly large or very small babies.

DIAMNIOTIC TWINS

Twins who each have their own separate amniotic sac, but not necessarily their own separate placentas.

DIAPHRAGM

The large muscle in the body that separates the chest cavity from the abdomen involved in inhaling and exhaling. During the latter months of pregnancy, pressure exerted by a baby on a mother's diaphragm can cause the mother a feeling of shortness of breath and episodes of breathlessness. The word also refers to a flexible contraceptive device for women made from a dome-shaped pouch that fits over the mouth of the uterus (cervix) to prevent sperm from entering the uterus to fertilize an egg.

DIASTASIS RECTI

When the muscles running down the center of the abdomen separate and move slightly to the side during late pregnancy. (See exercise recommendations on page 230.)

DIASTASIS SYMPHYSIS PUBIS (DSP) (See SYMPHYSIS PUBIC DYSFUNCTION [SPD])

DIASTOLIC BLOOD PRESSURE

The bottom number in a blood pressure reading, diastolic pressure is the pressure exerted between heartbeats when the heart is relaxed.

DICHORIONIC TWINS

Twins who each have their own separate amniotic sac and their own separate placentas.

DILATION (dilatation)

During pregnancy: the expansion of the opening of the mouth of the womb (cervix) and the passageway in its center (cervical canal) caused by the pressure of the baby's head or body as it descends the birth canal. Dilation is measured as the distance in centimeters from one side of the opening to the other (diameter). One centimeter equals about one-third of an inch. Ten centimeters means the cervix is wide open. This usually signals the onset of the pushing stage. Informally, dilation is measured as fingers, as in three fingers wide. (See discussion on pages 172–174.)

DILATION AND CURETTAGE (D&C, dilatation and curettage)
The stretching of the mouth and neck of the uterus (cervix) and scraping the lining of the uterus (endometrium) with an instrument called a curette. Often performed after a miscarriage in order to prevent an infection caused by incomplete removal of the products of pregnancy.

DILATION AND EVACUATION
A procedure of abortion done during the thirteenth to the twentieth week of pregnancy in which the cervix is gradually stretched open and the fetus is removed using both suction and curettage.

DILATION AND VACUUM CURETTAGE
A procedure used during an abortion that is done prior to 13 weeks of pregnancy. A mother's cervix is progressively stretched open, and then the contents of the pregnant uterus are suctioned out through a small tube using a vacuum device.

DIRECT-ENTRY MIDWIFE (See CERTIFIED NURSE-MIDWIFE)
A midwife who learns her skills through self-study, an apprenticeship, or at an independent midwifery school or college. Typically direct-entry midwives deliver babies at home, although some work in birth centers. States differ in the requirements for certification of direct-entry midwives.

DIURETIC
A drug or agent that increases urination.

DIZYGOTIC TWINS (fraternal twins)
Twins derived from two different eggs.

DOMINANT DISORDERS
Genetic (inherited) disorders transmitted from parent to child in which a single altered gene dominates (overrides) a normally functioning gene.

DOPPLER
A handheld ultrasound device that transmits the sounds of a baby's heart rate either through a speaker or into attached earpieces. The device can generally pick up heart tones after 12 weeks' gestation.

DORSAL PENILE NERVE BLOCK (DPNB)
An anesthetic injected into a baby boy's penis to help numb the pain of circumcision.

DOULA (pronounced doola) (See MONITRICE)
The word "doula" is derived from Greek, meaning trusted servant or woman's servant. A doula (almost always a woman) is a person who provides support and non-medical comfort coaching for mothers and their birth partners during birth. A doula has special training in the natural progression of labor. She may make suggestions on positions

to help to move labor along. Many doulas are certified through major childbirth education organizations. (See discussion on page 68.)

DOWN SYNDROME (Down's syndrome, trisomy 21) (See ALPHA-FETOPROTEIN TEST)
The most common type of chromosomal abnormality at birth, it is usually not inherited, but caused by a fetus having an extra copy of chromosome 21. As a mother's age goes up, her risk for giving birth to a baby with Down syndrome is increased. There are a number of physical characteristics for the syndrome: short stature, special facial structure with an extra fold at the outer corner of the baby's eyelids, and moderate mental retardation. The overall prevalence of the syndrome is one in eight hundred babies, but by the time a mother reaches ages 45, its prevalence is one out of every thirty-two babies. It can be detected by specific tests during pregnancy.

DTP VACCINATION
A vaccination for babies that protects them against diphtheria, tetanus, and pertussis (whooping cough).

DUCTUS ARTERIOSUS
An artery inside the unborn baby that permits incoming blood to bypass the lungs until they are ready to expand and begin the breathing process immediately after birth. The artery then closes.

DUE DATE (estimated date of delivery [EDD], estimated date of confinement [EDC])
An educated guess for the date your baby can be expected to be born. An average pregnancy lasts 280 days, or about 40 weeks measured from the first day of the expectant mother's last menstrual period, but normal pregnancies can last between 37 weeks to 42 weeks. Only about 5 of 100 babies are born on their due date, with most mothers giving birth within 2 weeks of the date. It is important in measuring the progress of pregnancy, the growth of the baby, and to determine the best timing for testing for fetal abnormalities. Note: First-time mothers (primiparas, primips, or nulliparous women, nullips) are likely to give birth later than mothers who have had more than one child.

DYSMATURITY SYNDROME
When a baby is born who appears malnourished with a long and lean body, an alert look on the face, lots of hair, long fingernails, and thin wrinkled skin. Often there can be meconium-stained amniotic fluid. The condition usually occurs in babies born more than 1 week after their due dates.

DYSPNEA
Difficulty breathing.

DYSTOCIA
A slow and difficult childbirth, which can be due to problems with the baby (unusually large, in the wrong position, stuck shoulders, abnormalities that make birth difficult or impossible, interlocked twins) or problems with the mother (a sluggish or malformed uterus, a small pelvis, a rigid cervix that will not open to allow the baby out). The treatment for dystocia depends upon the condition and can range from simply waiting for delivery to

occur naturally, giving medication to stimulate contractions, or performing a cesarean section to remove the baby from the mother's body.

DYSURIA
Pain during urinating.

E

ECLAMPSIA (See PREECLAMPSIA, PREGNANCY-INDUCED HYPERTENSION [PIH], and TOXEMIA)
A rare, life-threatening condition for mothers that can occur at any time between the twentieth week of pregnancy and the first week following birth. It is marked by coma and convulsive seizures, and it can be fatal if not treated. It is estimated that one out of every two hundred mothers who have preeclampsia (toxemia) will develop full-blown eclampsia. Currently, the only cure for eclampsia is giving birth, and the baby of a mother with the more severe form of the illness may have to have her baby delivered early in order to save her life.

ECTOPIC PREGNANCY (or tubal pregnancy)
When a fertilized egg implants itself some other place than the mother's uterine wall. The majority of these pregnancies occur in the fallopian tubes that conduct the egg to the uterus, but sometimes the pregnancy can occur in a mother's abdominal cavity, which can lead to life-threatening problems. Symptoms of an ectopic pregnancy include abnormal bleeding, severe abnormal pain, or shoulder pain.

Approximately one out of fifty pregnancies is ectopic. (See discussion on page 25.)

ECZEMA (atopic dermatitis)
A broad term for dry, itchy, inflamed skin, which can crack and become oozy. The first symptoms usually appear in babies during the first 3 months of life. The baby will have red, scaly skin, and red patches may appear on his cheeks that spread to scalp, arms, and legs. Babies with dry, sensitive skin or allergies to ingredients in formula, chemicals in detergents, fabric softeners, pollens, or house dust are more vulnerable to it. Sometimes creams, ointments, lotions, or moisturizers may help, as can steroids, but they should be used only under the guidance of a physician or skin specialist (dermatologist).

EDC (See ESTIMATED DATE OF CONFINEMENT)

EDD (estimated due date) (See DUE DATE)

EDEMA
Swelling of soft tissues as the result of excess fluid retention. Most pregnant women retain more fluid in their lower legs in the latter stages of pregnancy from pressure exerted on their circulatory systems by their babies and hormonal changes. Excess retention of fluid can also be an early sign of toxemia (preeclampsia), especially when it involves the hands and face. (See discussion of edema on page 148, and eclampsia on pages 412 and above.)

EFFACEMENT
The gradual thinning, shortening, and drawing up of the cervix in

preparation for birth. It is expressed in percentages, with 100 percent meaning totally thinned. For example, a mother may be told she is "40 percent effaced."

EFFLEURAGE
Light caressing of the abdomen using the fingertips that can be used during labor to help lessen the discomfort of labor contractions.

EGG (ovum)
The reproductive cell produced by the mother that is fertilized by the father's sperm, which forms an embryo that develops into a fetus and then a baby.

EJACULATION
When a man expels a white fluid, semen, from his penis, which contains sperm that seek out and fertilize a mother's egg during the process of sexual intercourse.

ELECTIVE INDUCTION (See INDUCTION)
Choosing to have labor started by drugs rather than on its own.

ELECTRONIC FETAL MONITOR (EFM)
An instrument used to record the baby's heart rate from moment to moment. It can be used as a test during pregnancy of the health of the baby or to monitor the baby during a mother's labor contractions. Monitoring can be continuous or periodic.

EMBOLISM
A blood clot that blocks circulation in a blood vessel to a part of the body, such as the lungs. Along with hemorrhage (excessive bleeding), and hypertension (high blood pressure), embolisms are one of the leading causes of maternal death during childbirth. Mothers who have a prolonged labor, who have a cesarean section, who are significantly overweight, or who have varicose veins are slightly more at risk of having blood clots. Common symptoms are tenderness around a vein, one-sided swelling, and pain in the leg near the ankle. A pulmonary embolism (pulmonary thrombosis) occurs when the clot travels to the lungs, causing sudden breathlessness and chest pain. This can result in respiratory collapse.

EMBRYO
The name for the fetus, or developing baby, up to 10 weeks of menstrual age, menstrual age being calculated from the first day of the mother's last period before pregnancy.

EMBRYONIC STAGE
The second through eighth weeks after conception.

EMLA CREAM
An anesthetic cream commonly used during circumcision to numb the tip of a baby's penis. It is applied to the skin of the penis in advance of circumcision and contains lidocaine and prilocaine. It may cause swelling and is not advised for use on mucous membranes. (See discussion of circumcision on pages 216–219.)

ENDODERMAL GERM LAYER (endoderm, entoderm)
Area of tissue in early development of the embryo that gives rise to other structures, including the digestive tract, respiratory organs,

vagina, bladder, and urethra (the tube that flows urine from the kidneys to the bladder).

ENDOMETRIOSIS
When the lining of the uterus (endometrium) is growing in the wrong place in the body such as in the abdominal cavity.

ENDOMETRITIS (See POSTPARTUM ENDOMETRITIS)

ENDOMETRIUM (endometrial tissue)
The lining of the inside wall of the uterus. (This lining sheds and flows out during a period.) The fertilized egg implants itself into this lining and takes early nourishment from it.

ENDORPHIN
Natural, morphine-like hormones made by the body that help to reduce pain and produce a feeling of calmness and peacefulness. Endorphins are secreted by a mother's body during labor.

ENEMA
Fluid flowed into the rectum for the purpose of clearing out the bowels. Enemas were formerly a standard procedure when laboring mothers were admitted to the hospital. They are seldom used now.

ENGAGED (engagement)
A laboring mother may be told that her baby's head has engaged. It means that a baby's head or other body part, such as the buttocks during a breech presentation, has moved down into the bones of the pelvis in preparation for birth. Also known as lightening, a mother will notice that the baby's position is lower and that she is able to breathe easier, but there may also be odd pains and a feeling of increased pressure to her bladder.

ENGORGEMENT
Swelling and hardening of a mother's breasts that occurs 24 to 48 hours after birth, whether or not a mother chooses to breastfeed. Nursing within an hour following birth and expressing milk can help to treat it. (See breastfeeding discussion on pages 238–246.)

ENTEROVIRUSES
A large family of viruses that live in the intestines and are responsible for many infections in babies and children. There are more than seventy different strains, which include the group A and group B coxsackieviruses, the echoviruses, polio, and hepatitis A, which can cause paralysis. Most children develop immunity to the most common forms and catch them only once. Typical symptoms include fever sometimes accompanied by stomachache, sore throats, or muscle aches. The viruses can live for days on surfaces at room temperature, and refrigeration and freezing do not kill them, but they are killed by disinfectants. Antibiotics are not useful in treating them. They are most often passed by human contact. Frequent hand washing can help to prevent them.

EPIDURAL (epidural anesthesia) (See BLOOD PATCH, SPINAL HEADACHE, and WALKING EPIDURAL)
A method for decreasing or eliminating pain during labor. It numbs a mother's body from the lower rib cage downward, but allows a mother to remain alert and awake, so she can watch the birth of

her baby. Medication is injected between two vertebrae of the lower backbone and into the epidural space of the spinal column. The tube (catheter) that is used for the procedure remains in place until after delivery. Epidurals are also used to provide anesthesia for a cesarean delivery. (See discussion on pages 189–192.)

EPISIOTOMY
A surgical incision into the tissue between the vagina and the rectum done for the purpose of widening a mother's birth outlet for the use of forceps or vacuum extraction or on the premise that it speeds up delivery or allows for better healing than a tear in the tissue. Afterward, your care provider will give an injection of a local anesthetic and stitch up the incision and any lacerations with dissolving stitches. Episiotomies are thought to contribute to more serious tearing and ruptures. (See discussion on page 179.)

ERB'S PALSY
(Erb-Duchenne paralysis)
When a newborn is paralyzed due to an injury of the network of nerves in the shoulder and neck that control the arms. The baby's arm will be limp. The condition usually goes away during the first 3 months of life, but on rare occasions, it can be permanent.

ERYTHEMA TOXICUM
A harmless red rash with small white bumps on the skin of newborns that happens in about 30 to 70 percent of babies. It appears within the second or third day of life and fades by the end of the first week.

ERYTHROBLASTOSIS FETALIS
A blood disease of newborns characterized by anemia (low blood cell count), jaundice (yellowing of the skin), enlargement of the liver and spleen, and generalized edema (swelling of the tissues). It can happen when a mother with Rh-negative blood carries a baby with Rh-positive blood.

ESTIMATED DATE OF CONFINEMENT (EDC)
(See DUE DATE)
Anticipated due date for delivery of the baby. Calculated from the first day of the last menstrual period.

ESTRIOL (See ALPHA-FETOPROTEIN TEST)
A hormone related to estrogen that is produced by the placenta. Lower-than-normal levels detected in a pregnant woman's blood may suggest a chromosomal abnormality.

ESTROGEN
A female hormone that regulates menstruation. The placenta also produces it during the first trimester of pregnancy to help sustain it.

EVIDENCE-BASED MEDICINE (EBM)
Medical practice based on the careful evaluation of well-designed research studies.

EXCLUSIVE BREASTFEEDING
Breastfeeding a baby without supplemental fluids, such as formula, or glucose water. Babies who are exclusively breastfed tend to be healthier than formula-fed babies. (See discussion on pages 238–239.)

EXTERNAL VERSION (external cephalic version, ECV)
A technique using external hand pressure on a pregnant woman's belly to turn a baby from a head upward (breech) to a head downward (cephalic) position in preparation for birth. Medication may be used to help the mother's uterus relax.

EXTRAUTERINE PREGNANCY (EUP) (See ECTOPIC PREGNANCY)
When a fertilized egg (ovum) implants itself in tissue outside of the uterus.

F

FACIAL PARALYSIS
Sometimes a baby may have a face that sags on one side as the result of damage to a nerve during birth, sometimes caused by the use of forceps. The paralysis requires no medical intervention and will usually disappear within a few days to several months. In rare cases, the damage may be permanent.

FACNM (Fellow of the American College of Nurse-Midwives)

FACOG (Fellow of the American College of Obstetricians & Gynecologists)

FAILURE TO PROGRESS (dystocia) (See DYSTOCIA)
A slow or stopped labor, often without a clear-cut reason.

FALLOPIAN TUBES
The tubes that carry eggs (ova) from the ovaries to the uterus. Fertilization often happens in the tubes, then the egg floats down to implant in the uterus. If the egg implants in the tube, it is called an ectopic pregnancy. These are the tubes that are tied (closed off) during female sterilization.

FAMILY-CENTERED CARE
Healthcare based on the philosophy of providing maximum support for the health, security, and well-being of mothers, fathers, and children. In birth centers or care provider offices this usually means that the mother can bring her partner and children along for health visits and the birth of her child, with the ability to keep them at her side during labor.

FAMILY PLANNING
The managing of fertility through a variety of options.

FASTING BLOOD SUGAR (See GLUCOSE TOLERANCE TEST)

FDA (Food and Drug Administration)
The FDA is the federal agency that oversees the safety of foods and drugs, including medications used by pregnant women and products used on babies such as baby food, formula, and creams. This agency sometimes recalls products that have been found to be harmful. The FDA currently does not compel any drug manufacturer to test the safety of medications on pregnant women (unless the drug claims specifically to be safe for pregnant women), which is why drug labels often instruct pregnant women to consult with a doctor before taking any medication.

FDLMP
First day of last menstrual period. It is used as the starting point for how

long pregnancy is expected to last and to calculate a mother's due date using a 40-week time frame.

FECAL INCONTINENCE
The inability to hold in bowel movements (and gas) that can sometimes be the result of tearing during labor usually from having an episiotomy, or deliveries using forceps or vacuum extraction. The condition is often temporary, and most mothers regain control of their bowels between 6 weeks and 4 months following birth, but the condition sometimes lasts longer. Kegel exercises may help. In the meantime, adult diapers may be useful. In rare instances, corrective surgery may be needed.

FELLOW
An individual who has completed an M.D. degree as well as a residency in a specialty such as obstetrics or pediatrics, and who is now taking advanced training, such as a fellow in perinatology or neonatology.

FERGUSON'S REFLEX
The release of oxytocin during the second (pushing) stage of labor triggered by the pressure of the baby's head on the tissues of the mother's lower body and mouth of her uterus (cervix). The reflex triggers the mother's urge to bear down. The reflex is more pronounced in labors without painkilling medication.

FERTILITY (BEING FERTILE)
Being able to conceive a baby.

FERTILITY MEDICATIONS
Medicines used to help mothers conceive by manipulating hormone levels and stimulating egg production. Currently, there are drugs approved by the FDA for this purpose, including Clomid, Gonal-F, and Pergonal.

FERTILIZATION
When sperm and egg join together.

FERTILIZATION AGE
Dating pregnancy from the actual date of fertilization (conception), rather than the medical practice of dating pregnancy from the first day of the last period. It is calculated as 266 days or 38 weeks.

FETAL ALCOHOL SYNDROME (FAS)
A series of non-genetic birth defects caused by a mother's drinking of alcohol during pregnancy. Not all children exposed to alcohol in the womb suffer from FAS, although even minimal drinking is now considered a threat to the baby's well-being. Currently, there is no way to predict the effects of alcohol on a baby. (See discussion on page 104.)

FETAL ANOMALY
Fetal malformation or abnormal development.

FETAL BLOOD SAMPLING (percutaneous umbilical blood sampling, PUBS, codiocentesis)
A test for fetal abnormalities in which blood is removed from a baby's umbilical cord while still inside the mother's womb. In less than 1 percent of cases, it can lead to fetal death.

FETAL COMPROMISE (See NONREASSURING FETAL STATUS)

FETAL DEATH IN UTERO (FDIU, intrauterine fetal death, stillbirth) (See STILLBIRTH)

FETAL DIAGNOSTIC TESTING
Tests conducted during pregnancy to ensure that the baby is alive and thriving. Tests include non-stress tests and contraction stress tests, biophysical profiles, amniocentesis, and ultrasound examinations.

FETAL DISTRESS (See NONREASSURING FETAL STATUS)

FETAL GROWTH RETARDATION (intrauterine growth restriction, or IUGR)
Inadequate growth of the fetus during the latter stages of pregnancy.

FETAL HEART RATE (FHR)
A baby's normal heart rate in the womb is between 120 and 160 beats per minute. The rhythm of a baby's heart rate during labor is considered an important way to measure whether the birthing baby is having a problem. Speeding up is called acceleration; slowing down is called deceleration. If a baby's heart rate slows to less than 100 beats per minute for a period of time, it is called bradycardia, or brady spell, and suggests that the baby may be having problems. It could indicate that the baby should be delivered quickly and receive extra attention after birth.

FETAL HEART TONES (FHT)
The sound made by a baby's heart that can first be detected as early as 10 to 12 weeks by ultrasound and between 18 and 20 weeks by an electronic fetoscope that transmits heart sounds using ear pieces similar to a stethoscope.

FETAL LOSS (fetal death in utero, stillbirth) (See STILLBIRTH)
When a baby dies inside the uterus during pregnancy. (See page 146.)

FETAL MONITOR
Device used to listen to and record a baby's heartbeat during pregnancy or labor. External monitoring uses a device fastened to a mother's abdomen; internal monitoring attaches to the baby's scalp through the mother's vagina.

FETAL MOVEMENT COUNTS (FMCS)
Healthy babies are usually very active inside the uterus. Most mothers don't feel their babies move until around twenty weeks of pregnancy. Beginning the twenty-seventh week of pregnancy, some healthcare providers request that mothers do periodic counts to measure how often their babies move within an hour. Ten times per hour is considered normal. If a mother has not felt her baby move all day (12 hours), or she becomes aware of a significant change in her baby's activity, then she should contact her healthcare provider.

FETAL PERIOD
The stage in a baby's growth following the first 10 weeks of gestation (embryonic period) until birth.

FETAL PULMONARY MATURATION
A baby who is born too soon may have lungs that don't function well. A number of tests are available to tell if a baby's lungs are mature enough for survival after birth which is an issue for preterm

(premature) births or when a baby needs to be delivered before 39 weeks of pregnancy for medical reasons. If the baby is suspected of having immature lungs, its mother may be given a course of drugs to help to promote lung maturation.

FETOPELVIC DISPROPORTION (cephalopelvic disproportion)
When a baby is so large that it may not be able to pass through the pelvis of the mother because of its size, when the mother has a smaller-than-normal pelvis, or a combination of these size mismatches. Disproportion is frequently cited as a reason for a cesarean section. A mother's pelvis is usually measured in the weeks prior to birth to detect any potential problems.

FETOSCOPE
A special cone-shaped stethoscope used for listening to a baby's heart. There are many types of fetoscopes available, although a regular stethoscope can also be used. Either type of monitoring device is able to detect a baby's heartbeat after about the eighteenth week of pregnancy.

FETOSCOPY
Passing a tiny tubular-shaped device, an endoscope, through the mother's abdomen into the amniotic cavity in order to take a biopsy of tissue or to perform a surgical intervention on the baby. This is only done when a condition threatens a baby's life and there is no effective treatment that can be performed after the baby is born.

FETUS
An unborn baby from the end of the eighth week of pregnancy until the moment of birth.

FEVER
When a person's temperature by mouth is elevated above normal: 98.6°F (37°C). Someone's temperature can also be taken rectally, by using a thermometer that goes in the ear, or by placing the thermometer in the crease of the underarm, with different numbers indicating what is normal. Fever associated with birth can be a serious sign that could indicate the mother has an infection. The baby may then have to undergo a series of tests to ensure that the infection hasn't been transmitted to him. (Baby fevers are discussed on pages 257–259.)

FEVER, PUERPERAL
When a mother has a fever during or after the process of birth. It could indicate an infection, or it could be one of the effects of an epidural.

FIBROID (myoma)
A non-malignant (non-cancerous) tumor on the uterus that may rarely affect pregnancy, particularly if it is near the amniotic sac or blocking the pathway for birth.

FIVE-POINT HARNESS
A child's car seat feature that refers to the number of straps. The five points refer to two straps for the shoulders, a strap for each side of the baby's waist, and a crotch strap for between the legs. Some rear-facing infant car seats have three-point harness systems (a strap for each shoulder, and for the crotch) which are thought to be less safe than those with five-point systems.

FOCAL POINT
A point of concentration in the room of a birthing mother that helps her

to maintain control during contractions.

FOLEY BULB (See FOLEY CATHETER)

FOLEY CATHETHER
A tube with an expanding pocket (balloon) inside that is most often used to drain the bladder, but the Foley catheter is sometimes inserted inside the mother's cervix in order to gradually soften and expand it during labor.

FOLIC ACID (FOLATE)
A member of the vitamin B-complex that increases a mother's metabolism, prevents a rare form of anemia, and is active in the formation of red blood cells and cell structures. Folic acid has also been found to help prevent certain malformations in the fetus, including spina bifida. (See discussion on page 163.)

FOLLICLES
Sacs in which eggs develop in a woman's ovaries.

FOLLICLE-STIMULATING HORMONE (FSH)
A hormone that stimulates the development of eggs in a woman's ovaries.

FONTANELS (soft spots)
Spaces between the hard bones of a baby's skull that allow the baby's head to compress during birth. As the skull's bones grow, the size of the fontanels shrinks. Normally, by 6 months of age, the fontanels become dense and fibrous, and they fuse into hard bone around 2 years of age.

FORCEPS
A spoon-shaped instrument with two blades and a handle designed to hold onto the sides of a baby's head to aid with delivery. Forceps can cause injury and are less frequently used now than in years past.

FORESKIN (prepuce) (See CIRCUMCISION)
A retractable skin covering that partially or completely covers the glans, or penis head, in a male baby. It is left intact when a baby is not circumcised, but removed by circumcision. In childhood and adulthood, the foreskin acts as a protective cover for a flaccid penis. (See discussion on page 215.)

FORMULA
An artificial substitute for human breastmilk usually made from specially processed cow's milk or soy protein and other added components. (See discussion on page 246.)

FRANK BREECH (See BREECH)
When a baby is positioned in the uterus with the buttocks first (nearest to the cervix) and legs stretched upward toward his chest.

FRATERNAL TWINS
Two babies that have developed from two different, separate fertilized eggs. The opposite of identical twins.

FRENULUM (FRENUM)
A connecting fold of membrane. One type is the elastic band of tissue under the head of a male infant's penis (glans) that connects to the foreskin, which is removed during most circumcision procedures. (See discussion of circumcision starting on page 216.) Another frenulum is the tissue in the center of the underside of baby's tongue, which, if

too tight, can interfere with breastfeeding.

FRIEDMAN LABOR CURVE
A widely followed chart for the normal progress of labor that measures cervical dilation over the duration of a mother's labor. The graph estimates that first-time mothers take approximately $6^1/_2$ hours to move from the latent to the active phase of labor with active labor lasting approximately $4^1/_2$ hours. The second pushing stage is estimated to last about an hour. The latent phase for mothers who have previously had a baby is 4.8 hours, and the active phase lasts about 2.4 hours, with the second, pushing stage taking only about half an hour.

FTP (See FAILURE TO PROGRESS)

FULL TERM
A baby is considered full term when he is born between the beginning of the thirty-seventh week and the end of the forty-second week.

FUNDAL HEIGHT
(McDonald measurement)
A measurement of the expansion of a pregnant uterus from the edge of the pubic bone to the top of the uterus (the fundus). After the first 20 weeks, the fundal height during pregnancy is generally equal in centimeters to the number of weeks a mother is pregnant, e.g., 32 centimeters at 32 weeks of gestation.

FUNDUS
The top of the uterus. It can be felt as a firm ridge by pressing downward on a mother's belly.

G

GALACTOCELE (plugged milk duct) (See MASTITIS)
A plugged milk duct inhibits milk flow in the breast. It can feel like a mass or firm nodules in the breast. A too-tight bra can cause it. Nursing a baby can help to dissolve the lump, or it can be suctioned out by a healthcare provider using a syringe.

GBS (See GROUP B STREPTOCOCCUS)

GENERAL ANESTHESIA (general anesthetic)
A drug used for surgery, so the patient is no longer conscious and feels no pain. It sometimes is used during an emergency cesarean, and it can be employed for a planned cesarean or a difficult vaginal birth. The delivery must occur quickly because this type of anesthetic can cross the placenta to the baby and may temporarily depress the baby's breathing. It is primarily used when speed is of the essence, such as when the circulation in a baby's umbilical cord has been blocked and his heart rate has begun to slow down; when there is severe, sudden bleeding that could endanger a mother's life (hemorrhage); or when an epidural or spinal anesthetic would not be safe for the mother.

GENES
A portion of a DNA molecule that is located on a chromosome that carries basic genetic information. Genes are the carriers of traits that are inherited from parents.

GENETIC
Determined by genes, such as inherited conditions.

GENETIC COUNSELING
Counseling for parents whose babies may have defects related to the baby's genetic makeup.

GENETIC DISORDER
A mental or physical problem that results from abnormal genes. It can happen by chance or be passed from parent to baby through an error in the parent's genes or chromosomes. (See discussion on page 108.)

GENETIC MARKER
An easily identified piece of DNA that is used to find the gene that may be inherited, whether normal or abnormal.

GENITAL HERPES
(herpes simplex)
A viral infection involving the genital area. It is important to know if a mother has herpes because of the danger of a newborn becoming infected during labor, which can have serious consequences.

GENITALS (genitalia)
Male and female sex organs.

GERMAN MEASLES
(See RUBELLA)

GESTATION
Another word for pregnancy: The length of time between the first day of a mother's final menstrual period before conception and delivery of the baby. Typically, the period of gestation is between 37 and 41 weeks from the first day after the last normal menstrual period, although the calculation of how long a mother has carried a baby is not always very accurate.

GESTATIONAL AGE
Baby's age measured from the first day of the last period: 280 days, or 40 weeks. It is 2 weeks longer than fetal age.

GESTATIONAL DIABETES
(See GLUCOSE TOLERANCE TEST)
A condition that develops during pregnancy when the expectant mother's body does not supply sufficient insulin for the demands of pregnancy. This leaves excessive amounts of glucose in the blood, potentially causing problems for both mother and baby. The increased level of blood sugar (glucose) can be detected in the urine and blood.

GESTATIONAL TROPHOBLASTIC DISEASE (GTD)
A rare condition that mimics pregnancy. It occurs when abnormal cells grow in the uterus at the site of the implanted egg. Hydatidiform mole is the most common form, occurring in one out of every fifteen hundred pregnancies. Choriocarcinoma, the cancerous variety, occurs in one of every twenty thousand to forty thousand pregnancies. Symptoms include faster-than-usual abdominal growth, severe nausea and vomiting, non-menstrual vaginal bleeding, fatigue and shortness of breath from anemia, and blood clots or watery brown discharge. Dislodged pieces of the tumor may resemble a bunch of grapes. GTD most often happens with very young (less than 17 years) or older women (30 to 40 years). It is treatable even in its late stage and has a 90 percent survival rate, although a medical specialist may be required.

GLANS
The bulbous, soft tip of the penis that is covered by the foreskin in an uncircumcised baby.

GLUCOSE
A form of sugar present in the blood that serves as the main fuel of the body.

GLUCOSE TOLERANCE TEST
(fasting blood sugar test)
(See GESTATIONAL DIABETES)
A blood test that measures the level of glucose in the bloodstream. The test is usually performed around 28 weeks of pregnancy. First, a fasting blood sugar reading is taken from a small blood sample. The pregnant woman is then asked to drink a heavily sweetened beverage. An hour later, blood is drawn to measure blood sugar levels. There may be additional tests in the hours that follow. High blood sugar levels may be a sign of diabetes mellitus, or gestational diabetes.

GLUCOSURIA
Glucose in the urine.

GONORRHEA
A highly contagious infection of the reproductive organs of men and women that is transmitted primarily through sexual intercourse. The incidence of gonorrhea during pregnancy is low, but it has been associated with miscarriages, low-birthweight babies, premature rupture of the amniotic sac, chorioamnionitis, and pelvic infections following birth.

GRAV1 (gravida 1, gravida one)
First pregnancy (pregnancy number one).

GRAVIDA (See MULTIGRAVIDA and PRIMIGRAVIDA)
Number of pregnancies.

GRIEF, STAGES OF
First identified by Dr. John Bowlby, a British researcher, it refers to stages that parents go through that are a part of the natural grieving process. The series of feelings, called phases, include numbness, yearning and searching, despair, and disorganization, followed eventually by hope and rebuilding.

GROUP-B STREPTOCOCCUS (GBS)
A bacterium found in the intestines and on the genitals of approximately one out of five pregnant women, who may not show any outward symptoms of colonization by the bacterium. It is the leading cause of serious neonatal infection of newborns and can affect the blood, spinal fluid, and lungs. It can be passed from mother to infant during delivery. Although only a small number of exposed babies develop serious complications, the infection can be fatal. You will likely be screened for GBS late in your pregnancy (see RVC [Rectal/Vaginal Culture]) and given an antibiotic such as penicillin during labor if you are found to carry the organism.

GROUP PRACTICE
A group of physicians and/or midwives who practice together in order to provide better around-the-clock coverage for their pregnant patients.

G.Y.N. OR GYN
Abbreviations for gynecologist.

H

HABITUAL ABORTION
Three or more consecutive, spontaneous miscarriages.

HEARTBURN (indigestion, sour stomach, gastroesophageal reflux, gastric reflux)

A burning sensation in the upper chest or throat caused by gastric juices being released upwards into the esophagus. Heartburn during pregnancy is thought to be caused by crowding of a mother's stomach by the growing baby, hormonal changes in the body, and eating excessive fat, caffeine, or spicy foods.

HEAT RASH (prickly heat, milaria rubra)

Pink bumps that appear on a baby's forehead under caps or visors, in body folds, or on the upper back, chest, and arms that are caused by the pores of sweat glands becoming plugged. The tiny pink bumps may form water blisters and can become itchy. Although heat rash is more common in warm weather, it can also occur when babies are overdressed in winter. Skin oils, lotions, and ointments can aggravate the condition. If the rash is accompanied by a fever, it may be a sign of chicken pox or a reaction to chicken pox vaccine. A healthcare provider may recommend a cleansing routine.

HEEL STICK

Pricking a baby's heel to obtain small amounts of blood for testing. The baby may have a big bandage on his heel afterward.

HEGAR'S SIGN

The softening of the area between the cervix and the body of the uterus that is a sign of pregnancy.

HELLP SYNDROME

A severe form of preeclampsia associated with significant risks for both mother and baby. HELLP stands for hemolysis (H), elevated liver enzymes (EL), and low platelet count (LP), which are measured by blood tests. Babies of mothers with HELLP Syndrome are more likely to be small for gestational age (SGA). Potential HELLP symptoms include pain in the upper right-hand side of the chest or stomach area, sometimes accompanied by nausea and vomiting. Mothers with HELLP are more likely to have anemia and cesarean deliveries, and are more at risk for heavy bleeding.

HEMATOCRIT (Hct, blood count)

The percent of blood cells in the total blood volume in a blood test. Important in diagnosing anemia.

HEMOGLOBIN

Pigment in red blood cell that carries oxygen to body tissues.

HEMOPHILIA

A genetically inherited blood disorder that disrupts the ability of the blood to clot. Persons having hemophilia may be labeled bleeders.

HEMORRHAGE, POSTPARTUM

Life-threatening bleeding from the uterus. If the bleeding doesn't stop, it may require a blood transfusion or other medical or surgical interventions, and, more rarely, a hysterectomy. Primary hemorrhage occurs within the first 24 hours after birth; secondary hemorrhage refers to excessive blood loss from the vagina between 24 hours and 6 weeks after birth.

HEMORRHOIDS (PILES)

Swollen blood vessels around the anus that can become inflamed and painful. Sometimes they bleed. They can be caused by constipation during pregnancy, lightening when the baby settles more deeply into the pelvis, or the pressure of the baby or childbirth on the veins of the rectum. (See discussion on page 129.)

HEPARIN LOCK (hep-lock)
A capped-off intravenous (IV) line usually placed on the back of a mother's hand or forearm that can be used later should medications or fluids be needed.

HEPATITIS B
A serious infection of the liver caused by a virus that typically is transmitted through sexual intercourse or exposure to an infected person's blood. It can be transmitted from mother to baby during the process of birth, unless the baby receives preventive medication following delivery and is then vaccinated against it. People at high risk for contracting this disease, including expectant mothers, should be vaccinated against hepatitis B, and it is currently recommended that all newborns be vaccinated too.

HERNIA
A protrusion of an organ or part of an organ into surrounding tissues.

HERPES SIMPLEX
(See GENITAL HERPES)

HIP DYSPLASIA
When the top of a baby's thigh bone (the femoral head) is badly positioned in or is dislocated from the socket of the pelvis (acetabulum).

HIV (HUMAN IMMUNODEFICIENCY VIRUS)
HIV is a sexually transmitted disease that causes AIDS (acquired immunodeficiency syndrome). The virus attacks the body's immune system, causing a loss of resistance to various infections. HIV may circulate in the bloodstream many years before the symptoms of AIDS appear. It is transmitted through contact with blood, semen, vaginal secretions, and, more rarely, through human breastmilk. Mothers with HIV are most often infected through heterosexual contact with an infected partner or through drug use. Twenty to 30 percent of babies born to untreated mothers with HIV will get the infection during pregnancy or during labor and delivery, but with therapy, only 1 to 2 percent of infants who are born to an infected mother will acquire HIV from the mother.

HOMAN'S SIGN
When a mother feels pain in her calf when her foot is flexed upward. The sign, along with swelling and tenderness in one leg following birth, may indicate a mother could have thrombosis, a clot forming in her leg.

HORMONE
A chemical secretion produced in the body to stimulate or slow down the function of various organs or body systems.

HUMAN CHORIONIC GONADOTROPIN (hCG)
(β-human chorionic gonadotropin, β-hCG)
A hormone produced by the embryo as measured in pregnancy tests. It stimulates the secretion of estrogen and progesterone for maintaining pregnancy. It doesn't appear to play a role in the second and third trimesters of pregnancy but is

thought to be related to nausea and vomiting during early pregnancy.

HUMAN GENOME
An individual's entire collection of genes.

HUMAN PLACENTAL LACTOGEN
Hormone of pregnancy produced by the placenta found in a mother's bloodstream. It plays a role in the body's processing of blood sugar (glucose).

HYALINE MEMBRANE DISEASE (See RESPIRATORY DISTRESS SYNDROME [RDS])

HYDATIDIFORM MOLE (See GESTATIONAL TROPHOBLASTIC DISEASE [GTD])
An abnormal pregnancy in which there is no fetus, only the abnormal growth of the placenta.

HYDRAMNIOS (See AMNIOTIC SAC)
Greater than normal amount of fluid in the amniotic sac.

HYDROCEPHALUS (hydrocephaly)
The collection of an abnormal amount of fluid in the brain, causing an enlargement of a baby's skull. It can be caused by spina bifida. Putting a small tube, called a shunt, inside the baby's head after birth will allow the fluid to be drained.

HYPERBILIRUBINEMIA (jaundice) (See BILIRUBIN and JAUNDICE)
An excess of bilirubin in the blood.

HYPEREMISIS GRAVIDARIUM (See MORNING SICKNESS)
Ongoing, extreme nausea and vomiting during pregnancy that can lead to serious dehydration in mothers. It requires medical intervention.

HYPERGLYCEMIA (See DIABETES, GESTATIONAL DIABETES, and GLUCOSE TOLERANCE TEST)
Having too much blood sugar (glucose) in the blood. Usually a sign of diabetes or gestational diabetes.

HYPERKALEMIA
Greater-than-normal levels of potassium in the blood that can be caused by the excessive vomiting of hyperemesis gravidarium.

HYPERPIGMENTATION
The darkening of skin color. During pregnancy, this is most common in the nipples and areola of the breasts, the vagina, and the area surrounding the rectum. It is thought to be a side effect of pregnancy hormones, which make the body's skin cells produce more pigment.

HYPERTENSION (See PREGNANCY INDUCED HYPERTENSION)
High blood pressure. If it occurs for the first time in the second half of pregnancy, it is called pregnancy-induced hypertension. Hypertension is a significant cause of problems in both mothers and babies, complicating about 10 percent of all pregnancies.

HYPERTHYROIDISM
Elevation of the thyroid hormone in the bloodstream.

HYPERVENTILATION
When a mother breathes too fast

and too many times per minute. It can cause symptoms of tingling, dizziness, and numbness in the hands.

HYPOTENSION
Low blood pressure. It can affect the delivery of oxygen to the baby through the placenta. Sometimes it occurs with epidural analgesia.

HYPOTHYROIDISM
Low or inadequate levels of thyroid hormone in the bloodstream.

HYPOVOLEMIA
(See HEMORRHAGE, POSTPARTUM)
Lower than normal blood volume often due to bleeding.

HYPOXIA
A lack of sufficient oxygen. A baby may suffer hypoxia during labor if his mother's blood pressure falls or his umbilical cord gets compressed.

HYSTERECTOMY, PERIPARTUM
(See HEMORRHAGE, POSTPARTUM)
The removal of the uterus. It may done during the period surrounding birth in order to save a mother's life when there is uncontrollable bleeding.

I

ICEA
Stands for a nonprofit childbirth education organization, the International Childbirth Education Association.

IDENTICAL TWINS
(monozygotic twins)
Twins formed from the division of a single egg into two separate fetuses.

IMMUNE SYSTEM
The protective system of the body that fights the invasion of what it interprets as foreign substances such as bacteria, viruses, or fungi.

IMMUNIZATION
An injection that makes the body resistant to a certain virus or bacteria, such as hepatitis or the flu. When a body is exposed to a virus, its immune system will create fighters (antibodies) to eliminate the germ. If the body is exposed again, disease-fighting cells will recognize the bug and destroy it. Vaccines are made from killed, weakened, or genetically altered forms of a virus or bacteria, which activate the immune system to protect the body should it be exposed to virus later on. (See discussion on page 256.)

INCISION
The cut made to open the body during surgery using a sharp knife (a scalpel).

INCOMPETENT CERVIX
(See CERCLAGE)
A cervix that dilates painlessly, without contractions, and may not be able to hold a baby inside.

INCOMPLETE ABORTION
(See DILATION & CURETTAGE)
A miscarriage (losing the pregnancy naturally or through medical intervention) in which part, but not all, of the uterine contents are expelled. The remaining tissue can lead to infection or bleeding and needs to be removed.

INCONTINENCE
(See STRESS INCONTINENCE and URINARY INCONTINENCE)
The body's inability to hold in urine

or feces. Sometimes incontinence is related to vaginal births, although many women who have it have never given birth.

INCUBATOR (ISOLETTE)
A small bed often made out of clear plastic for newborns that maintains an even temperature to keep the baby warm. Incubators are often used with vulnerable premature and low-birthweight babies.

INDUCTION (Induction of labor, IOL)
Using artificial means to start labor. Medical induction is the use of drugs to cause the uterus to contract. Amniotomy is a form of induction by the breaking of the bag of waters in order to trigger labor. Sweeping the membranes induces labor by stimulating the release of hormones from the cervix.

INEVITABLE ABORTION (See MISCARRIAGE)
Pregnancy complicated with bleeding and cramping in which a miscarriage, the loss of the pregnancy, cannot be prevented.

INFANTICIDE
The purposeful killing of a baby.

INFECTION
An illness caused by the invasion of bacteria, viruses, or fungi. Infections often are signaled by a fever.

INFORMED CONSENT
Being given full information about a medical procedure or medication including benefits and known risks to enable a patient to make a decision about whether or not to agree to undergo it. In some cases, a patient may be asked to sign a form to provide a record that she has been fully informed of the potential consequences of a decision. Informed consent ensures that a patient is given adequate information by a healthcare provider and to protect the healthcare provider from a potential legal action should a patient later claim she was not properly informed about the risks or side effects of procedures or medications.

INFUSION
The injection of a substance into a vein.

INHALATIONAL PNEUMONITIS
A rare and serious lung infection resulting from an unconscious patient inhaling stomach contents or acids during general anesthesia. The reason why, as a precaution, some healthcare providers feel mothers should not drink or eat during labor.

INSULIN
A hormone made by the pancreas that enables the body to use glucose in order to create energy for the body.

INTESTINAL MOTILITY
Movements of the intestines that force food from the stomach to the rectum. Increased levels of progesterone and other hormones during pregnancy can slow down the speed with which food moves through the stomach and intestines. This may contribute to nausea, vomiting, heartburn, and constipation.

INTRACRANIAL HEMORRHAGE (ICH)
Bleeding inside or on the surface of the brain. In newborns, it can be related to trauma during birth, infection, prematurity, and many other factors.

INTRAPARTUM FEVER (puerperal fever)

Fever occurring in a mother during labor and delivery. It can be caused by an infection of the lining of the uterus, the fluid surrounding the baby, a urinary tract infection, an oncoming cold, or viral or other infectious illness. It may also be caused by epidural analgesia during labor.

INTRAUTERINE GROWTH RETARDATION (IUGR, intrauterine growth restriction)

When a baby grows more slowly than normal during pregnancy.

INTRAVENOUS CATHETER (IV) (See IV)

A small needle or hollow tube (catheter) inserted into a vein in order to administer fluids or medications.

INTRAVENTRICULAR HEMORRHAGE (IVH)

Bleeding inside the brain, in the ventricles of the brain. In babies, usually related to prematurity.

IN UTERO

Within the uterus.

IN VITRO FERTILIZATION

The fertilization of an egg by a sperm conducted outside of the uterus and then implanted back into the body to grow.

INVERTED NIPPLES (flat nipples)

Normal nipples stick out from the areola, particularly when they are stimulated or become cold. Inverted nipples do not protrude out of the areola or become erect. Partially inverted nipples (dimpled or folded) will not protrude when stimulated but can be pulled out manually by the fingers, while a severely inverted nipple will retract more deeply into the areola when it is squeezed, making it level or recessed from the areola. The condition may affect a baby's latching on for breastfeeding, but correct positioning of the baby to the breast may help. (See breastfeeding positioning information on pages 240–244.)

INVOLUTION

The process of the uterus returning to its normal size after birth.

IRON DEFICIENCY ANEMIA

A common condition of pregnancy, it is produced by not getting enough iron in the diet and can be treated with iron supplements, usually pills.

ISCHIAL SPINES (See STATION)

Two bony knobs on the inside of the pelvis that are located at its narrowest point. The spines can be felt by hand and are used to gauge how far down a baby's head has moved during birth.

ISOIMMUNIZATION (See Rh FACTOR)

The development of immune fighters (antibodies) in a mother's body most commonly when she has Rh-negative blood cells and her baby has Rh-positive blood cells. It can be prevented with the administration of Rh immunoglobulin.

ISOLETTE (incubator)

A small, enclosed bassinet used for extremely premature babies to help supply them with oxygen, keep them warm, and protect them from outside germs.

IUD (intrauterine device)

A small contraceptive device made

of plastic or metal that is implanted in a woman's uterus to interfere with the passage of sperm reaching an egg. It may also discourage the implantation of a fertilized egg, if fertilization has managed to occur.

IV (Intravenous) (See INTRAVENOUS CATHETER)

Intravenous literally means "into a vein," and it is a method for providing fluid or infusing drugs into the body. Fluid is injected or dripped from a plastic bag suspended from a stand through a long tube and into a catheter inserted and taped onto the back of one hand, or along the forearm. IVs are used during labor and birth to prevent dehydration and can also be used to administer Pitocin, a drug that strengthens and increases the number of contractions. IV risks include fluid overload in the mother, or redness and swelling at the insertion site.

IV SITE (SEE IV)

The place where an IV enters the skin, usually the back of the hand or in the forearm.

J

JAUNDICE (neonatal jaundice, icterus neonatorum)

In the first few days after birth, more than half of full-term babies and about 80 percent of premature babies who are otherwise healthy develop a yellowish discoloration of their skin and the whites of their eyes, called jaundice. While some babies are jaundiced at birth, most develop it during the second or third day of life. It is not a disease, and in most cases,

means a baby's liver simply isn't mature enough to process a substance called bilirubin, which is created as the body recycles old or damaged red blood cells. It is not painful for the baby, but should the levels of bilirubin become too high (see KERNICTERUS), it can cause brain damage. Usually jaundice disappears within 1 to 2 weeks. Your healthcare practitioner may want to monitor your baby and may recommend the use of special treatment lights or sunlight to help the body break down the excess bilirubin. (See discussion on page 238.)

JPMA (Juvenile Products Manufacturers Association)

The trade organization for the makers of products for babies and young children. Products certified by the JPMA will have a sticker showing they adhere to voluntary safety standards that require testing of their product lines for safety and durability.

K

KANGAROO CARE (wearing your baby)

Modeled after how a mother kangaroo holds her baby (a joey) next to her bare chest in her pouch, it is the practice of giving babies skin-to-skin contact to help in soothing and nurturing them.

KAROTYPE

A picture of chromosomes from a cell that is enlarged and grouped for study.

KEGEL EXERCISES (Kegels)

Named after Dr. Arnold Kegel, these are a form of exercise that calls for the repeated contracting and releasing of the muscles that surround the anus and vagina and those used to stop urination. It's done to tone up the pelvic floor during pregnancy, to strengthen these muscles for childbirth, and to help control post-birth urine leaks (urinary incontinence) some mothers experience after giving birth.

KERNICTERUS (See JAUNDICE)
A rare complication of jaundice in which the base of the baby's brain and portions of the spine become invaded by excess bilirubin during the second to eighth day of life with serious consequences.

KETONES (KETOSIS)
Ketones are substances in the body produced by the body's fat processing (metabolism). Ketosis is the incomplete metabolism of fatty acids that can be caused by a lack of sufficient carbohydrates in the body or by diabetes mellitus. Ketosis can be tested in the urine.

L

LABIA
Literally means lips and refers to the two sets of skin folds that protect a woman's genitals. The outer set has pubic hair, the inner set does not.

LABOR
The act of giving birth beginning with the onset of periodic, rhythmical contractions, through the dilation of the cervix, the emergence of the baby, and the expelling of the placenta (afterbirth).

LABOR, BACK
(See BACK LABOR)

LABOR, LATENT (latent phase)
The early stage of labor that is characterized by regular contractions and slow dilation and effacement of the cervix that lasts about 8 hours for first-time mothers, but is shorter for mothers who have given birth before. Typically, it ends when the cervix is approximately 4 centimeters dilated and has reached complete (100 percent) effacement. (See centimeter chart on page 173.)

LABOR, OBSTRUCTED
When labor slows or stops, and delivery may not be achieved without medical intervention, such as a cesarean delivery.

LABORING DOWN
A medical practice that allows a mother with an epidural to hold back from pushing until she has the urge to do so, or until certain signs of readiness appear, such as the position of the baby low in her body (at least one centimeter below the ischial spines), his head rotation, and the pulling back of the mouth of the uterus (cervix) during contractions.

LABOR SUPPORT PERSON
(See DOULA)
Sometimes refers to a doula, or it can mean an inexperienced, untrained friend or relative whom you have chosen to accompany you through labor.

LACERATIONS
A laceration is any sort of tear. In pregnancy, lacerations refer to tears in the opening of the vagina that occur during birth. The seriousness

of the tear is usually expressed in degrees. A first-degree laceration is minor, involving only the superficial layers of skin. A fourth-degree laceration is the most serious, involving several layers of flesh to the rectum. It is more likely to occur with the use of episiotomies, forceps deliveries, and vacuum extractions.

LACTATION
Another word for breastfeeding or milk making.

LACTATION CONSULTANT
A person trained in advising mothers and medical personnel about breastfeeding.

LACTOSE INTOLERANCE
Some people, especially non-Caucasians, have symptoms such as bloating, diarrhea, gas, and indigestion after drinking milk or eating dairy products due to a lack of sufficient amounts of a certain digestive enzyme. (If you have this problem, note that milk is not the only source of calcium during pregnancy.)

LA LECHE LEAGUE (LLLI)
An international nonprofit organization that provides information and support for expectant and breastfeeding mothers through trained leaders and monthly in-home group meetings, state level conferences, and bi-annual international conferences. It also provides a Web site and a national, toll-free information line. (See Resources.)

LAMAZE INTERNATIONAL
An international organization to help parents preparing for childbirth. Its theories were initially developed by Dr. Ferdinand Lamaze

based on the concept that the body and breathing control could help to control the experience of pain during labor and delivery. Lamaze has moved far beyond breathing instructions. Trained instructors teach mothers and supporting partners about the processes of pregnancy, birth, and baby care, and offer a variety of relaxation techniques to help allay fear and cope with discomfort during the different stages of labor.

LAMINARIA
Small rod-shaped pieces of dried seaweed, which, when placed within the mouth of the uterus (cervix), gradually cause it to widen for birth (dilate).

L&D (or LD)
Stands for labor and delivery. An L&D nurse specializes in helping mothers during the process of labor and delivery.

LANUGO
Soft, downy hair that covers the body of a baby in the uterus. Some babies are born with the hair.

LAPAROSCOPY
The viewing of the inside of the abdomen, such as the ovaries and fallopian tubes, using a viewing instrument (laparoscope) inserted through a small incision in the belly.

LARGE FOR GESTATIONAL AGE (LGA) (See MACROSOMIA)
A newborn weighing more than 90 percent of babies that are the same gestational age—approximately $9\frac{3}{4}$ pounds or more for a full-term newborn.

LCSW (See GRIEF, STAGES OF)
Stands for licensed clinical social

worker. The skills of a social worker may be used to assist parents in planning for their baby's special needs or to help them in coping with the shock and grief of baby loss.

LDR (labor and delivery room)
Refers to the room where mothers labor and give birth in a hospital. They may then be transferred to a private or semi-private room until discharge.

LDPR (labor delivery postpartum room)
Refers to a room where mothers labor, give birth and stay until they are discharged from the hospital.

LENGTH OF STAY (LOS)
How long a patient stays in the hospital before going home. Current insurance practices usually allow a mother giving birth vaginally a 2-day stay, and those having cesarean sections, 3 to 4 days.

LEOPOLD MANEUVERS
The way a midwife or obstetrician positions his hands to tell the position of a baby inside the mother's abdomen. The baby's head will feel hard and round and will move in response to a gentle push. The baby's rump feels larger than the head and bulkier and does not move much in response to pressure. The practitioner will then press in with his hands on the sides of the abdomen to tell the direction of the baby. The back of the baby will feel smooth and hard. The front will have both soft and hard bumps that move in response to pressure. Fingers are used to locate the baby's brow to determine if the head is well flexed and how low the baby has dropped into the pelvis.

LETDOWN (let-down reflex, milk-ejection reflex)
A letdown happens when the stimulation of a baby's sucking, the action of a breast pump, or a mother's images of breastfeeding cause hormones in a mother's body to stimulate her breasts to flow milk into ducts inside the breast so it flows toward the nipple. Sometimes milk will drip from the nipples, or even spew out in a steady stream.

LEUKORRHEA
White or yellowish discharge from the vagina that does not itch.

LEVATOR ANI
The major muscle that helps to hold up a mother's pelvic floor and prevent loss of stool from the rectum.

LIE
Position of a baby during labor in relation to the mother's body. Longitudinal lie refers to a baby's body being parallel to the mother's spine. Transverse lie refers to a baby's lying crosswise.

LIGHTENING
When a baby moves lower and deeper into the pelvis in the weeks prior to the onset of labor.

LINEA NIGRA
A brownish or blackish line that runs from the top of the pubic bone to the belly button during pregnancy. It becomes more noticeable during the latter part of pregnancy.

LISTERIOSIS
A rare illness (only about four hundred cases of listeria are reported for pregnant women each

year in the United States), listeriosis is caused by bacteria that may be found in certain foods such as unpasteurized milk products, undercooked poultry, and prepared meats, including hot dogs and sandwich meats, soft cheeses, raw vegetables, and shellfish. Its symptoms are similar to the flu and can include fever, chills, headache, aches and pains, and sore throat. Samples of fluids from a mother's vagina, cervix, and blood and the baby's amniotic fluid may be checked if a provider is concerned a mother may have the disease. Listeriosis can also be transmitted during the baby's travel down the birth canal. It can lead to life-threatening blood infections and meningitis in the newborn.

LITHOTOMY POSITION
A position traditionally used in labor which places a woman on her back with her legs and feet spread apart with her knees bent. While it gives easy access for the provider to the head of the baby as it delivers, it can be an uncomfortable and ineffective position during the pushing (second) stage of labor. Patients can ask to try other positions, such as squatting or lying on the left side. (See discussion of labor positions on pages 182–184.)

LMP (also LNMP)
Stands for last menstrual period or last normal menstrual period. It's shorthand term for the way pregnancy is dated, which is from the first day of normal menstrual bleeding prior to getting pregnant.

LOBI
Stands for low-birthweight infant.

LOCAL ANESTHESIA (a local)
Any anesthetic injected to numb a small area on the body, usually lidocaine or novocaine. If a mother is given an episiotomy, she may be given a local while the incision is stitched up.

LOCHIA
Vaginal discharge after delivery. It resembles a heavy period that lasts for about six weeks after birth. (See discussion on page 222.)

LOW-BIRTHWEIGHT BABY (LOW BIRTHWEIGHT INFANT, LBWI)
A baby weighing less than 5 pounds, 8 ounces at birth. These babies have a greater chance of health problems. A very tiny, premature baby is referred to as an extremely low-birthweight baby (ELBW). (See discussion of premature delivery on pages 220–222.)

LYMPHATIC SYSTEM
A series of glands, nodes, and vessels in the body that filter a clear or milky fluid called lymph. The body uses the lymphatic system to carry waste products away from the tissues and back into general circulation for removal from the body.

M

MACROSOMIA
When a baby is larger than average (e.g., 9¾ pounds). Sometimes a very large baby is related to a mother's having diabetes or a baby's being born later than its due date. A large newborn may also result from having a large parent. Sometimes a baby's size in relation to its mother can cause problems during and after delivery.

MAGNESIUM SULFATE

A medication sometimes used in an attempt to prevent premature birth. Also used for women with preeclampsia to decrease their chance of having a seizure (eclampsia).

MAGNETIC RESONANCE IMAGING (MRI)

A diagnostic tool, an MRI can be used to obtain a closer and clearer image of the baby (or a mother) than ultrasound. The procedure is non-invasive and is similar to getting an X-ray, but it uses a magnetic field and radio waves to create an image.

MALPRESENTATION (MALPOSITION)

When a baby's head or body is in an abnormal position during birth.

MAMMARY GLANDS

Milk-producing glands of the breast.

MANA (Midwives Alliance of North America)

An organization of midwives, student/apprentice midwives, and persons supportive of midwifery that works to promote basic competency in midwives, and develops guidelines for their education. MANA offers legal, legislative, and political information and resource referrals for midwives. (See Resources.)

MANEUVERS OF LEOPOLD (See LEOPOLD MANEUVERS)

MARIJUANA (cannabis, joint, or weed)

Like alcohol and tobacco, marijuana use during pregnancy has been linked to low-birthweight and premature babies. Studies have shown that it can be associated with slow embryo growth and spontaneous abortion in the early stages of pregnancy. Symptoms such as excessive trembling and withdrawal-like irritability in newborns have also been associated with heavy marijuana use by the mother.

MASK OF PREGNANCY (See CHLOASMA)

MASTITIS

Inflammation of the breast with redness and tenderness in an area of the breast accompanied by fever, mastitis is usually caused by bacterial infection. It most often occurs to breastfeeding mothers. Sometimes there may be a discharge of pus. Treatment includes gentle massage, moist, warm compresses, nursing heavily on the affected side, and rest. In some instances, antibiotics may be recommended.

MATERNAL AND CHILD HEALTH NURSING

A field in nursing that specializes in the health of women, their partners, and their babies and children. It focuses on the problems associated with giving birth and rearing children.

MATERNAL-FETAL MEDICINE

A medical subspecialty of obstetrics that offers training in advanced fetal diagnosis, such as targeted ultrasound, skills in special surgeries, and interventions for fetuses prior to birth, such as transfusions, genetic counseling for parents, and management of severe pregnancy complications.

MATERNAL-FETAL MEDICINE SPECIALIST (MFM, perinatologist)

A fully trained medical doctor and obstetrician/gynecologist who has undergone three additional years of training in the management of special conditions during pregnancy such as high-risk pregnancies. He or she also cares for pregnant women that had medical conditions prior to their pregnancies, who develop medical or surgical problems during their pregnancies, or who carry a fetus with a problem.

MATERNAL MORTALITY RATE

The number of mothers who die during pregnancy or within 42 days after birth in the United States, expressed as the number of deaths per 100,000 live births. The cause of death must be related to or aggravated by the pregnancy or its management. The rate excludes accidental, or nonpregnancy-related causes of death. The most common causes for maternal death are hemorrhage, embolism, and pregnancy-induced hypertension (eclampsia). The overall maternal mortality rate for 2000 was 9.8 deaths per 100,000 live births. The mortality rate for African-American mothers was 22 per 100,000, or roughly three times higher than for Caucasian mothers (7.5 per 100,000).

MATERNITY NURSING (perinatal nursing)

The field of nursing that focuses on the care of childbearing women and their families during pregnancy, childbirth, and the first 4 weeks afterward.

M.D.

Medical Doctor, Doctor of Medicine.

MEATUS

The outer opening of the urethra through which urine passes.

MECONIUM

The first bowel movements of a newborn. The BM can be dark green or yellow in color and tarry in consistency; it consists of cells, mucus, and bile. Once meconium has cleared the baby's system, his bowels will become softer and turn to green, and then to yellow, custardy stools if the baby is breastfed. The appearance of heavy meconium staining during the process of birth may indicate that a baby is in distress.

MECONIUM ASPIRATION (See ASPIRATION)

MECONIUM STAINING

When meconium stains the amniotic fluid. It sometimes indicates a baby is in trouble (non-reassuring status fetal distress).

MEDICAL GENETICIST

A physician who specializes in genetic disorders.

MEMBRANES

Refers to amnion and chorion that make up the amniotic sac, which contains the fluid in which a fetus floats inside the uterus.

MENINGITIS

A serious infection of the membranes of the brain or spinal cord that can result in disability or death, especially in infants and children.

MENINGOMYELOCELE

A congenital defect of the central nervous system of the baby. The covering of the spinal cord and sometimes the spinal cord itself protrude through an opening or defect in the vertebral column.

MENSTRUAL CYCLE
The monthly change in a woman's reproductive organs as they prepare the uterus for implantation if the egg is fertilized by a man's semen. A typical cycle lasts 28 days and is counted from the first day of a woman's period to the first day of her next period. The ovaries usually release an egg approximately 2 weeks into the cycle.

MERCURY
A toxic substance that can harm an unborn baby's brain or nervous system. Found in high concentrations in certain fish, including shark, swordfish, king mackerel, or tilefish. Current recommendations include limiting the ingestion of these fish to two servings a week and taking a DHA (fish oil) supplement as an alternative source for omega-3 fatty acids thought to play a role in fetal brain development.

MFM (See MATERNAL-FETAL MEDICINE)

MICROCEPHALY
A birth defect in which the baby's brain fails to develop to a normal size.

MIDWIFE
A person with professional experience and/or training to provide health services and care for pregnant women during pregnancy, labor, and birth and immediately after birth. Midwives also assist in family planning.

MILIA
Harmless, tiny white spots on a newborn's nose, forehead, and cheeks that originate in the oil glands that disappear in the first few weeks of life. No treatment is needed.

MISCARRIAGE (spontaneous abortion)
The spontaneous loss of a pregnancy before the fetus can survive outside the uterus. Most miscarriages occur in the first trimester of pregnancy. They happen in 15 to 20 percent of all pregnancies. The causes of miscarriage are not completely known, but more than half of those that occur during the first trimester of pregnancy are caused by problems with the fetus's chromosomes. Other causes may be an infection in the uterus; the mother's hormonal imbalance; chronic disease, such as poorly controlled diabetes; or the chronic and heavy use of cigarettes, alcohol, or certain recreational drugs.

MISOPROSTOL (Cytotec)
A drug used to soften the cervix and to induce labor.

MISSED ABORTION
During the first 20 weeks of pregnancy when an embryo or fetus dies but stays in a mother's uterus for 4 weeks or more afterward. Eventually, the mother will have a heavy, long period that releases the products of the pregnancy. Some women choose to have a dilation and curettage or to take medications in order to avoid heavy bleeding by encouraging the total expulsion of the products of the pregnancy.

MM (MILLIMETERS)
A measurement of size used, for example, in measuring the embryo or fetus during sonograms. There

are 10 millimeters in a centimeter and 25.4 millimeters in an inch.

MN
Master of Nursing.

MOHEL
A person of the Jewish faith who is legally certified and religiously ordained to perform circumcisions.

MOLAR PREGNANCY (See GESTATIONAL TROPHOBLASTIC DISEASE)

MOLDING
The temporary reshaping of a baby's head in order to pass through the birth canal.

MONGOLIAN SPOTS (blue-gray macules)
A birthmark of slate-blue discolorations resembling bruises that are commonly found on the lower back of newborns, particularly those of African, Indian, Asian, or Mediterranean descent. These marks are not signs of abuse, nor are they associated with mental retardation, as some people believe. They usually, but not always, fade during the preschool years, and no treatment is required.

MONILIA (moniliasis) (See YEAST INFECTION)
A yeast infection. (See discussion on page 153.)

MONITOR
In medical terminology, a machine to record vital body signs such as heart rate, breathing, and body temperature, or the length of contractions. Monitors can also be devices used to listen to baby sounds at home (nursery monitor) or to keep tabs on baby breathing (apnea monitor).

MONITRICE
A specially trained nurse who is usually hired by a doctor, a woman, or a couple to provide support, nursing care, and assessment during labor.

MONOZYGOTIC TWINS (See IDENTICAL TWINS)
Twins conceived from the splitting of one egg into two eggs.

MONS PUBIS (hairy mound)
The hair-covered, fatty pad over the top of a woman's pubic bone.

MONTGOMERY'S TUBERCLES (Montgomery's glands)
The small, goose pimple–like gland openings that supply lubrication to the areola (dark part) of the breast and alter the pH of the skin to discourage growth of bacteria.

MORNING SICKNESS (See HYPEREMESIS GRAVIDARIUM)
Nausea and vomiting, usually occurring during the first 13 weeks of pregnancy. Although this is called morning sickness, it can strike any time during the day or night. Severe morning sickness, called hyperemesis gravidarium, when a mother can't keep down liquids or food, can cause serious dehydration and requires medical intervention. (See discussion on pages 29–30.)

MORO REFLEX
A primitive, preprogrammed reaction (reflex) seen in newborn babies, usually in response to noise or movement, such as tilting the baby's head backward. The baby will react by flinging its arms and legs wide open and will stiffen, usually followed by crying. The reflex normally disappears

spontaneously by 4 months of age. (See page 226.)

MORULA
A fertilized egg about 3 days following conception that consists of a cluster of thirteen to thirty-two cells. It moves down the fallopian tube to implant in the uterus.

MOTOR DEVELOPMENT
The way in which a baby's muscle skills become more sophisticated over time.

MOXIBUSTION
A traditional Chinese treatment to promote a baby's changing position near the time of birth from a head up (breech) position to a head down position. Herbs are burned to stimulate acupuncture points on the mother's body.

MSAFP (maternal serum alpha fetoprotein) (See ALPHA-FETOPROTEIN TEST)

MSCN (MSN)
Master of Science in Nursing.

MSD (mean sac diameter)
The size of the amniotic sac (bag of waters) that is usually measured by ultrasound during the early first trimester before the fetus is visible.

MSW
The letters after a person's name signify that he has a master's degree in social work.

MUCOUS MEMBRANES
The moist surfaces lining the vagina, rectum, mouth, nose, and throat.

MUCUS PLUG (See SHOW)
A jellylike plug that serves to seal off the neck of the uterus (cervix) during pregnancy. It is chunky and can be pinkish, white, or clear. When it is discharged, it indicates that the cervix is starting to efface (pull up and become thinner) and dilate (spread open). Usually mothers discover it within hours or days of starting labor, but sometimes labor may not start for as long as several weeks after it appears.

MULTIGRAVIDA
A person who has previously been pregnant. She may have aborted or delivered a viable baby.

MULTIPARA (multip)
A woman who has had more than one baby in the past weighing at least 500 grams or 20 weeks old, regardless of whether the baby has lived or not. Sometimes written as para II, or para III, depending upon the number of births. A grandmultipara is a woman who has delivered five or more times.

MULTIPLE PREGNANCY (multiple gestation)
When a mother is carrying more than one baby inside. Babies will initially be labeled as Twin A, Twin B, etc., depending upon which baby is anticipated to be born first.

MUTATION
A non-inherited genetic disorder that happens when an egg, sperm, or embryo undergo spontaneous changes.

MYOMETRIUM
The muscle layer of the uterus that does much of the work of labor.

N

NAEGELE'S RULE
A simple method for estimating a mother's expected due date. It

works best if the mother has regular 28-day cycles with ovulation on day 14. From the mother's first day of her last period, add 7 days, subtract 3 months, and add 1 year.

NARCOTICS

Drugs that reduce pain and anxiety by acting on the central nervous system. Common brand names are Nubain and Demerol. These drugs are sometimes used during birth, though they're not sufficiently powerful to totally eliminate pain. They are often used to "take the edge off" pain. Narcotics can be administered by mouth, as an injection, by inhalation, or through an IV. They may cross the placenta and, rarely, temporarily depress a baby's breathing after birth, which is treated by medication. Note that narcotic drugs can cause constipation, which can be very uncomfortable after birth.

NASW

National Association of Social Workers. The abbreviation after a name is used to signify that the social worker has been approved for practice by the national organization.

NATURAL ALIGNMENT PLATEAU

A period of time during labor when the cervix stops dilating although contractions continue. It often ends with a rapid dilation of the cervix.

NATURAL CHILDBIRTH (normal childbirth)

Childbirth without medical interventions, such as the use of analgesics, sedatives, or anesthesia. Mothers who choose natural childbirth rely more on personal encouragement and support during labor and birth than medical technology and obstetrical interventions. Bradley and Lamaze, for instance, are considered natural, or normal, childbirth methods. Proponents of natural birth use the term "hospital birth" to denote the opposite.

NAUSEA (See MORNING SICKNESS and HYPEREMESIS GRAVIDARIUM)

NEONATAL

Means near the time of birth—the period from the time the baby is born until it reaches 4 weeks of age. The term may also be used in titles of nurses and physicians specializing in dealing with problems of babies around the time of birth, e.g., neonatal nurses who specialize in the care of sick babies in the neonatal intensive care unit (NICU—sometimes pronounced nick´-ewe); neonatal nurse practitioners who specialize in training in the management of newborns and can perform some procedures usually done by physicians; and neonatologists, physicians who specialize in the care of premature babies and those with medical or surgical problems.

NEONATAL ABSTINENCE SYNDROME (baby drug withdrawal)

Babies whose mothers are addicted to heroin, barbiturates, amphetamines, or other drugs inherit their mothers' drug dependence. A baby may appear normal at birth but begin to show extreme irritability, constant crying, poor feeding, vomiting, diarrhea, respiratory problems, tremors, hyperactivity, and seizures within 8 to 10 hours after birth. The baby may be medicated temporarily and placed in a dim room to help her weather the withdrawal.

NEONATAL CLINICAL NURSE SPECIALIST
A registered nurse with a master's degree who is a specialist through study and supervised practice in care of newborns.

NEONATAL DEATH
Death of a live-born infant any time between birth and 28 days.

NEONATAL INTENSIVE CARE UNIT (NICU, pronounced nick´-ewe)
An intensive care unit just for newborns where babies who are born too early or have special medical needs are taken after birth. Babies in NICU may have been premature or show signs of physical problems, such as breathing problems or fever. NICUs are staffed with specialists trained to care for babies with special needs. Some hospitals also have step-down units for babies needing long-term care who are not well enough for regular nursery care.

NEONATAL MORTALITY RATIO
The number of deaths of babies prior to 28 days of life per 1,000 babies. The primary causes of neonatal mortality are prematurity, low birth weight, and birth defects. In the year 2000, the U.S. neonatal mortality rate was 4.6 per 1,000 live births.

NEONATAL NURSE PRACTITIONER (NNP)
A registered nurse with clinical expertise in the nursing care of newborns. He can conduct assessments and diagnoses and manage caseloads of newborn patients in collaboration with physicians.

NEONATE
Another word for newborn.

NEONATOLOGIST
A physician specializing in pediatrics with advanced training in the care of sick newborns. Neonatologists often head neonatal intensive care units.

NEONATOLOGY
A specialty field in medicine and nursing for the care of premature and sick newborns that have special medical needs.

NESTING INSTINCT (nesting)
Many pregnant mothers feel a strong urge to prepare for their new babies as the time to go into labor nears. A nesting mother-to-be may feel an uncharacteristic surge of energy that she spends cleaning the house or organizing things. It's important, though, to consider conserving energy for the upcoming work of giving birth.

NEURAL TUBE DEFECT (NTD) (See ANENCEPHALY, HYDROCEPHALUS, and SPINA BIFIDA)
Any of a group of birth defects related to the fetal brain and spine.

NEWBORN
Another name for a baby between birth and 1 month of age.

NFTD
Stands for normal full-term delivery.

NICOTINE
A substance found in tobacco that can be potentially harmful to the fetus.

NICU (pronounced nick'-ewe)
(See NEONATAL INTENSIVE
CARE UNIT)

NIPPLE CONFUSION
When newborns drink formula from
an artificial nipple, they may adapt
sucking patterns that interfere with
suckling at their mothers' breasts.

NIPPLES, INVERTED (See
INVERTED NIPPLES)

NONREASSURING FETAL
STATUS (fetal distress)
A term that indicates concern that a
baby is not receiving sufficient
oxygen from the placenta. The baby
may not move for a period of time
or have a slower-than-normal
heartbeat (60 to 80 beats per minute
instead of a heart rate greater than
140).

NON-STRESS TEST (NST)
A way of measuring fetal activity in
the uterus when there is a concern
that the baby may not be thriving.
An instrument strapped around a
pregnant mother's abdomen
measures the fetal heart rate. The
mother is directed to push a button
each time she feels the baby move,
which is recorded on a paper. The
fetus's heart rate is expected to rise
when the mother senses movement.

NOTOCHORD
A rod of cells that appears in the
sixth week of gestation that will
eventually become your baby's
spinal cord.

NPO (*Nil per Oram* [Latin])
Literally translated as nothing by
mouth, the term refers to a medical
order that restricts someone from
eating and drinking to protect from
vomiting and aspirating

regurgitated matter into the lungs
during general anesthesia (being
put to sleep for surgery). The policy
of preventing pregnant women
from eating and drinking during
labor is now no longer universally
accepted unless there is a problem
during labor.

NUCHAL TRANSLUCENCY
In the first 15 weeks after conception, fetal skin is very thin and
semi-transparent from the fluid that
gathers between the fetus's skin and
underlying structures. When the
baby has a chromosomal disorder,
fluid tends to be increased.
Excessive fluid is detected by
ultrasound of the baby's neck
(nuchal) area.

NULLIPARA
(nullip, nulliparous [adj.])
A woman who has never delivered a
viable baby.

NURSE-MIDWIFE
A nurse with special training and/or
certification for assisting with birth
(labor and delivery). Nurse-
midwives can perform most of the
same tasks as physicians including
delivering a baby and most have a
backup physician in the event of an
emergency requiring surgical
intervention, such as a cesarean
delivery.

NURSE PRACTITIONER
A nurse who has completed a
master's degree or post–master's
degree program in a specialty and
is certified to practice by the
appropriate professional
organization, such as obstetrics or
neonatal medicine. Nurse
practitioners can diagnose medical
conditions, treat them, prescribe

medications, and offer medical advice to families, but they do not deliver babies.

O

OB/GYN (Obstetrics & Gynecology)
Stands for obstetrics and gynecology (pronounced guy-nuh-kology).

OBSTETRIC EMERGENCY
A rare, severe, life-threatening condition related to pregnancy or delivery that requires urgent medical intervention to prevent the likely death of the mother or baby. Major signs of an obstetric emergency during pregnancy, birth, or within 6 weeks after giving birth include the following: heavy bleeding, high fever, convulsions, loss of consciousness, or severe blood loss (hemorrhage).

OBSTETRICIAN (An OB or an OB/GYN, an obstetrician gynecologist)
A physician with special training in providing medical care for women who are pregnant and giving birth. An OB can perform surgery, such as c-sections, if needed, or operative vaginal deliveries using forceps or vacuum extraction. Often, obstetricians also specialize in the reproductive health of women of all ages. In that case, they are often called by the initials of their specialty: an OB/GYN.

OBSTETRICS
(See OBSTETRICIAN)
The branch of medicine dealing with the management of pregnancy, labor, and the postpartum period (the first 42 days after birth).

OBSTRUCTED LABOR
(See DYSTOCIA)
When labor doesn't progress at a normal, steady pace. The formal, medical term is dystocia.

OLIGOHYDRAMNIOS
Abnormally low amount of fluid in the baby's amniotic sac during pregnancy.

OMPHALOCELE
A birth defect involving a failure of the abdominal wall to form at the place where the umbilical cord attaches to a baby's belly. If this occurs, the baby's intestines are usually protruding out of its belly into a sac. It can be repaired surgically after delivery.

OPERATIVE VAGINAL DELIVERY
Assisting the process of birth with the use of forceps or vacuum extraction when a mother's or baby's health is compromised during the process of labor or if the mother is having difficulty pushing the baby out. Medical terms are used to describe how deeply inside the mother forceps or vacuum extraction are applied. High or midpelvis refers to reaching into the highest point in the mother, followed by low, and outlet forceps deliveries when the baby is lower in the mother's birth canal or its scalp is already visible.

OPHTHALMIA NEONATORUM
A severe newborn eye infection of the lining of the eye and eyelids that occurs within the first 10 days of life acquired by an infection of a mother's birth canal at the time of delivery. Gonorrhea is responsible for the great majority of cases, but it can also be caused by a staph

infection, strep, and chlamydia. All states in the United States require that babies receive eye medication soon after birth to protect them from the blindness that may result from these infections.

OTITIS MEDIA
The medical name for a middle ear infection, an infection behind the eardrum.

OVARIAN CYST
A swelling of the ovary from fluid. It is most common in women after they start having periods and before they go through menopause. Most ovarian cysts are harmless.

OVARIES
The part of a woman's reproductive system that produces and releases eggs and secretes the hormones estrogen and progesterone into the bloodstream.

OVULATION
The release of an ovum (egg) from the ovary, which usually occurs around the middle of the menstrual cycle, or 14 days from beginning of the last period.

OVUM
A human egg.

OXYTOCIN (PITOCIN)
A natural, and sometimes synthetic (manmade) hormone used to artificially start labor (called induction) by making the uterus contractions stronger. Its natural form in the body causes the uterus to contract and is involved in the let-down of breastmilk.

OZ (OUNCE)
A measure of weight. There are 16 ounces in a pound.

P

PA (Physician's Assistant)
Stands for physician's assistant, a person certified to provide basic medical services under the supervision of a licensed physician.

PALPATION
To feel with the hand, as in pressing down upon or massaging a mother's belly in order to determine the baby's position.

PARACERVICAL BLOCK
Local anesthetic for the cervix (the mouth of the womb).

PARTURITION
The giving of birth. Birthing mothers are sometimes called parturients.

PATENT DUCTUS ARTERIOSUS
A heart defect in newborns in which a part of the heart, the ductus arteriosus, stays open, causing excess blood flow into the lungs and potential heart failure.

PATIENT-CONTROLLED ANALGESIA (PCA)
A mechanical pump used to allow a mother to control the administration of painkilling medication (analgesia) according to her need for pain relief. The pump regulates the amount of analgesia a mother receives over a period of time to prevent overdosing.

PCA (SEE PATIENT-CONTROLLED ANALGESIA)
Stands for patient-controlled analgesia.

PEDIATRICIAN
A physician with special training in the care of healthy and sick infants and children.

PELVIC FLOOR MUSCLES (See KEGEL EXERCISES)

A group of muscles inside the base of the pelvic bones that help to support the vagina, uterus, bladder, urethra, and rectum. These muscles also help to prevent leaking urine or bowel movements (incontinence).

PELVIMETRY (See PELVIS, CONTRACTED)

Measurements taken by a healthcare provider using hands, an X-ray, or CT scan to determine the dimensions and proportions of a pregnant woman's pelvic bones in order determine if there is adequate space for a baby to pass through during labor and delivery.

PELVIS

The basin-shaped bones at the bottom the spinal column that connect the hip bones to the body. A baby must journey through the narrowest portion of the pelvis in order to be safely born. The size and shape of the pelvis are important measurements taken prior to birth. The pelvis bones are joined by ligaments that can stretch the pelvis by as much as one-third during birth, especially when a squatting position is used or the mother is in an upright position.

PELVIS, CONTRACTED

Narrow pelvic bones in a mother that could conceivably interfere with the birth process. In severe cases, a cesarean delivery may be advised.

PERCUTANEOUS UMBILICAL BLOOD SAMPLING (PUBS)

A test for fetal problems in which blood is removed from the umbilical cord while the baby is still inside the mother's womb.

PERINATAL

The period shortly before and after birth. It is defined by various sources as beginning with the completion of the twentieth to the twenty-eighth week of pregnancy and ending anywhere between the seventh and twenty-eighth days following delivery.

PERINATAL DEATH

Death of a fetus occurring after the birth of a live baby between the time it weighs at least 500 grams, or between the twentieth and twenty-eighth completed weeks of gestation and up through the seventh to twenty-eighth day after delivery.

PERINATOLOGIST (MFM, Maternal-Fetal Medicine Specialist)

A fully trained medical doctor and obstetrician/gynecologist who has undergone three additional years of training in the management of special conditions during pregnancy such as high-risk pregnancies. He cares for pregnant women who had medical conditions prior to their pregnancies, who develop medical or surgical problems during their pregnancies, or who carry a fetus with a problem.

PERINEAL SUTURES

Stitches used to sew up tears or cuts made in a woman's perineum. (See EPISIOTOMY and discussion on page 179.)

PERINEUM

The tissues and muscular structures that surround the vagina.

P.G. (Preggo, Preggers)
Slang for being pregnant. "I'm P.G.," or "I'm preggo."

PHENYLKETONURIA (PKU)
A condition in babies found at birth in which the body lacks a specific enzyme that can lead to abnormal metabolism and, when untreated, could result in brain damage.

PHOSPHATIDYL GYLCEROL
A substance in the family of chemicals called surfactants that is present when fetal lungs are mature. If a baby's lungs are immature (prior to 38 weeks of pregnancy), surfactants may not present in sufficient quantities, which will affect a baby's ability to breathe after birth.

PHOTOTHERAPY
A treatment for babies with jaundice. These bright lights, called bililights, help babies breakdown bilirubin in their blood. Excessive levels of bilirubin are the cause of neonatal jaundice.

PHYSIOLOGIC ANEMIA OF PREGNANCY (See ANEMIA)
Anemia during pregnancy caused by an increase in the amount of plasma (fluid) in the blood compared with the number of cells in the blood.

P.I.
Stands for premature infant.

PICA (pronounced pye-ka)
The strong urge by some pregnant women to eat nonfood items such as clay, ice, laundry starch, cornstarch, plaster, or dirt. It is thought to be related to anemia.

PITOCIN (See OXYTOCIN)
A synthetic form of oxytocin.

PITUITARY GLAND (See SHEEHAN'S SYNDROME)
A gland located in the center of the front of the brain that produces a variety of hormones that have many jobs, including signaling the breasts to produce milk in a mother. A mother's pituitary gland may be affected by hemorrhage.

PLACENTA (See AFTERBIRTH)
A red, round fleshy organ resembling a large piece of liver about 6 to 7 inches in diameter at birth. It forms and grows alongside the baby inside and is fastened to the side of one wall of the uterus with tiny, fingerlike projections called villi. The placenta extracts oxygen and nutrition from the mother's blood and transfers it to the fetus's blood. The expelling of the placenta after a baby is born is known as the third stage of labor.

PLACENTA ACCRETA
When the placenta slightly invades the muscles of the uterus during pregnancy, making it difficult to remove after birth. Sometimes with this condition, the placenta will not separate, and a removal of the uterus is necessary after delivery of the baby in order to stop the mother from bleeding.

PLACENTA INCRETA (See PLACENTA ACCRETA)
When the villi of the placenta penetrate deep into uterine muscles.

PLACENTAL ABRUPTION (placenta abruption)
When the placenta separates from the uterus wall prior to the delivery of the baby.

PLACENTAMEGALY
When the placenta undergoes

abnormally large growth during pregnancy.

PLACENTA PERCRETA
(See PLACENTA ACCRETA)
When the villi of the placenta penetrate completely through uterine muscles.

PLACENTA PREVIA
When the placenta is abnormally positioned over the mouth of the uterus (cervix), it can result in serious bleeding during mid- or late pregnancy. Even though placenta previa may be noted on an ultrasound during the first two trimesters of pregnancy, it may not actually cover the cervix by the time labor begins. If it doesn't move out of the way, a cesarean delivery may be necessary.

PNEUMONITIS, INHALATIONAL
(See INHALATIONAL
PNEUMONITIS)

POLYCYTHEMIA
When a newborn's red blood cell count (hematocrit) reaches such a mass that the blood is too thick to flow through her body. In newborns it may be associated with low blood sugar, sluggishness, poor feeding, jitteriness, possibly seizures, respiratory distress, and blood clots. The baby's blood may be thinned through a special transfusion. Potential causes are intrauterine growth restriction, a mother's diabetes mellitus, asphyxia, some medications taken by mothers, smoking, and pregnancy at a high altitude. The blood condition can result in neonatal jaundice.

POLYDACTYLY
When a baby is born with extra fingers or toes.

POLYHYDRAMNIOS
An excessive amount of amniotic fluid during pregnancy.

POLYP
A small growth of tissue in the lining of the uterus or the intestines. It is usually harmless during pregnancy.

PORT WINE STAIN
A birthmark that appears as a patch of reddish-blue skin. Your healthcare provider should evaluate it since it is sometimes associated with genetic problems.

POSITIONAL APNEA
Refers to interrupted breathing that may occur in a premature or low-birthweight baby as the result of being placed in a sharply angled, nearly upright position, such as that provided by a rear-facing infant seat. If a baby is suspected of having positional apnea, a healthcare practitioner may suggest ways to pad the car seat or recommend that a flat infant bed be used that is designed specifically for restraining a small baby in a fully reclined position while riding in the car.

POSTDATE PREGNANCY
(See POSTTERM PREGNANCY)
A pregnancy that lasts longer than 42 weeks of gestation.

POSTDURAL HEADACHE
(spinal headache)
A headache that results when the needle used to place an epidural catheter for epidural analgesia accidentally punctures the covering of the spinal cord, causing seepage of spinal fluid into the epidural space. It is less common due to the increased sophistication of the procedure

including the use of better needles for the injection of painkilling liquid into the epidural space (the space outside the sac that covers the spinal cord).

POSTERIOR PRESENTATION (occiput posterior)
When the back of the head of the baby presses on the back of the mother. A baby's being in this position can play a part in back labor and may make it more difficult for the mother to push the baby out.

POSTMATURE PREGNANCY
A pregnancy that lasts longer than 42 weeks.

POSTNATAL PERIOD
The time following delivery, usually between birth and 10 to 28 days, when mothers and babies are carefully watched for complications.

POSTPARTUM
After delivery.

POSTPARTUM DEPRESSION (PPD)
PPD can set in any time during the year after a baby is born. It affects 10 to 15 percent of new mothers and is more serious and prolonged than baby blues. It requires professional help.

POSTPARTUM ENDOMETRITIS (See INTRAPARTUM FEVER)
Swelling and infection in the inner layer of the uterus following birth. Its symptoms are a fever, a uterus that is tender to the touch, discharge from the vagina that is foul-smelling, and a change in blood cells due to infection. It is treated with a strong course of antibiotics. The infection occurs in approximately 1 to 3 percent of women who have given birth

vaginally and between 10 and 30 percent of women following cesarean sections. It remains one of the leading causes of death from cesarean section, although the aggressive use of antibiotics has made that occurrence extremely rare.

POSTPARTUM HEMORRHAGE (See HEMORRHAGE, POSTPARTUM)

POSTPARTUM PSYCHOSIS
Mental illness that is precipitated by pregnancy and birth. It is rare and affects approximately 0.1 percent of new mothers (or about one out of one thousand women). It can happen any time during the first year after childbirth and is marked by a break with reality that resembles bipolar disorder. Symptoms may include hallucinations (seeing things that aren't there) and delusions (believing things that aren't true). Professional intervention is needed.

POSTPARTUM THYROIDITIS
Fluctuating thyroid function after childbirth. Symptoms may include fatigue, anxiety, emotional ups and downs, and feelings of weakness and tiredness. It is not usually associated with a painful or tender thyroid gland, which is located in the center of the neck.

POST-TERM GESTATION (See POST-TERM PREGNANCY)

POST-TERM PREGNANCY (post-mature pregnancy, post-term gestation)
A pregnancy that lasts beyond 42 weeks from the first day of the mother's last period. About 95 percent of babies born after 42 weeks are normal, though the risk

of a poor pregnancy outcome increases the longer a woman's pregnancy extends beyond this time. Between 3 and 12 percent of all pregnancies last beyond the forty-second week of gestation, or 294 days. Many cases of post-term pregnancy are simply the result of inaccurate estimations about a baby's age, but when pregnancy is prolonged, labor may be induced.

POST-TRAUMATIC BIRTH DISORDER (post-traumatic stress disorder)
Severe emotional turmoil following birth experienced by some women whose births were complicated or who have perceived that mistakes were made during their deliveries. It is more common in women who had previous emotional vulnerabilities prior to giving birth, such as a history of emotional, physical, or sexual abuse. Symptoms include feelings of panic when nearing the place where the birth occurred; obsessive thoughts about the birth; feelings of numbness and detachment; disturbing memories of the birth experience; nightmares; flashbacks; and unexplainable sadness, fearfulness, anxiety, or irritability.

PRECIPITOUS BIRTH
Labor and delivery that lasts less than 3 hours.

PREECLAMPSIA (toxemia) (See ECLAMPSIA)
A complication of pregnancy that occurs after the 20th week of pregnancy. Sometimes it can be silent with no outward symptoms, but a mother will have protein in her urine and high blood pressure. Physical symptoms include rapid weight gain and swelling in fingers, face, and ankles from fluid retention. A mother may also experience odd vision problems such as blurring or headaches. The causes of preeclampsia are not completely understood, but poor nutrition and genetic predisposition are thought to be contributors. Preeclampsia (toxemia) left untreated can turn into seizures (eclampsia) and could lead to coma and possibly death.

PREGNANCY GINGIVITIS
Pregnant women often have swollen red gums that are tender to the touch and bleed easily. This condition is thought to be caused by hormonal changes in the body plus the buildup of a bacterial film on the teeth. Swelling generally starts during the second month of pregnancy and reaches a peak during the last month and a half before birth. The condition can last from 3 to 6 months after delivery and can be mild or severe depending upon the condition of gums prior to pregnancy. Effective dental hygiene, including frequent brushing and flossing, and having the teeth cleaned, is thought to be an important treatment for the condition.

PREGNANCY-INDUCED HYPERTENSION (PIH)
A condition of pregnancy marked by high blood pressure that occurs after 20 weeks of pregnancy.

PREMATURE BABY (PREEMIE)
A baby that comes early, that is, one that is born before 37 weeks of gestation.

PREMATURE LABOR (See PRETERM LABOR)

PREMATURE RUPTURE OF MEMBRANES (PROM) (See AMNIOTOMY)

When the bag of waters ruptures prior to going into labor so that fluid drains from the vagina. Often labor soon ensues after this happens, but if it doesn't, there is a risk of complications or infection that may be controlled using antibiotics and delivery of the baby.

PRENATAL

Means before birth. Prenatal checkups refer to a mother getting regular exams throughout her pregnancy.

PRENATAL CARE

Medical care during pregnancy that includes assessing a mother's risk and interventions to help reduce the risk of a poor pregnancy outcome.

PREPUCE

The foreskin, the fold of skin that naturally covers the tip (glans) of the penis. Circumcision surgically removes it.

PRESENTATION

The part of the baby that will deliver first. Cephalic presentation is head first; breech presentation is the buttocks or leg.

PRESENTING PART

The part of the baby's anatomy that delivers first, usually the skull, but it could be an arm, or the buttocks or a leg in a breech presentation.

PRETERM BABY
(premature baby)

A baby born before 37 weeks of pregnancy, regardless of weight.

PRETERM DELIVERY
(PTD, preterm birth)

Delivery of a baby prior to 37 weeks of completed pregnancy that happens in 5 to 16 percent of all deliveries. Currently, PTD can rarely be predicted, prevented, or effectively treated. Some factors thought to contribute to preterm delivery include infection, abnormalities in the baby or uterus, problems with the placenta, bleeding caused by pregnancy, multiple gestation (twins, etc.), premature rupture of the amniotic sac (bag of waters), and hydramnios (too much fluid in the amniotic sac). But in one-third to one-half of the cases, there is no known cause for PTD.

PRETERM LABOR

Labor that happens after 20 weeks of pregnancy, but before the end of the thirty-seventh week. It includes regular contractions occurring at intervals 10 minutes apart or less for at least an hour, accompanied by changes in the cervix.

PRICKLY HEAT (See HEAT RASH)

PRIMAGRAVIDA
(pronounced pry-me-grav-ida)

A woman who is pregnant for the first time.

PRIMIPARA (PRIMIP, PRIMY)

A woman who has given birth for the first time to a baby or babies, alive or dead, weighing at least 500 grams from a pregnancy that has lasted at least 20 weeks.

PRODROMAL LABOR
(false labor)

Another term for Braxton-Hicks contractions or any contractions that happen before actual labor sets in. Sometimes it is called false labor, though it is a legitimate form of preparation that the uterus goes through prior to giving birth. (See discussion on page 95.)

PROGESTERONE
A hormone that keeps the uterus from contracting and promotes the growth of blood vessels in the wall of the uterus.

PROGNOSIS
A prediction about the course of a disease and its outcome. A poor prognosis means that a mother, or baby, may not be expected to do well (or survive).

PROLACTIN
A hormone that is involved in the production of breastmilk. Called the mothering hormone, prolactin together with oxytocin are thought to be partly responsible for the strong feelings of attachment that mothers have toward their babies. During pregnancy, prolactin speeds the growth of breast tissues in preparation for breastfeeding.

PROLAPSED CORD (prolapse)
When a loop of a baby's umbilical cord slips down below the body and into the birth canal during birth.

PROLONGED LABOR
A labor lasting more than 18 to 24 hours.

PROLONGED PREGNANCY
A pregnancy that lasts longer than 40 weeks of gestation.

PROMETHAZINE
An antihistamine given by injection, often with a narcotic, to counteract nausea and relieve pain during the early stages of labor.

PROSTAGLANDINS (PGE-2)
A hormone sometimes used as a drug to ripen and soften an unready cervix in order to induce labor. It is not recommended for use with mothers who have certain forms of heart disease or severe asthma.

PROTEIN
Proteins are chains of amino acids that are required to repair and build the body tissue especially needed for fetal growth. Common sources of protein for pregnancy are milk, eggs, cheese, fish, meat, beans, tofu, and some vegetables. (See dietary recommendations on pages 160–161.)

PROTEINURIA
When protein is found in the urine. Sometimes a sign of preeclampsia.

**PROTRACTED LABOR
(See LABOR, OBSTRUCTED)**
A labor that lasts longer than expected.

PRURITIS GRAVIDARIUM
Itching during pregnancy.

PUBIC SYMPHYSIS
The front part of the pelvis. The bony ridge at the top of the pubic symphysis is used for measuring the growth of the uterus up into the abdominal area.

PUBOCOCCYGEUS MUSCLE (PC)
One of the muscles of the pelvic floor. This muscle is tightened when doing Kegel exercises.

PUDENDAL BLOCK
A type of pain relief frequently used just prior to delivery. It is injected through the walls of the vagina to numb the vaginal area.

**PUERPERAL FEVER
(See PUERPERAL SEPSIS)**

PUERPERAL SEPSIS (puerperal fever, puerperal infection) (See INTRAPARTUM FEVER)

A maternal infection around the time of childbirth that can be a cause of maternal death if it is not treated in time.

PUERPERIUM

A period of time following delivery that lasts about 6 to 8 weeks when a mother's reproductive organs and body gradually return to the prepregnancy state. The uterus undergoes involution, a remarkable reduction in size. There is also a discharge of blood and other fluids, called lochia, for 4 to 6 weeks following pregnancy.

Q

QUICKENING

The moment a mother first feels her baby move. The sensation is similar to a slight flutter or gas bubbles in the belly. While ultrasound can often pick up fetal movement around the eighth week of menstrual age, most mothers don't detect it until about the eighteenth to the twenty-second week. If the placenta has attached to the front of the uterus, a mother may not experience a baby's movement until the fetus is larger.

R

RDS (See RESPIRATORY DISTRESS SYNDROME)

RECALL

Baby products routinely undergo federally mandated recalls or corrective actions when serious safety flaws are discovered. Unsafe products may be removed from the marketplace, or they may simply be furnished with new components to make them safer. Cribs, strollers, toys, and other baby products are recalled by the U.S. Consumer Product Safety Commission (CPSC), car seats by the National Highway Traffic Safety Administration (NHTSA), and baby formula and cosmetics by the Food and Drug Administration (FDA). (See Resources, and discussion on pages 276–280.)

RECESSIVE DISORDER

A genetic disorder that is transmitted to a child when both parents are carriers of defective genes.

RECTUM

Lower part of the large intestine about 5 inches (12.7 cm) in length that connects from the colon to the anus, the outward opening for bowel movements.

RECTUS ABDOMINUS (See DIASTASIS RECTI)

The two muscles that run parallel to one another down the front of the abdominal wall, on each side of the belly button to the pubic bone. During pregnancy, the muscles and the tissues that connect them stretch to accommodate a mother's expanding belly, sometimes causing the muscles to draw apart.

RECURRENT ABORTION

When a mother has lost two or more babies to miscarriages.

RED BLOOD CELLS

Cells in the blood that carry oxygen and carbon dioxide to and from the tissues of the body.

REGIONAL ANESTHESIA
Numbing of just the lower part of a mother's body during labor, in contrast to general anesthesia, which puts the mother totally to sleep.

RELAXIN
A hormone produced by a pregnant mother's ovaries and uterus during the latter months of pregnancy. It is thought to play a part in the loosening of the ligaments holding the joints together and may play a part in the ability of the pelvic bones to expand during birth.

RESIDENT
A physician who has completed an M.D. degree and is in the process of training in a specialty under the supervision of experienced specialists, such as obstetricians or pediatricians.

RESPIRATORY DEPRESSION
Slowed or shallow breathing that can be caused by medications that a mother is taking. It may occur temporarily when a mother hyperventilates (breathes too fast) during birth.

RESPIRATORY DISTRESS SYNDROME (RDS, hyaline membrane disease)
A lung condition occurring in some premature babies when their lungs don't completely expand or expand imperfectly. It can be caused by the lack of a surfactant in the airway. Treatments include giving the baby oxygen and administering a surfactant.

RETAINED PLACENTA
When the placenta (afterbirth) remains in the uterus for 30 minutes or more after birth. Action is usually taken to remove the placenta at that time to help lower the risk of infection and heavy bleeding (hemorrhage).

RETINOPATHY OF PREMATURITY
(ROP, retrolental fibroplasia)
An eye condition that can develop in very premature newborns. In milder cases, a premature baby's eyes will recover, but if the baby is very immature, the blood vessels within the retina may not have had adequate time to grow, and the baby may be visually impaired or blind.

RETRACTION
The unique muscle process in the uterus by which its muscle fibers shorten after each contraction.

RETROLENTAL FIBROPLASIA
(See RETINOPATHY OF PREMATURITY)

RETROVERTED UTERUS
(tipped uterus, tilted uterus)
Normally the uterus is suspended in a straight up-and-down position, or it tips slightly forward toward the abdomen. A retroverted uterus tips or tilts backward, pointing toward the spine. The condition is usually inherited, but pregnancy can also cause the uterus to tilt backward when the ligaments holding the uterus stretch or relax. In most cases, the uterus will return to a forward-facing position after childbirth. The condition can sometimes result in painful sex.

RHESUS ANTI-D GAMMA GLOBULIN INJECTION
(Rh IMMUNOGLOBULIN [RhIg], RhoGAM)
An injection given to Rh-negative pregnant woman at 28 weeks of

pregnancy, or at the time of an amniocentesis, to prevent the development of antibodies that could be harmful to the baby. If the baby is Rh-positive, the injection will be given again within 72 hours following birth.

Rh FACTOR (Rh blood factor)
A protein found in the blood serum. If a mother has this substance, she is considered Rh-positive; if she does not have it, she is Rh-negative. (Rh stands for rhesus.) An Rh-negative mother carrying an Rh-positive baby may produce antibodies against the fetus that attack the fetus's blood. Rh incompatibility requires special care during pregnancy. (See discussion on page 140.)

Rh IMMUNOGLOBULIN (RhIg) (See RHESUS ANTI-D GAMMA GLOBULIN INJECTION)

RhoGAM (See RHESUS ANTI-D GAMMA GLOBULIN INJECTION)

RINGER'S LACTATE SOLUTION
A special salt solution used in an IV (intravenous tube) designed to replace the body's fluid loss. Its main ingredients are sodium, potassium, and calcium balanced with chloride and lactate.

ROOTING
Instinctive head and mouth movements of a baby (reflexes) that help him in finding his mother's nipple. A baby will turn his head toward the nipple, open his mouth, and extend his tongue to enclose the nipple for nursing.

ROUND-LIGAMENT PAIN
Pain caused by ligaments stretching on the sides of the uterus during pregnancy.

RSV (Respiratory Syncytial Virus)
RSV infects nearly all children by the time they reach age 2. It usually causes mild coldlike symptoms, but in premature babies with vulnerable lungs, the infection can be serious and potentially fatal. Babies are more at risk of catching RSV if they are in child care, have school-age siblings, or are exposed to tobacco smoke.

RUBELLA (German measles, 3-day measles)
A highly contagious form of measles causing a red rash that is usually mild, which can cause severe damage to a fetus if contracted during the early months of pregnancy.

RUPTURE OF MEMBRANES (breaking of waters, amniotomy) (See ARTIFICIAL RUPTURE OF MEMBRANES)
The membranes make up the amniotic sac, the tissue-like balloon where the fetus floats inside the uterus during pregnancy. It will rupture naturally during the process of labor, or sometimes earlier, or it may be intentionally ruptured to start labor. If the waters rupture and labor doesn't start right away, the baby's umbilical cord could come out first, cutting off his oxygen supply. Also, mother and baby may be more vulnerable to infection.

RVC (rectal/vaginal culture) (See GROUP B STREPTOCOCCUS)
A test to determine if a mother is carrying Group B Strep during pregnancy or labor.

S

SAC (See AMNIOTIC SAC and MEMBRANES)

SCAN (See ULTRASOUND)
Another term for an ultrasound examination or a sonogram. (See discussion on pages 149–150.)

SCIATIC NERVE
The largest nerve in the body, it is the diameter of the little finger. It runs from the spinal column down the legs and provides sensation and movement to the back of the thighs, the lower parts of the leg, and the soles of the feet.

SCIATICA (pinched nerve) (See SCIATIC NERVE)
During pregnancy, pressure from the baby or inflammation to the sciatic nerve can cause pain, burning, tingling, numbness, or electric shock–like shooting sensations that follow the path of the nerve. The mother's changing positions, such as lying on the opposite side from the pain, doing gentle stretching exercises, or elevating one leg can sometimes bring relief.

SCM (State Certified Midwife)

SDMS
Member of the Society of Diagnostic Medical Sonographers, persons trained to perform ultrasound tests.

SEMEN
White fluid containing sperm from a man's penis that fertilize an egg (ovum), which causes pregnancy. Semen is ejaculated (spewed out) during sex.

SEPSIS
The presence of infection in the blood.

SEXUALLY TRANSMITTED DISEASE (STD)
An infection transmitted primarily through sexual contact between a man and a woman. Syphilis and gonorrhea are two STDs that can seriously harm unborn babies.

SHEEHAN'S SYNDROME (postpartum pituitary necrosis)
When a mother's pituitary gland dies as the result of severe bleeding (hemorrhage) following childbirth. Symptoms are a cessation of periods, shrinking of the genitals, and premature aging.

SHOULDER DYSTOCIA
When a baby's shoulders become entrapped in the bones of the mother's pelvis following the delivery of his head. It is rare and can be life-threatening for the baby.

SHOW (bloody show)
A discharge from the vagina of a jellylike mucus plug that serves to seal off the neck of the uterus (cervix) during pregnancy. It is chunky and can be pinkish, white, or clear. Show indicates that the cervix is starting to efface (get thinner) and dilate (open). Usually mothers discover show within hours or days of starting labor, but sometimes labor may not begin for as long as several weeks after it appears.

SICKLE-CELL ANEMIA
A genetic disorder that occurs in families of African descent that causes red blood cells to be crescent shaped, rather than round, and to clump in small capillaries so that the body has trouble getting adequate oxygen from the blood. The result is anemia, fatigue,

delayed growth, and development and episodes of severe, debilitating pain.

SICKLE-CELL TRAIT
A disorder in which a mother carries the trait of sickle-cell anemia, but her red blood cells have a normal lifespan. Presence of the trait for sickle-cell anemia is not sickle-cell disease itself.

SKIN-TO-SKIN CONTACT
Allowing a newborn to lie chest-to-chest on her mother's body in order to help with mother/baby bonding, breastfeeding, and maintaining the baby's body temperature.

SLEEP APNEA (Obstructive Sleep Apnea– OSA) (See also APNEA and POSITIONAL APNEA)
Some pregnant women develop breathing problems as the result of physical changes during pregnancy, such as changes in the upper airway, increased nasal congestion, and pressure from the baby on the mother's lower chest. Symptoms can be breathing irregularity, snoring and restlessness during sleep, and exhaustion after awakening. Treatment includes adequate hydration, nasal strips, adopting a semi-upright position, and, for serious cases, the use of a mask attached to a ventilation machine to offer a continuous air supply. Some premature babies also suffer from sleep apnea.

SLIUP (SINGLE LIVING INTRAUTERINE PREGNANCY)
A single, live pregnancy in the womb.

SMALL FOR GESTATIONAL AGE (SGA)
A newborn that is less than the smallest 10 percent of babies of a similar gestational age. It may mean that the baby is not growing as well as it should, that a mother's due date hasn't been calculated accurately, or simply that a baby is taking after his small parents.

SMEGMA
A white, curdlike substance that forms under the folds of an uncircumcised boy's foreskin and in the folds of a girl's vagina. It serves to moisturize and lubricate delicate genital tissues. Smegma has antibacterial and antiviral properties to protect from infection, so there is no need to try to wash or wipe it off.

SMFM
An abbreviation for the organization Society of Maternal-Fetal Medicine.

SONOGRAM (See ULTRASOUND)
An ultrasound image of your baby inside your uterus. (See discussion on pages 149–150.)

SONOGRAPHER (ultrasound technologist, scanner)
The person who performs an ultrasound (sonogram) examination.

SONOLOGIST
A physician specifically trained to perform ultrasound examinations and to interpret their findings.

SPECULUM
A plastic or metal device used to spread a woman's vaginal opening in order to make viewing the mouth of the womb (cervix) easier.

SPIDER VEINS (spider nevi, telangiectasias, angioma)
Small red or blue blood vessels that

appear close to the surface of the skin during pregnancy. They resemble the branching pattern of a tree or a spider web with short jagged lines and appear on the nose or cheeks, or sometimes on the back, chest, or arms. They usually disappear by 6 weeks after delivery.

SPINA BIFIDA
A defect in the spine of a fetus that results in the failure of the vertebra to fuse. It can occur anywhere along the spine, but most often the condition happens at the base of the back or lower spine. In some cases, folic acid deficiencies in the mother can result in this condition.

SPINAL ANESTHESIA (spinal block) (See EPIDURAL)
A spinal block is similar to an epidural. An anesthetic injected into the spaces surrounding the spinal cord to numb the lower half of the body. After the numbing medicine is put in the mother's back, an anesthetic medicine is injected; however, the tube is not left in place as in an epidural. The spinal lasts for a limited time, and it is usually done shortly before birth. Sometimes it may cause a mother's blood pressure to drop, and this may be treated with intravenous (IV) fluids and medication.

SPINAL HEADACHE (See BLOOD PATCH)

SPONTANEOUS ABORTION
Another name for miscarriage, the loss of a baby during the first 20 weeks of pregnancy.

SPONTANEOUS LABOR
Labor that starts on its own without the use of medical augmentation, such as drugs that cause the uterus to contract (induction) or the artificial rupture of the membranes.

SPONTANEOUS MISCARRIAGE (spontaneous abortion)
When the body discharges a baby before the baby is ready to be born.

STAGES OF LABOR
Labor is divided into three stages. The first stage is from the onset of labor until the cervix, the mouth of the uterus, is completely thinned (effaced) and stretched open (dilated). The second stage is the pushing stage, during which the baby is ejected from the uterus. It lasts from full dilation of the cervix until the baby is born. The third stage lasts from the birth of the baby until the placenta and membranes have been expelled. (Stages of labor are discussed starting on page 171.)

STATION
The location of a birthing baby's head in relation to the ischial spines, small bony knobs inside the pelvis. The location of the baby's presenting part is measured in centimeters. A baby above the ischial spines is said to be at a minus station using numbers to indicate the exact location (–3, –2, –1). The baby is said to be at the 0 (zero) station if the presenting part is level with the spines. Positive numbers (+1, +2, +3) indicate that the baby's head is below the ischial spines and therefore closer to being born.

STEM CELLS
A basic blood cell, or mother cell, found in a baby's umbilical cord blood that can reproduce and give rise to different blood cell lines of

distinct characteristics and appearance. Cord blood stem cells make red blood cells for carrying oxygen, white blood cells for fighting infections, and platelets for clotting blood. Stem cells have been used experimentally to help in treating patients with leukemia and other blood disorders.

STEP-DOWN NURSERY
Where babies are sometimes sent after being discharged from the neonatal intensive care unit (NICU), but before they are moved to a standard nursery. The care in a step-down nursery is less intensive than in the NICU, but more specialized than nurseries for healthy newborns.

STILLBIRTH (intrauterine death, intrauterine stillbirth, intrapartum death, or intrapartum stillbirth)
When a baby dies inside its mother or during the process of being born. The exact cause of a baby's dying is often difficult to pinpoint, although research shows that stillbirth happens more often in pregnancies with multiple babies, to mothers who smoke, to those with previous cesarean sections, and to those who are over 35 years of age. (See discussion on page 146.)

STILLBORN (STILLB.)
Born dead.

STORK BITE
A red birthmark that is flat and whitens on touch. It usually appears on the back of the neck, but can also appear on the face. The mark may gradually fade, or it may be permanent but only show up when a person blushes, becomes excited, or gets hot.

STRAWBERRY MARK (nevus vaculosus)
A raised red birthmark with a rough surface that may be present at birth or not appear until days or weeks later. The mark usually goes away on its own, but if constant chafing irritates it, surgical removal may be recommended.

STREPTOCOCCUS, GROUP B (See GROUP-B STREPTOCOCCUS)

STRESS INCONTINENCE
Being unable to hold in urine (urinary incontinence) or bowel movements (fecal incontinence) when sneezing or coughing. Pelvic floor exercises (Kegel exercises) can sometimes help to alleviate this problem. Some mothers may experience these conditions after forceps or a vacuum delivery. The condition may be temporary, or surgery may be required to correct it.

STRETCH MARKS (STRIAE)
Areas of the skin that are stretched by rapid weight gain during pregnancy often found on the abdomen, breasts, buttocks, and legs. They resemble rippled stripes that are lighter than normal skin, and usually disappear after pregnancy.

SUDDEN INFANT DEATH SYNDROME (SIDS, pronounced sids, like kids)
A sudden, unexplained death of a baby less than one year of age, and the leading cause of death in babies after 1 month of age. Most deaths occur between 2 and 4 months of age, and more happen in colder months. Babies placed to sleep on

their stomachs are much more likely to die than those placed on their backs. African-American babies are twice as likely to die of SIDS than white babies, and Native-American babies nearly three times more likely to die from it. The U.S. Consumer Product Safety Commission recommends that all babies be placed on their backs for sleep. (See SIDS warning on page 233.)

SUPINE HYPOTENSION (supine hypotensive syndrome)
When the pressure of the pregnant uterus compresses a large blood vessel, the inferior vena cava, impeding the return of blood to the heart, which results in a drop in blood pressure (hypotension), a speeding up of the heart rate (tachycardia), and, possibly, fainting. A mother's upper body should always be kept at a raised angle, or she should be placed on her left side to allow the weight of the uterus to move away from the great vein.

SURFACTANT
A slippery substance covering the inner lining of the air sacs inside the lungs so they can expand normally during breathing. Premature babies may need to be given a surfactant to enable their lungs to function.

SWEEPING OF THE MEMBRANES
Inserting a gloved finger up into the rim of a mother's cervix in order to free the baby's membranes from their attachment at the rim of cervix. It is used to encourage the onset of labor. The procedure can be painful and cause minor bleeding.

SYMPHYSIS PUBIC DYSFUNCTION (SPD)
Pain in the pubic area during pregnancy or following birth caused by a misalignment of the pelvis or gaps in the alignment of the front pubic bones caused by their stretching apart during pregnancy or after birth. Diastasis symphysis pubis (DSP) is the name for the problem in its most severe form when the bones of the pelvis actually separate or tear apart. Lifting one leg at a time or parting the legs can be extremely painful and interfere with putting on clothes, getting out of a car, climbing stairs, and other everyday activities. Using pillows and supports and gentle stretching exercises using an exercise ball may be of some help.

SYNDACTYLY (syndactylism)
When a baby is born with webbed fingers or toes.

SYPHILIS
A sexually transmitted disease (STD) that can affect an unborn baby.

SYSTOLIC BLOOD PRESSURE (See BLOOD PRESSURE)
The first number in a blood pressure reading, it is the highest blood pressure produced by the contraction of your heart.

T

TACHYCARDIA
Rapid heartbeat. For an unborn baby, that can mean 160 bpm (beats per minute) or more. Causes include oxygen starvation (hypoxia), maternal fever, maternal

hyperthyroidism (hyperactive thyroid), and certain drugs that affect the nervous system.

TACHYPNIA
(transient tachypnia)
Abnormally fast breathing.

TALIPES (CLUBFOOT)
A foot deformity that affects babies in 1 out of 1,000 births and is more common in boys than girls. The baby's foot is held in a drawn-up, turned-in position that will require orthopedic correction at some point. Positional clubfoot is when a newborn's feet are turned inward because of pressure inside the uterus. It goes away without treatment.

TAY-SACHS DISEASE
One of a series of inherited genetic disorders common among Ashkenazi Jews. The enzyme needed to break down certain lipid fats is absent, resulting in physical and mental retardation, enlargement of the head, and eventually death.

TENS (Transcutaneous Electrical Nerve Stimulation)
A device that applies low-level electrical stimulation to the nerves in a mother's back that can help to mask her sensation of pain.

TERATOGEN
A drug or agent that can cause abnormal fetal development or physical deformities when a woman is exposed to it during pregnancy.

TERATOLOGY
The study of the effects that drugs, medications, chemicals, and other exposures may have on babies during pregnancy. A drug will be termed teratogenic if it is known to cause changes in a baby's body during pregnancy.

TERBUTALINE SULFATE
(Brethine)
An asthma medication sometimes used to slow down or stop labor contractions during preterm labor by relaxing the smooth muscles of the body (the uterus contains smooth muscle).

TERM (See FULL TERM)
The length of pregnancy, usually measured in weeks.

TERMINATION
Another word for abortion, or the purposeful ending of a pregnancy, perhaps because of detected abnormalities.

THALASSEMIA
Group of inherited disorders of hemoglobin formation, which result in a decrease in the amount of hemoglobin formed. This can cause severe anemia and require blood transfusions.

THREATENED ABORTION
When symptoms show that a pregnancy may not be able to continue because of bleeding or other problems. A threatened abortion may go on to become a miscarriage (spontaneous abortion).

THROMBOPHLEBITIS
(thrombosis) (See EMBOLISM)
Inflammation of a vein associated with a blood clot (thrombus).

THRUSH
Monilial or yeast infection occurring in the mouth or mucous membranes of a newborn infant. It appears as milky, white patches on a baby's tongue that cannot be wiped off.

TLC (tender loving care)
Refers to giving babies gentle, loving attention. Example: "All babies need lots of TLC."

TOCOLYSIS (See TOCOLYTICS)
When contractions are stopped during premature labor with the use of medication.

TOCOLYTICS (See TOCOLYSIS)
Drugs, including magnesium sulfate and beta-mimetic agents designed to reduce involuntary contractions in smooth muscles, such as the uterus. A mother who has gone into premature labor may be given a tocolytic by injection in an attempt to make her uterus stop contracting (tocolysis) so pregnancy can continue. There is little evidence to demonstrate that these drugs have succeeded in reducing the rate of preterm births or the death of premature babies, but they may succeed in stopping labor for a short period of time, at least 48 hours. Their use is not recommended after 34 weeks of pregnancy, and many tocolytics have side effects that may affect mothers with serious physical problems, such as heart or kidney disease.

TOL (See TRIAL OF LABOR)

TONIC NECK REFLEX
A built-in baby behavior (reflex). During sleep, the baby's head is turned to one side with one arm bent behind the head and the other arm extends in front of the face in a fencing position.

TOP
Stands for medical termination of pregnancy, an abortion.

TORSION
Twisting.

TORTICOLLIS (wryneck)
When a baby's neck is stiff on one side as the result of birth trauma so that his head is pulled to one side of the neck and his chin to the opposite side. Although the problem may not show up at birth, within 2 weeks a small lump can be felt in a muscle of the neck. Parents may be given exercises to help stretch the baby's neck, and physical therapy may be recommended. Rarely, surgery may be required.

TOXEMIA (See PREECLAMPSIA)

TOXOPLASMOSIS
An airborne protozoa (*Toxoplasma gondii*) found in cat feces that can also be caught from contaminated raw or rare meat, from unwashed fruits and vegetables, or from gardening without gloves. The infection can affect unborn babies, but most mothers have already developed immunity to it from prior infection. The disease is not serious unless a mother catches it for the first time during pregnancy. Exposure can cause blindness, mild retardation, and hearing loss in unborn babies. Some children may develop brain or eye problems years after birth. Most healthcare providers routinely test to see if a mother is at risk.

TRANSITION STAGE
The period of time at the end of the first stage of labor when the cervix dilates from 8 to 10 centimeters prior to the second stage of labor. It is often a short but challenging time marked by irritability or confusion for the mother.

TRANSVERSE LIE (See EXTERNAL VERSION)

When a baby lies crosswise in the uterus prior to birth, which can cause the shoulder to present first. A healthcare provider may attempt to turn the baby externally by applying pressure to put it in a more favorable position for birth. (See discussion on page 88.)

TRAUMA

An injury or a wound. Birth trauma can refer to physical injury to the baby as a result of delivery, or the term is sometimes used to refer to profound psychological damage from the birth experience that could remain a part of a person's memories even into adulthood.

TRIAL OF LABOR (TOL, trial of labor after cesarean section) (See vaginal birth after a cesarean)

Choosing to enter into labor after having had a prior cesarean in an attempt to have a vaginal birth, rather than undergoing a second (or subsequent) cesarean prior to the start of labor, called an elective cesarean.

TRICHOMONAS VAGINITIS

Inflammation of the vagina caused by a parasitic protozoan that causes itching and a profuse, bubbly, yellow discharge.

TRIMESTER

Pregnancy is divided into three parts: up to 14 weeks for the first trimester, 14 to 27 weeks for the second trimester, and 28 weeks until delivery, the third trimester. Stated as: "I am in my second trimester of pregnancy."

TUBAL PREGNANCY (See ECTOPIC PREGNANCY)

When a fertilized egg stays in the fallopian tube instead of traveling down to the uterus to implant.

U

ULTRASOUND (ultrasonography)

A device that uses high-frequency sound waves to produce a picture of a baby's body. It shows the position and size of the baby and the placenta, the baby's heartbeat, breathing, and body movements. It can also be used to measure the amount of amniotic fluid. Level II ultrasound is a closer look at the fetus in search of structural and anatomic abnormalities. (See discussion on pages 149–150.)

UMBILICAL CORD

The flexible, cordlike structure that connects a baby at the navel with the placenta, which, in turn, is attached to the uterus. It contains two umbilical arteries and one vein that transport blood, oxygen, and nutrients to the baby and carry away waste products and carbon dioxide.

UMBILICAL CORD BLOOD BANKING (See CORD BLOOD BANK)

Harvesting and storing stem cells from the blood of a baby's umbilical cord following birth, usually for a fee. It may offer promising therapies in the future, especially for family members who may need a transplant of stem cells in order to overcome serious diseases, such as leukemia, but at this time the procedure and the uses for stem cells are still in the experimental phase.

UMBILICAL STUMP
The leftover portion of a baby's umbilical cord that dries up and falls off a few weeks after birth. Sometimes the stump can get infected, causing the belly button area to turn red and ooze pus. Antibiotics may be necessary to prevent the spread of infection (umbilical sepsis).

UMBILICUS (NAVEL)
Another word for belly button.

UNDESCENDED TESTICLES (cryptorchidism)
Failure of a baby boy's testicles to descend into the scrotum through the small, inguinal canal at the time of birth. More common in premature boys. It usually resolves itself in time.

UNRIPE CERVIX (See CERVICAL RIPENING and CERVIX, RIPE)

UPT
Urine pregnancy test.

URETER
The tube that transports urine from the kidneys to the bladder.

URETHRA
The tube that transports urine from the bladder to the outside of the body.

URGE TO PUSH
An inborn body reaction (reflex) at the end of labor that gives the mother an overwhelming urge to bear down in order to push the baby out.

URINARY INCONTINENCE (UI) (See CONTINENCE, INCONTINENCE, and KEGEL EXERCISES)
When a woman accidentally urinates while sneezing or coughing.

Pelvic floor exercises can help alleviate this problem, and usually healthcare providers will give instructions. (Some mothers may experience fecal incontinence, the inability to hold in a bowel movement following childbirth.)

URINARY SPHINCTER (See URINARY INCONTINENCE)
A tight ring of muscle at the neck of the bladder that helps to hold in urine and support the muscles of the pelvic floor.

URINARY TRACT INFECTION (UTI)
Urinary tract infections (UTIs) occur when bacteria or other infectious organisms invade the organs that produce urine and transport it out of the body—the urethra, bladder, ureter, or kidneys. There may be no symptoms, or symptoms could include a frequent and urgent need to urinate (every 30 to 60 minutes), burning or painful urination, or blood in the urine. UTIs are more common during pregnancy, and, untreated, they can lead to a kidney infection that could contribute to early labor. (See discussion on page 154.)

US
Ultrasound.

USCPSC (or CPSC) (See CPSC)

UTERINE ATONY
When the uterus becomes flaccid and soft, lacking in normal tone and strength. When this occurs after the birth of the baby, there is a danger of heavy blood loss to the mother at the site where the placenta was attached.

UTERINE HYPERSTIMULATION (TACHYSYTOLE)

Defined as more than five uterus contractions per 10 minutes, and sometimes as more than seven contractions over 15 minutes. Although it can sometimes happen during non-medicated (spontaneous) labor, it is more common during the induction or augmentation of labor, such as with the use of oxytocin (Pitocin) or misoprostol (Cytotec).

UTERINE INERTIA

When contractions become sluggish or come to a stop during labor.

UTERINE INVERSION

When a mother's placenta fails to separate from the wall of the uterus during the third stage of labor so that part of the uterus comes out of the vagina. Women who have had several babies, who have had long labors, or who have been given magnesium sulfate, a drug that lowers blood pressure and acts as a muscle relaxer, are more at risk for the problem. Pulling on the baby's umbilical cord in an attempt to deliver the placenta can also cause inversion. An attempt may be made to manually reposition the uterus back in the body, or, in more serious cases, surgery may be required to put it back in place.

UTERINE INVOLUTION

The return of the uterus to normal size following birth.

UTERINE RUPTURE

When scar tissue from previous obstetrical surgery, such as a cesarean section, ruptures during the process of birth. The most common sign of rupture is a slowing down of the baby's heartbeat, or an undetectable heart rate accompanied by a labor that fails to progress. A uterine rupture can be life threatening.

UTERUS

A hollow, muscular, pear-shaped organ where a fertilized egg implants, it serves to nurture a growing baby during pregnancy. Its muscular walls help push the baby out during birth. While a non-pregnant uterus is about 3 to 4 inches long and weighs about 3 ounces, at the time of birth it will weigh approximately 2 pounds.

UTI

Urinary tract infection.

V

VACCINATION (immunization, shots) (See IMMUNIZATION and VACCINE)

Another word for immunization to help prevent diseases. (See discussion on page 256.)

VACCINE (See IMMUNIZATION and VACCINATION)

A preparation containing killed or weakened living microorganisms that cause the body to form protective fighter (antibodies) against that type of organism. Once that happens, the person is protected from catching the disease, either permanently or for a period of time. (See discussion on page 256.)

VACUUM EXTRACTION (vacuum-assisted birth) (See CAPUT SUCCEDANEUM)

A procedure using a device similar to a suction cup that attaches to the baby's head, guiding it through the birth canal during delivery. It causes temporary swelling on the baby's scalp.

VAGINA
The canal, or birth canal, that leads from the uterus to the opening between the labia.

VAGINAL BIRTH
Birth of the baby through the birth canal, versus a c-section, which is the birth of the baby through an opening in the abdomen.

VAGINITIS (See BACTERIAL VAGINOSIS)
A vaginal infection with a number of causes. Symptoms may include unusual discharge that may be green, yellow, or strong smelling; redness; soreness; or itching around the vagina.

VALSALVA MANEUVER
Encouraging a mother in her second (bearing down) stage of labor to hold her breath while pushing down with the diaphragm. The maneuver is thought by some healthcare providers to be outdated and potentially harmful to the baby, because of the potential for decreasing a mother's heart output and lowering her blood pressure, which could diminish blood flow and oxygen to the baby. (See discussion on page 179.)

VARICOSE VEINS
Blood vessels (veins) that are dilated or enlarged, most often in the calves of the legs.

VBAC (pronounced vee back) (See TRIAL OF LABOR)
Stands for vaginal birth after cesarean section, and refers to giving birth through the birth canal (vagina) after having undergone one or more cesarean sections with previous babies. Pre-VBAC, or trial of labor (TOL) after a cesarean, allows a mother to enter into normal labor with close monitoring to see whether it is safe for her to deliver vaginally rather than having to undergo another cesarean. There is a rare risk of a life-threatening uterine rupture during a VBAC from the scar of a prior cesarean.

VENEREAL DISEASE (See SEXUALLY TRANSMITTED DISEASE)

VENTRAL WALL HERNIA
A protrusion of the contents of the body of the fetus, usually its abdominal organs, sometimes discovered during an ultrasound examination.

VERNIX (vernix caseosa)
A thick, protective white or yellowish cream produced by an unborn baby's skin that protects the skin while the baby floats in the amniotic fluid. It is often wiped off immediately after birth, but can also be gently massaged into the baby's skin. It has antibacterial properties.

VERSION (See EXTERNAL VERSION)

VERTEX PRESENTATION (See PRESENTATION)
The typical, chin-against-the-chest position of a baby being born headfirst.

VIABLE
Able to live. A baby mature enough to survive outside the womb.

VILLI (chorionic villi)
The villi attach the placenta to the

mucous lining of the uterus so that nutrients from the mother's blood can flow to it and the baby.

VITAMIN K
All newborns routinely receive injections of vitamin K, which encourages the liver to produce blood-clotting agents to assist a baby's immature liver and to prevent excessive bleeding. Excessive vitamin K in a baby's bloodstream can lead to jaundice.

VULVA
A woman's external genital organs. The vulva includes the labia (the lips around the opening of the vagina) and the clitoris (a small knob of tissue at the opening of the vagina that helps a woman achieve orgasm during sexual intercourse).

W

WALKING EPIDURAL
The administration of an epidural that allows a mother to maintain sensation in her legs so that she is able to stand for periods of time, although she may be asked to wear monitors for herself and her baby.

WEIGHT GAIN DURING PREGNANCY
A steady pattern of weight gain is important for a baby's growth. Unusual weight gain, more than 2 pounds in 1 week, may be an early sign of preeclampsia. Failure to gain weight, on the other hand, may signal growth problems for the baby. At the time of birth, a baby weighs only about 7.5 pounds of the 24–28 pounds that a mother typically gains. The placenta weighs 1 pound;

amniotic fluid, 2 pounds; the uterus, 2.5 pounds; breast tissue, 3 pounds; increased blood volume, 4 pounds; a mother's fat stores, 4 to 8 pounds.

WHARTON JELLY
A jellylike substance on the umbilical cord that is thought to protect the vessels of the cord and to prevent kinking.

WIC
Women, Infants, and Children Supplemental Nutrition Program, which provides counseling, formula, and food supplementation for low-income mothers and children.

WITCHES' MILK
Small amounts of white, milky discharge from a newborn's swollen nipples due to stimulation of the male or female baby's breast tissue by high levels of female hormones. The swollen nipples should not be massaged, which may introduce infection. The swelling will disappear within 2 weeks as the hormonal levels drop.

WOMB
Another name for the uterus.

Y

YEAST INFECTION (Candida infection, Monilia, moniliasis)
A vaginal infection common during pregnancy, its symptoms are intense itching, bright red coloration, and a white discharge that smells like baking bread. Consult your healthcare provider before undertaking any over-the-counter treatment. Babies can also have yeast infections. If it occurs in a

baby's mouth, it is called thrush and is a white, milky patch that cannot be rubbed off.

YOGA, PRENATAL
A form of stretching exercise designed to help mothers remain limber.

Z

ZINC OXIDE
A thick white cream used in diaper rash products to protect baby's skin and aid in healing.

ZYGOTE
A fertilized egg from the union of sperm and ovum that will soon begin to divide and grow.

Endnotes

1 Your Pregnancy Week by Week

1. "The Association of Folate, Zinc and Antioxidant Intake with Sperm Aneuploidy in Healthy Non-smoking Men," *Human Reproduction* 23, no. 5 (2008): 1–9.
2. *Wien Klin Wochenschr* 113, no. 23–24 (December 17, 2001): 942–946.
3. *Journal of Maternal-Fetal Neonatal Medicine* 22, no. 10 (October 2009): 843–848.
4. *Obstetrics & Gynecology* 112, no. 5 (November 2008): 1067–1074.

2 What (and What Not) to Worry About

1. *Reproductive Toxicology* 19, no. 4 (March–April 2005): 453–458.
2. "Nitrous Oxide for Pain in Labor—Why Not in the United States?" *Birth* 34, no. 1 (March 2007): 3–5.
3. *British Medical Journal* 342 (June 14, 2011):d3403 doi: 10.1136/bmj.d3403.
4. "Racial Disparities in Stillbirth Across Gestation in the United States," *American Journal of Obstetric Gynecology* 201 (2009): 496.

3 Managing Your Nutrition

1. Dietary Reference Intakes for Thiamin, Riboflavin, Niacin, Vitamin B6, Folate, Vitamin B12, Pantothenic Acid, Biotin, and Choline, "A Report of the Standing Committee on the Scientific Evaluation of Dietary Reference Intakes and its Panel on Folate, Other B Vitamins, and Choline," Subcommittee on Upper Reference Levels of Nutrients, Food and Nutrition Board, Institute of Medicine, 1998.
2. *Journal of the National Cancer Institute* 93, no. 14 (2001):1088–1095.
3. "Outbreak of Norovirus Infection Among River Rafters Associated with Packaged Delicatessen Meat, Grand Canyon, 2005," *Clinical Infectious Diseases* 48, no. 1 (January 1, 2009): 31–37.

4 Birth

1. "Listening to Mothers: Report of the First National U.S. Survey of Women's Childbearing Experiences," survey conducted for the Maternity Center Association by Harris Interactive." New York: Maternity Center Association, October 2002.

5 You and Your Baby

1. *Pediatrics* 103 (1999): 686–693.
2. "Rates of Selected Neonatal Male Circumcision-Associated Severe Adverse Events in the United States, 2007–2009," XVIII International AIDS conference, Vienna, Austria.
3. Ibid.
4. *Pediatrics* 105, no. 1 Supplement (January 2000): 246–249.
5. *Zhonghua Nan Ke Xue* (National Journal of Andrology) 14, no. 4 (April 2008): 328–330.

Index

Copper, 159, 165
Cough syrup, 117
Couvade syndrome, 52, **370**
Cradle cap, 251, 254, **370**
Cradles, 311–312
Cramps. *See also* Afterpains; Round ligament pains: leg, 57, 58, 65, 70, 134, 167; menstrual-like, 2, 19, 23, 24, 25, 116, 175, 204; muscle spasms and, 134; stomach/abdominal, 113, 120, 126, 170, 196. *See also* Nausea and vomiting (mother); uterine, 88, 99, 196, 208. *See also* menstrual-like
Cravings. *See* Foods
Crib mobiles, 274, 331
Cribs, alternatives to, 310–312
Cribs and crib mattresses, 274, 306–310
Cribs, portable, 312
Crown-to-rump length, 38, 48, 54, 58, 73, 79, **370**
Crying, 234–238; colic and, 235–237, 259, **367–368**; excessive, 237; overwhelmed by, 237; reasons for, 234–235; responding to, 232, 234, 235–236; shaking baby precaution, 237; sleeping and, 232–233, 234, 235; strategies for reducing, 235, 236–237; in womb, 40
Custody, single motherhood and, 142–143
Cystic fibrosis, 27, 108, 118, **371**

D&C. *See* Dilation and curettage (D&C)
Dehydration: baby, 203, 238, 240, 242, 250, 260; breastfeeding during pregnancy and, 111; caffeine and, 102, 112; defined, **371**; headaches from, 37, 128; mother, pregnancy and, 6, 15, 29, 32
Deli meats, 118
Delivery. *See* Birth; Labor
Dental care, 35
Depo-Provera, 109
Depression, antidepressants and, 118–120. *See also* Postpartum depression (baby blues)
DHA (docosahexaenoic acid), 161–162
Diabetes: defined, **372**; gestational, 66–67, 97, 103, 136, 160; LGA and, 210; pre-existing, 11; reducing risk of, 161; testing for. *See* Glucose tolerance test
Diaper bags, 312–313
Diaper-changing tables, 303–306
Diapers, 313–317; buying, 274; changing, 224–225; disposables, 316–317; fabric reusable, 314–315; services, 315–316; system type options, 313–314; traveling

with baby and, 267; weekly/lifetime use, 313
Diaphragm: of baby, 40, 93; defined, **372**; of mother, 63, 184–185; valsalva maneuver and, **428**
Diarrhea: baby, 238, 260; breastfeeding baby and, 225, 238; gas, bloating and, 126. *See also* Gas references; labor and, 90; mother, 29, 120
Dichorionic twins, **372**
Diet. *See* Foods; Nutrition; Vitamins and minerals
Dilation: checking/monitoring, 93, 94, 172–174; by labor stage, 174, 176; measuring, 173
Dilation and curettage (D&C), 24, **373**
Dilation and evacuation, **373**
Dilation and vacuum curettage, **373**
Direct-entry midwife (DEM). *See* Certified professional midwife (CPM)
Discharge. *See* Vaginal discharge
Disgust, experiencing, 13, 19
Dizygotic (fraternal) twins, 199, **373**
Dizziness, 13, 18, 19, 20, 25, 62, 70, 163, 206
Dogs, 120–122
Doppler devices, 33, 102, 136, 172, **373**
Doulas (labor assistants), 11, 68
Down syndrome, 34, 39, 103, 105, 124, 354, **374**
Dreaming: baby, 60, 72, 80; during pregnancy, 122
Drooling (mother), 19, 144
Drugs, neonatal abstinence syndrome, **403–404**. *See also* Cocaine; Medications
Due date. *See also* Post-date pregnancies: approaching, 84; definition and other terms for, **374**; induction and, 86, 93. *See also* Induction; this book and, 1
Dysuria, **375**. *See also* Urination, painful

Ear infections, 259–260
Echinacea, 122
Ecstasy pills, 123
Ectopic (tubal) pregnancy, 17, 19, 25, 109, 110, 197, 366, **375**
Eczema, 73, 132, 254–255, **375**
Edema, 148, 149, **375**
Effacement, 94, 174, **375–376**
Eggs, raw, 139
Electric and magnetic fields (EMF), 123, 124
Electric blankets, 5, 123, 124
Electronic fetal monitor (EFM), 172, **376**
Electronic toys, 333

deli food precaution, 118; eating out, 21; keeping journal of, 14–15, 35, 126, 160; nutritionists and, 37–38, 220, 221; organic, 168; poorly handled, pregnancy precaution, 5; safety, 169–170; to stimulate labor, 97

Footprints, development of, 62

Foreskin, circumcised. *See* Circumcision

Foreskin, intact, 215, **383**

Formula. *See also* Bottle feeding: bowel movements and, 225–226; constipation and, 238; cost, compared to breastfeeding, 271; dehydration and, 242; heating, 247, 249; hospital mixed messages, 204; introducing, 245–246; preparing, 247; samples and coupons, 204, 221; saving money on, 247; traveling with baby and, 267; types and qualities, 246–247

Frank breech, **383**. *See also* Breech presentation (birth)

Fraternal (dizygotic) twins, 199, **373**

Front carriers, 267, 271

Fuzziness, mental, 13

Games, for newborns, 227

Gardening, 126

Gas (baby), 233, 234

Gas (mother), 19–20, 39–40, 41, 126, 161, 196. *See also* Bloating

Gear. *See* Baby gear

Gender of baby, 16, 32, 36, 49–50, 105

General anesthesia, 188, **384**

Genetic defects and conditions, 11, 27, 49, 50, 93, 108, 115. *See also* Birth defects

Genitals, of babies, 33, 36, 215–216, **385**. *See also* Circumcision

Genitals, piercing, 139

GERD, 250

German measles. *See* Rubella (German measles)

Germs, 5

Gestational age: appropriate for, **357**; defined, **385**; large for (LGA), 210–211, 385, **395**; small for (SGA), 86, 210, 233, 385, **419**

Gestational diabetes, 66–67, 97, 103, 136, 160

Gestational Trophoblastic Disease (GTD), **385**

Gingko biloba, 127

Glucose tolerance test, 66, **386**

Glycolic acid, 127

Grief, 147, **356**, **386**. *See also* LCSW (licensed clinical social worker)

Group B strep (GBS), 81, 127, **386**

Habits, journaling about, 14–15

Hair (baby), 43, 54, 78, 81, 88, 251. *See also* Lanugo

Hair, changes in (mother), 12, 17, 32, 36, 127–128, 223

Hair products, 127

Handprints, development of, 62

Hands, development of, 26, 32, 63

Hands, of newborn, 214

Headaches, 128; from bed rest, 107; caffeine and, 113; dealing with, 128; from epidurals, 181, 192, 208, 360–361; high altitudes and, 130; hydration and, 6, 37, 160; migraine, 128; post-dural puncture (PDPH) or spinal, 192, 360–361, **410**; postpartum, 203, 208, 223; preeclampsia precaution, 81, 412; swelling and, 148; when to contact healthcare provider, 81, 90, 203, 208, 223

Head, of baby: compacting for birth, 87–88; control of, facial expressions and, 226–227; newborn neck and, 213; position during birth. *See* Presentations; soft spots (fontanels), 209, **383**; too large to fit through pelvis (CPD), 150, **364**

Healthcare, baby, 255–262; about: overview of, 255; colds and infections, 259; diarrhea, 238, 260; ear infections, 259–260; emergency life support, 260–262; fevers, 237; fevers and, 254, 256–259, 267, 303; illnesses and treatments, 256–260; immunizations, 256; researching medical information, 338; RSV and, 259, **417**; state-mandated screening tests, 255–256; taking temperature, 257–258; thrush, 260; Web sites, 348–349

Healthcare providers. *See also* Prenatal care; *specific provider types*: about: overview of, XI–XII; asking questions, 14; changing, indicators for, 51; doctors vs. midwives, 7–10; finding pediatrician, 46–48; first visit to, 27–28; frequency of visits, 70, 84; good, characteristics of, 7; importance of, XII; making appointments with, 3–4, 6; questions to ask, 10–11, 28; questions to ask yourself about, 11–12; seeking advice of, XII; telling about pregnancy, 6; types of, pros and cons, 7–10

Herbal tea, 130

Heartburn, 44, 52, 62, 63, 112, **387**

Heart rate: increased blood volume and, 36–37, 52; of mother, 41, 129; of newborn, 200, **361**

management, at hospital, 172; monitoring progress, 172–174; oxytocin release and, 180; pain and pain management, 88; prodromal (false), 91, 95, 97, **413–414**; "purple pushing," 179; relaxin effects before, 84, **416**; "ring of fire" and, 177; starting, 90; stimulating, things to try, 96–97; support during, XII, 67–68, 71, 182; trial of, 150, **425**; urge to push, 177, 178, 179, 181, 191, **426**; water breaking before, 85, 90–91, 172

Labor assistants. *See* Doulas (labor assistants)

Labor pain, 180–192; afterpains, 181, 204, **354**; conscious relaxation for, 187–188; coping with, 180–181; hypnotherapy for, 185–186, 340; making sounds for, 188; massage for, 182; medication for, 188–192. *See also* Epidurals; *specific medications*; movement and positioning for, 182–183; prayer for, 187; relaxation breathing for, 184–185; sterile water injections for, 186–187; water birth and, 186; without drugs, 181–188

Labor stages, 171–180; about: overview of, 171–174; stage 1, 174–176; stage 2, 176–179; stage 3 (birth), 180; stage 4 (after birth), 206–208

Lactation consulting, 9, 48, 65, 203, 204, 205, 247, 288, **395**

Lactose intolerance, 126, **395**

La Leche League, 65–66, 238, 240, 347, **395**

Lanugo, 43, 51, 78, 211, **395**

LCSW (licensed clinical social worker), **395–396**

Leg cramps, 57, 58, 65, 70, 134, 167

Legs, restless, 58

Lifestyle. *See also* Babies; Postpartum life: adjusting, 4–6, 14; journaling habits, 14–15; parenting styles/situations Web sites, 350–351

Life support, emergency, 260–262

Lifting, heavy, 129

Lightening, 82, **396**

Light-headedness, 20, 223. *See also* Dizziness

Litter, cat, 5, 114

Local anesthesia, 188, **397**

Lochia, 222–223, **397**

Losing baby, 340–341. *See also* Miscarriages; Stillbirth

Lymphatic system, 148, **397**

Macronutrients, 158–159

Magnesium, 35, 58, 65, 77, 134, 149, 158, 159, 167

Magnesium sulfate, **398**

Magnetic fields, 123

Manganese, 159, 166

Manicures, 69, 132–133

Marching game, 227

Marijuana, 133, **398**

Massage, 69, 82, 132, 133, 151, 175, 182, 323

Maternal-fetal medicine specialist (MFM), 93, 99, 194, **399**. *See also* Perinatologists

Maternity clothes, 45, 72–73, 92; good and bad buys, 72–73; minimizing restriction, 74, 149; reducing swelling, 149; second trimester, 44–45; support hose, 73, 74, 151; third trimester, 72–73; underwear, 30, 45, 72, 73, 92, 154. *See also* Bras; to wear home, 92; Web sites for, 350

MDMA (ecstasy), 123

Meconium, 83, 91, 172, 186, 201, 225, **399**

Medical information, searching for, 338

Medications: for baby, 267; breastmilk and, 244; narcotics, 75, 175, 181, 190, **403**; pregnancy and, 4

Meditation, 188

Membranes, stripping or sweeping, 96, **422**

Mental health tips, 21–22. *See also* Emotions; Stress

Mercury, 5, 55, 125, 137, 147, 148, 257, **400**

Mice. *See* Rodents

Microwaves, 134

Midwife. *See also* Healthcare providers: CNM, 8–9, **364**; CPM/DEM, 9–10, **370**, **373**; doctors vs., 7–10; questions to ask, 10–11; questions to ask yourself about, 11–12

Miscarriages, 23–25; age over 35 and, 103; air travel and, 103; alcohol and, 104; amniocentesis and, 105; bleeding and, 23; caffeine and, 5, 102, 112–113; causes of, 23; conception and, 23; CVS and, 35, 115, 116; defined, 23, **400**; early, 20; ectopic pregnancies and, 25; EMFs and, 123; feelings associated with, 24; hot baths, saunas, heating pads and, 5; multiple, precautions, 22, 30; nausea and, 26, 29; responding to, 23–24; Rh screening and, 140; risk, before heartbeat detected, 13; sexual activity and, 141; smoking and, 144–145; solvents, paints and, 137; support for, 25, 340–341; symptoms of, 23; timing of, 20, 23

Misoprostol, 24, **400**

Mobiles, 274, 331
Mold, 134
Molding, of head, 87–88, **401**
Mongolian spots, 211, **401**
Monilia, moniliasis. *See* Yeast infections
(*Candida albicans*, Monilia, moniliasis)
Monitors, 274, 319–321
"Monkey see, monkey do" game, 227
Monozygotic (identical) twins, 199, **401**
Mood swings, 6, 18, 19, 33, 44, 113, 163, 223
Morning sickness, **401**. *See also* Nausea and
vomiting (mother)
Motor development, 147, **402**
Movements, fetal, 49, 53, 61. *See also* Kicks,
baby; Quickening
Mucus plug. *See* Show (bloody show or
mucus plug)
Muscle spasms, 134
Music, baby and, 52–53

Name, last, 143
Naming baby, 62–63
Naps, 14
Nasal sprays, 116–117
Nausea and vomiting (baby), 247, 249–250,
257
Nausea and vomiting (mother): about:
overview of, 18–19; caffeine and, 31, 112;
coping strategies, 30–31; drug-induced,
181, 189, 191; easing, 18, 40, 42, 44, 163;
epidurals and, 191, 192; miscarriage and,
26, 29; partner experiencing, 52; severe
vomiting, 90; upside to, 29; vitamins
and, 18–19, 31, 157, 163; when to contact
healthcare provider, 29
Neck, of newborn, 213
Neonatologists, 220, **404**
Nesting, 83, **404**
Neural tube: defects, 105, 108, 115, 117, 124,
129, 131, **404**; development of, 17, 18, 20;
supplements to avoid defects, 159, 163, 164
Niacin (B3), 159, 163
Nicotine, 133
NICU (neonatal intensive care unit), 64–65,
69, 205, 207, 210, 220–221
NICU support site, 350
Nipple confusion, 240, **405**
Nipples: for bottles. *See* Bottle feeding; of
newborns, 214; piercing, 139; rooting for,
207, 226, 242, **417**; sore, help for, 243;
stimulating, to induce labor, 96
Nitrous oxide, 134–135
Nonreassuring fetal status (fetal distress),
193, **405**

Non-stress tests, 97–98, **405**
Nosebleeds, 49, 135
Nose, of newborn, 213
Nuchal translucency, 34, 50, 149, **405**
Nursing pillow, 240–241, 274
Nutrition. *See also* Carbohydrates; Fiber;
Foods; Protein; Vitamins and minerals:
about: overview of, 157; about: overview
of text, X; balanced diet, 157, 159, **359**;
blood sugar, mood and, 58; calories and
weight gain, 159–160; DHA, 161–162;
eating right, 14; pregnancy menu, 158;
vegetarian and vegan diets, 5, 164, 168

Obstetricians. *See also* Healthcare
providers: pros and cons, 8; questions
to ask, 10–11; questions to ask yourself
about, 11–12
Odors, offensive, 2, 13, 31
Omega-3 fatty acids, 6, 55, 125, 159, 161, 162
Omega-6 and -9 fatty acids, 161–162
Opiates, 135
Organic food, 168
Organizing things, 33, 72, 74–75, 89
Otitis media, 259–260, **407**
Ovaries (baby), development of, 32, 36,
53, 59
Overdue babies. *See* Post-date pregnancies
Ovulation, 1, 15, 16, **407**
Oxytocin, 180, 191, 195, 239, **407**
Oysters, 136

Pacifiers, 250–251, 267, 274
Packing, for hospital, 91–92
Pain. *See also* Labor pain; *specific types/
locations of pain*: relief alternatives,
60, 339–340; shooting, 137; talking with
healthcare provider about, 59–60
Paint and painting, 61, 137, 307
Paint, body, 70
Palm trick, 227
Palsies, **361**, **364**, **378**
Pantothenic acid, 159
Parenting Web sites, 350–351
Partner: childbirth classes and, 43;
fatherhood Web sites, 349; postpartum
period, 227–229; relating to baby,
228; role in childbirth, 71; roles and
responsibilities, 228–229; showing
pregnancy symptoms, 52; talking to baby,
62; telling about pregnancy, 6
Partogram. *See* Cervicogram (partogram)
PCB (polychlorinated biphenyl), 137
Peanuts, 138

Radiation and X-rays, 5, 33, 103, 104, 114, 123, 134, 152–153
Rashes, 253–255, 267
Rattles, 214, 227, 331–332
Recovery: from c-sections, 86, 88, 196–197, 203, 205, 222; guidelines and expectations, 202–205, 222–224; planning for, 76
Rectum, 257, **415**
Reflexes, of newborns, 226
Reflexology, 182
Regional anesthesia, 188, **416**
Registry, baby, 77
Relaxation techniques: Bradley Method and, 188, 344, **361**; breathing, 184–185; conscious relaxation, 187–188
Relaxin, 84, **416**
Reptiles, 140
Resources, 338–352. See also Web sites; books and magazines, 338–339; searching for medical information, 338
Rest. See also Sleep and naps (mother): bed rest, 107; pregnancy and, 6
Retained placenta, 24, **416**
Retardation, intrauterine growth, 199, **392**
Rh screening, 140
Riboflavin (B2), 159, 162–163
"Ring of fire," 177
Risk ratios, 38–39
Rockers, gliders, and footstools, 274, 322–323
Rodents, 5, 114, 169
Round ligament pains, 32, 52, 84, **417**
RSV (respiratory syncytial virus), 259, **417**
Rubella (German measles), 27, **417**
Rupture of membranes, 85, **417**. See also Amnion (amniotic sac), breaking; Water breaking
Rupture of membranes (ROM), 85
Rupture, uterine, 99, **427**

Safety gates, 275, 323–325
Saline nasal sprays, 116–117
Saunas, 5, 140. See also Hot tubs
Scented products, 30
Sciatic nerve pain (sciatica), 54, 68, **418**
Seat belts, car, 35–36, 104
Selenium, 159, 164–165
Self-tanning sprays, 141
Senses, development of, 52–54, 66
Sex: conception and. See Conceiving/ conception; drive, 51–52, 141; first trimester, 32, 40, 141; increased pleasure, 19; orgasms, 45, 97, 141, 152; positions, 141; safety of, 141; second trimester, 42,

51–52, 141; to stimulate labor, 96–97; third trimester, 96–97, 141; vibrators and, 152
Shaken baby syndrome, 237
Sheets and bedding, 274
Shoes, 40, 130
Shopping for gear. See Baby gear; *specific gear*
Show (bloody show or mucus plug), 26, 84, 87, **418**
SIDS (sudden infant death syndrome), 145, 231, 233, 245, 251, 311, 312, **421–422**
Single motherhood, 141–143
Sit-ups, 143, 230
Skiing, 143
Skin (baby): bathing, 251–253, 285; clothes and, 298; development of, 43, 51, 54, 60, 61–62, 78; newborn, 211–212, 238; protecting, 267; rashes, 253–255, 267; yellow, 238
Skin (mother): changes in, 17, 32, 42, 61; glycolic acid and, 127; home facial for, 69; irritations, 73; stretching, 61; vitamin D for, 164
Skin-to-skin contact, 200, 220, 235, **419**
Sleep and naps (baby), 230–233; bedding sets and, 272; bed sharing, 231, 232; bottle feeding in bed, 250; clothing for, 300; crying and, 232–233, 234, 235; hours per day, 230; safety precautions, 231–233; SIDS and, 145, 231, 233, 245, 251, 311, 312, **421–422**; traveling options, 267–268; where to sleep, 230–231
Sleep and naps (mother): after epidurals, 190; excessive sleep, 22, 119; first trimester, 14, 19, 22, 31, 35; importance of, 22; nausea and, 31; newborns and, 222, 230–233; positioning and problems, 66, 144; second trimester, 66; stillbirth and, 66, 144; third trimester, 72, 99; whenever possible, 22
Sleep apnea, 233, **419**
Sleep sacks, 300, 303
Slings, 271, 325, 326
Smegma, 216, **419**
Smell, sense of, 2
Smoke, household, 302, 417
Smoking, 144–145; in bed, 231, 233; breastfeeding and, 244–245; dangers of, 4, 74, 144–145, 153, 233; marijuana, 133, **398**; miscarriage and, 24; quitting, 4, 11, 14, 74, 145; radiated tobacco and, 153; secondhand, 4, 231; vitamin C and, 164
Soft carriers, 228, 235–236, 271, 275
Soft spots. See Fontanels

Sonograms, 34, 41, 149, **419**
Spermicides, 109
Spider veins, 151, **419**
Spina bifida, 115, 135, **420**
Spinal anesthesia (block), 188–189, **420**
Spinal headaches, 192, 360–361, **410**
Spitting up vs. vomiting, 249–250. *See also* Vomiting
Stationary exercisers, 275
Stillbirth, 23, 66, 86, 98, 103, 144, 146–147, 340–341, **421**
St. John's Wort, 145
Stork bites, 211, **421**
Strawberry marks, 212, **421**
Stress: depression, antidepressants and, 118–120; effects of, 147; labor without drugs and, 181–188; lower, during birth, 182; reducing, 22, 147, 188. *See also* Massage; Yoga; of what to do/not do, 101
Stretch marks, 43, 69, 70, 149, 204–205, **421**
Stripping membranes, 96
Stroller/car seat combos, 295
Strollers, 267, 271, 275, 327–331
Sun shields, 266
Support: for crying baby, 237; emotional, 237; during labor, XII, 67–68, 71, 182; for miscarriages, 25; postpartum, planning for, 54, 86
Surfactants, 66, 409, 416, **422**
Sushi, 147–148
Swallowing, baby beginning, 57
Sweeping of membranes, 96, **422**
Swelling, 59, 148–149, 195, 196, 203, 208, 222
Swimming, 37, 74, 149
Swings, 275, 280–282
Syphilis, 27, **422**

Talipes (Clubfoot), **423**
Tanning, 149
Tanning sprays, 141
Tea, herbal, 130
Teethers, 275, 331–332
Temperature, taking, 257–258
Termination, **423**. *See also* Abortion
Testes, development of, 32, 33, 36, 58, 83
Tests. *See also specific tests*: diagnostic, about, 140; newborn, state-mandated, 255–256; post-date pregnancies, 95; pregnancy, results, 2–3, 17; prenatal, 34–35, 38–39, 108; risk levels, 50; screening, about, 140
Thermometer, taking temperature with, 257–258

Thrush, 243, 260, **423**
Torticollis, 213, **424**
Toxoplasmosis, 27, 114, **424**
Toy boxes, 332
Toys and play equipment, 275, 331–333. *See also* Play yards
Traveling: air travel, 103–104, 265–268; with baby, 265–268; high altitudes and, 130; products to ease, 297–298; what to pack, 266–268
Trial of labor, 150, **425**
Trimester, defined, **425**
Trimester, first, 12–41; about: overview of, 12–15; weeks 2 and 3, 12–16; week 4, 16–17; week 5, 18–20; week 6, 20–22; week 7, 26–28; week 8, 28–31; week 9, 32–33; week 10, 33–36; week 11, 36–38; week 12, 38–40; week 13, 40–41
Trimester, second, 42–69; about: overview of, 42–43; week 14, 43–45; week 15, 45–48; week 16, 48–50; week 17, 51–52; week 18, 52–53; week 19, 53–54; week 20, 54–56; week 21, 57–58; week 22, 58–60; week 23, 60–61; week 24, 61–63; week 25, 63–66; week 26, 66–68; week 27, 68–69
Trimester, third, 69–100; about: overview of, 69; week 28, 69–71; week 29, 71–73; week 30, 73–76; week 31, 76–77; week 32, 78; week 33, 79–80; week 34, 80–81; week 35, 81–82; week 36, 82–83; week 37, 83–85; week 38, 85–88; week 39, 88–92; week 40, 92–97; week 41, 96–100
Tubal pregnancy. *See* Ectopic (tubal) pregnancy
Tubal sterilization (ligation), 109–110
Twins and multiples, giving birth to, 199–200

Ultrasound, 5, 23–24, 26, 28, 33, 34, 35, 41, 49–50, 115–116, 146, 149–150, **425**
Umbilical cord, 36; belly button and, 201, 215, 238; clamping and cutting, 201; cleaning stump, 201, 215; drying and withering, 201
Urethra, 74, 154, **426**
Urinary incontinence. *See* Incontinence
Urinary tract infections (UTI), 27, 30, 73, 112, 154, 216, 217, **426**
Urination: catheters and. *See* Catheters; epidurals and, 181; frequent, 91, 154, 176; painful, 30, 90, 153; problems with, reporting, 203, 222
Uterine hyperstimulation, 99, **427**
Uterine rupture, 99, **427**

Uterus: afterpains, 181, 204, **354**; of baby, 59; Braxton-Hicks contractions and, 45–46; conception and. *See* Conceiving/conception; contracting. *See* Contractions; diagrams showing, 29, 39, 50, 55, 62, 87; fibroids in, 124, **382**; keeping sealed, 26. *See also* Show (bloody show or mucus plug); labor and. *See* Labor; monitoring growth, 55, 60; oxytocin increasing tone of, 239; pains around front and side. *See* Round ligament pains; pressuring bladder, 19, 72, 74; pressuring blood flow, 66; pushing into abdomen, 41; shrinking, after birth, 206, 207, 229; size and position, 27, 32, 34, 41, 49, 52, 55, 57, 62, 63, 80, 85, 113; topping pelvic bones, 37

Vaccinations. *See* Immunizations
Vagina: immediately after birth, 203; of newborn, 216; wart near (condyloma), **368**
Vaginal birth after cesarean (VBAC), 10, 51, 150–151, 193, 345, **428**
Vaginal changes, 151
Vaginal discharge, 30, 52, 59, 85, 87, 120, 146, 153–154, 215, 222–223
Vaginal discharge (newborn), 215
Vaginal infections, 30, 154, **358**. *See also* Yeast infections (*Candida albicans*, Monilia, moniliasis)
Vaginitis, 30, 153–154, **428**
Varicose veins, 151, **428**
VBAC. *See* Vaginal birth after cesarean (VBAC)
Vegetarianism and veganism, 5, 164, 168
Vernix, 54, 90, 211, **428**
Vibrators, 152
Villi (chorionic villi), 16, **428–429**. *See also* Chorionic villus sampling (CVS)
Vitamin A, 159, 162
Vitamin B. *See* B vitamins
Vitamin C, 159, 164, 166, 167, 202, **429**
Vitamin D, 4, 6, 125, 159, 164
Vitamin E, 159, 167
Vitamin K, 159
Vitamins and minerals, 157–167. *See also specific vitamins and minerals*; appropriate amounts of, 4; macronutrients, 158–159; nausea and, 18–19, 31, 157, 163; prenatal vitamins, 11, 18, 26, 28, 31, 58, 111, 134, 157, 158, 162–164; RDAs, 158–159
Vomiting: baby, 247, 249–250, 257; mother.

See Nausea and vomiting (mother); as sign of labor, 90; spitting up vs., 249–250

Walkers and exercisers, 333–335
Water birth, 59, 186, 344, 346
Water breaking, 85, 90–91, 98, 172
Water injections, for pain, 186–187
Water intake, 6, 14, 31, 32, 36–37, 39, 70, 80, 159, 160, 176
Weaning, 245–246
Web sites, 339–352; alternative pain relief options, 339–340; baby loss, stillbirth, miscarriage, 340–341; birth defects, 343; birth information, 343–346; breastfeeding, 347; child health, 348–349; fatherhood, 349; maternity/breastfeeding wear, 350; parenting styles/situations, 350–351; pregnancy, miscellaneous, 351–352; pregnancy, special circumstances, 352; products and product safety, 342–343
Week-by-week development. *See* Trimester *references*
Weight (baby, newborn), 209–211
Weight (baby, prenatal): birth experience and, 87–88; breastfeeding and, 111; estimating, 87; gain guidelines, 112; by trimester weeks. *See* Baby size and development
Weight (mother): BMI and, 136, **361**; calories and, 159–160; feeling baby move and, 49, 61; gaining/amount of, 35, 57, 61, 64, 78, 79, 84, 159–160; increased fluid levels and, 36–37; losing after delivery, 223; overweight or obese, 136, 160, 361
Weight training, 152
What (and what not) to worry about, 101–155. *See also specific items*; about: overview of, X, 101–102; alphabetical listing of. *See Table of Contents*
Wipes or washcloths, 267, 272, 274
Work. *See* Job (work)
Worrying, 17, 29–30, 39, 57–58. *See also* What (and what not) to worry about

X-rays. *See* Radiation and X-rays

Yeast infections (*Candida albicans*, Monilia, moniliasis), 30, 59, 131, 153, **429**. *See also* Thrush
Yoga, 15, 37, 55–56, 65, 155, 185, **430**

Zinc, 158, 159, 167
Zinc oxide, 267, **430**
Zygotes, 16–17, 110, **430**